PLEASE RETURN TO
VI AT SILVERSTONE
23005 N. 74TH STREET
SCOTTSDALE, AZ 85255

D0040380

An Alphabet of
Good Health
in a Sick World

An Alphabet of
Good Health
in a Sick World

Martha M. Grout, M.D., M.D. (H)
Mary Budinger

An Alphabet of
GOOD HEALTH
in a Sick World

THIRD PRINTING

cover art and design by
Lucy Swerdfeger, B.F.A.
The Three Pillars depiction by Alex Swerdfeger

Published by

NEW MEDICINE PRESS
6137 East Mescal Street
Scottsdale, Arizona 85252-5418

Alphabet of Good Health.com
NewMedicinePress.com

Paperback — $ 24.95 — 978-1-932842-54-8

E-book — $ 12.99 — 978-1-932842-55-5

Published in the United States of America

*To all who are willing to look
for the door in the ceiling.*

Table of Contents

Epilogue

PREFACE

Martha M. Grout, M.D., M.D. (H)

There is a story crying to be told. Never before in our history have we seen so much chronic illness in so many people at such a young age. For the first time in centuries we are facing a world in which our children's generation has a shorter predicted lifespan than our own generation.

Many people walk through my doors looking to find out what is wrong with them. They have seen a dozen doctors, they have undergone two dozen tests, nothing appears to be wrong, and yet they feel terrible. Sometimes their symptoms are so debilitating, they can barely hold a job. Usually they are on a slew of medications – something to lower cholesterol (which has never been proven to cause heart disease), something for the fatigue and muscle pain caused by the cholesterol-lowering medication's "side effect" of gumming up the cellular waste-disposal system, something for the high blood pressure caused by the need for more fuel because cells are drowning in cellular trash… My heart goes out to these walking wounded. They often did exactly what their insurance company told their doctors to tell them to do, and after all that time and money, they are still in search of an answer. Conventional medicine has failed them because too often it is looking in the wrong places.

For example, doctors will readily enough do a fasting glucose test – and insurance will pay for it – but if your glucose is high, it's way too late. By then you have a disease with a label, you are given a drug to increase the muscle sensitivity to insulin (in theory), and you are "managed" until such time as you might have renal failure. For some reason, the fasting *insulin* test is rarely done. That's unfortunate because it is far more helpful to people in the long run. It can tell if you are losing the ability to control glucose metabolism years before you actually develop diabetes.

i

In America, we treat illness as though it is an enemy to be vanquished, rather than the body's cry for help. Our mindset appears to be that of the warrior, whose tools are those that slash, burn, and poison. In war there is generally a good deal of collateral damage – the side effects of drugs and surgery, the reduced quality of life because symptoms are just being managed instead of being solved. Allopathic medicine is a hammer, and pretty much sees only nails.

Allopathic medicine = conventional, Western medicine. Seeks to manage symptoms rather than restore fundamental well being.

I have a different view of illness; as paradoxical as this may seem, I think it is our friend. I treat illness as if it were the body's best effort at telling us that something needs to be addressed. If our blood pressure is high, there is some reason for it. Perhaps we are stressed beyond our capacity to function, and our body is raising our blood pressure internally to provide adequate nutrients and oxygen to the brain and critical organs. Or perhaps we are eating so many sweets that our muscles cannot tolerate the sugar load, our pancreas can no longer keep up with the demand for insulin to keep the blood sugar low, and thus our blood sugar rises. If our cholesterol is high, perhaps our liver is unable to break it down, or perhaps our demand for stress hormones (of which cholesterol is a precursor) is high, or maybe our arteries are damaged by our stiff red blood cells and require a cholesterol bandage for repair.

Our bodies, like our brains, really do their best to let us know when something is out of balance. The first sign is generally some form of an energetic imbalance. The information systems – electrical impulses generated by neurotransmitters, inflammatory cytokines, hormones, etc. – become distorted and misfire. We may not be able to measure that change in a conventional laboratory, but we can see it with energetic scanning devices that measure the bioelectric field. In the physical realm, patients begin to experience symptoms – anxiety, insomnia, brain fog, or perhaps just a vague sense of malaise. For these, they are usually prescribed antidepressants and sleeping pills.

If we do not modify our behavior (eat vegetables instead of potato chips, reduce our stress levels, change jobs, go back to school, forgive that person who hurt us and move on), then we begin to develop the second level of signs – functional symptoms which begin to interfere with our lives. We see high blood pressure, high fasting insulin, anxiety, depression, abdominal pain, low back pain, etc. There still is no organ damage, but the body is calling for change with a louder voice. Now we are prescribed pills which interfere with our body's protective mechanisms – antihypertensives, anti-inflammatories, narcotics.

If we suppress or ignore the functional symptoms, then we begin to develop signs of actual organ damage – stroke, heart attack, diabetes, inflammatory bowel disease, disc herniation, etc. At some point, we may have to go on kidney dialysis. We may be hospitalized with a heart attack or congestive heart failure.

Looking at the body as the enemy and treating it with brute force is one way to do it. It strikes me as being cruel in an unthinking sort of way.

Is the body the enemy? Are bacteria really all bad? Do even molds not serve some useful function in the world? It really comes down to a question of balance. In our bodies we have both inflammatory and reconstructive pathways. They are in balance with each other – up-regulated and down-regulated, according to the need. We, as physicians, need to be very careful when we interfere with those pathways. We lower cholesterol levels without realizing that we are also stopping the synthesis of a molecule (CoQ-10) which is crucial – did I say crucial? – to the function of our cellular energy factories, the mitochondria. We give antibiotics to treat pneumonia without realizing that we are killing off many of the beneficial bacteria whose existence in the gut is crucial to our own well-being.

The history of American medicine is heavily sprinkled with stories of people who made breakthrough discoveries, but were called quacks by their peers for decades, then awarded the Nobel Prize in medicine.

One famous "quack" was Dr. Ignaz Semmelweis. In the 1840s, he recognized that doctors were somehow transmitting infection from one maternity patient to another – they carried "something" from one delivery room to another. Despite his extraordinary success by simply cleaning his hands before going from one room to the next, he was met with intense ridicule and ostracism. Semmelweis' claims were said to lack scientific basis.

"Great spirits have often encountered
violent opposition from weak minds."

ALBERT EINSTEIN

As you are about to read in this book, homeopathic medicine was the predominant form of medicine in America until about the 1920s when the influence of the pharmaceutical industry kicked into gear. This is why many homeopathic physicians like myself really dislike calling what we do "alternative medicine." But we understand the marketing forces that shaped where we are today.

Homeopathic medicine = focuses on the resolution of dysfunction to produce a cure through the use of bio-energetic medicines.

The use of so-called Bioenergetic Medicine is a great example of the resistance to old and new ideas. Aura photography is considered "woo-woo," a nice parlor trick, by some. And yet its principles are based in the sound science of quantum physics. Measurement of electrical energy in the meridians was done first in the 1950s – meridians which some maintain do not exist, but which have been used to excellent effect in Oriental Medicine for the past 3500 years. Electroacupuncture (EAV), developed by Dr. Reinhold Voll, also uses frequencies, but is derided by conventional medicine as quackery.

Yet, conventional medicine uses frequencies all the time. X-rays, such as CT scans and mammography, use energy to see an image of the body's structure. EKG machines measure the electrical impulses of the heart. The EEG (electroencephalogram) measures the electrical output of the brain. Electromyography measures the nerve impulses to our muscles.

Crisis medicine in America is among the best in the world. If you've been in a traffic accident, a hospital is exactly where you want to be. But most medicine today is not that. Eight of ten times that a patient goes to see a doctor it is because they have a chronic illness – ADHD, asthma, allergies, arthritis, autism, cancer, chronic fatigue, diabetes, fibromyalgia, high blood pressure, Lyme, inflammatory bowel, leaky gut, lupus, multiple sclerosis, Parkinson's disease, etc. And far too many times after too many tests, patients feel the system has let them down.

Patients do not all fit the same mold. In terms of the individual patient, statistics are worthless. I can predict the likelihood of something happening statistically, but I cannot predict that something will happen with any certainty to any given individual unless I know their genetics and all about them. The "scientific method" would have us believe that the human race is sufficiently homogenous that we all fit within a bell-shaped curve of probabilities, and can be treated accordingly. Do you really want to play roulette with your health? Perhaps the biggest difference between allopathic medicine and alternative medicine is the mindset of the bell shaped curve versus individuality. The "correct dose" is what works for the individual patient, not what works for a large group of people with 90% accuracy. What if you are among the 10%? What if you are part of the smaller group at the outer edges of the bell curve?

The American Society of Clinical Oncology, for example, still recommends against genetic testing for most cancers and recommends only the standard cancer therapy protocols, which have only convention and placebo-controlled double blind studies to draw on as a rationale for choosing them. To do genetic testing of circulating tumor cells is considered "fringe" medicine – although it is done in Europe as a matter of routine. Blood levels, as another example, can only deal with population "norms", not with individual requirements. Some people require huge doses of vitamin B12 or folic acid because they have a particular defect in the gene which codes for the MTHFR (methylene tetrahydrofolate reductase) enzyme. In conventional medicine these patients are called "outliers" (outside the normal parameters). In alternative medicine, physicians realize that as long as a person takes sufficient B12, he or she can function normally. But no blood level is going to tell us to which category our patients belong. For this reason, practitioners of functional medicine test whether someone has enough stores of B12 to carry out the necessary metabolic processes. "Alternative" medicine? Or simply good medicine?

Functional medicine = the intersection between allopathic and alternative medicine; personalized medicine that deals with primary prevention and underlying causes for serious chronic disease, instead of merely the symptoms.

Convention has its uses – sort of like ballast. Ballast helps to keep a ship weighted down so the wind does not blow it over. But ballast is also something to be jettisoned when the waves start to wash over the deck. And, if we may carry the analogy a little further, that is indeed what is happening to our children and grandchildren right now. We are in the midst of an epidemic of autism, ADHD, pediatric obesity, childhood cancers, adult chronic illness and type 2 diabetes, the likes of which have never been seen before in recorded history.

Frances Pottenger, Jr., M.D., was a California physician who conducted a study from 1932 to 1942 that became known as the "Pottenger Cat Study". More than 900 cats were studied. He found that a natural feline diet produced generation after generation of healthy cats. But an unnatural diet – which for cats means cooking their food – caused each successive generation to be less healthy than the last. By the third generation, the kittens were too sick to reproduce. The cats suffered from most of the degenerative diseases encountered in human medicine and died out by the fourth generation.

Is this beginning to sound familiar? Our great-grandparents may have died of infectious diseases, but chronic illness was virtually unknown. They ate fresh food and meat that was not laden with chemicals, antibiotics and hormones. Then we began to eat differently. "Better living through chemistry" was the way to go. Now we spend our last years dying of renal failure, diabetes, heart disease, cancer or Alzheimer's dementia. Those who should be at the peak of their productive years are on multiple medications to prevent diabetes and heart disease, and one in six children is suffering from some diagnosed mental illness. Men have erectile dysfunction at 40 or even 30. Young men have low testosterone levels. Pharmaceutical companies are making "chewable Lipitor®" for our children as young as age four. What is wrong with this picture?

I am saddened to see intelligent, caring and skillful physicians persecuted by their state medical boards for pursuing something more than the narrow allopathic standards of care.

I am not the only physician to be concerned about where conventional medicine has taken us. An allopathic surgeon, R.D. Wolcott, M.D., writes in an online interview:[i,ii]

> I take it you are familiar with evidence-based medicine? It's the increasingly accepted approach for making clinical decisions about how to treat a patient. Basically, doctors are trained to make a decision based on the most current evidence derived from research. But what such thinking boils down to is that I am supposed to do the same thing that has always been done – to treat my patient in the conventional manner – just because it's become the most popular approach. However, when it comes to chronic wound biofilms, we are in the midst of a crisis – what has been done and is accepted as the standard treatment doesn't work and doesn't meet the needs of the patient.
>
> Thus, evidence-based medicine totally regulates against innovation. Essentially doctors suffer if they step away from mainstream thinking. Sure, there are charlatans out there who are trying to sell us treatments that don't

work, but there are many good therapies that are not used because they are unconventional. It is only by considering new treatment options that we can progress.

The public is demanding change. And little by little, their demands are being heard, even by the establishment. Acupuncture, for example, is practiced in some hospitals, and even in some cancer care centers – but still pretty much only to treat the side effects of chemotherapy.

I spent almost 30 years as a physician in hospital emergency rooms. I was an allopath, an ER Doc. Still am an allopath – I have an M.D. license. But when the day came that I saw that the options for patients were too limited, and I was specifically instructed by my hospital administrator and ER Director NOT to refer patients outside the bounds of traditional allopathic medicine, I had to step out of the box. I just could not practice medicine in such a very limited way, when I knew that there were sometimes better options. I came to Arizona because the state legislature had listened to patients' demands and had established the Board of Homeopathic and Integrated Medicine Examiners. The license granted by that board allows Medical Doctors and Doctors of Osteopathy to take advanced studies and qualify (by taking an examination) to utilize approaches to medicine that often are not taught in conventional medical schools. We homeopathic physicians have the ability to practice medicine within a broader standard of care. For example, patients come to me after surgery for intravenous vitamin C and glutathione to flush out the anesthesia and speed the healing process – anesthesia is necessary but toxic and very much worth flushing out. Medical schools don't teach this, but why not? It helps patients recover much faster.

The word "doctor" comes from the Latin word "docere" meaning "to teach." Good medicine requires that we do that. People who come to me already know the answers won't come in the form of a simple pill. They want to know what went wrong and how to fix it. By not taking insurance, I have been able to free myself from the ten minute appointment structure so I actually have time to teach. My patients learn that food is information to their body, and to their genes. They learn how environmental pollutants chisel away at their health and what they can do to limit that. With this book, I begin to share that with you.

I saw a movie once where the main character, a gladiator, said something to the effect that what we do here on earth echoes in eternity. He probably wasn't thinking about genetics, but I was when I heard it. The food and environmental pollution we encounter each day tweaks our genes in ways that will be passed down for generations to come. The field of epigenetics is turning upside down what we in medicine thought we knew about genes and inheritance. What my grandmother ate makes a difference in who I am and how my body works. Fascinating to consider, isn't it? And it brings whole new meaning to the term "family practice." If we want a world in which our children's generation has a *longer* lifespan than our own generation, then I, as a doctor, need to do what I can to teach how our world impacts our health and that of those who come after us.

Welcome to the journey.

---

[i] Wolcott RD, Rhoads DD. A study of biofilm-based wound management in subjects with critical limb ischaemia. *J Wound Care.* 2008 Apr;17(4):145-8, 150-2, 154-5.

[ii] http://bacteriality.com/2008/04/13/wolcott/ downloaded on August 14, 2010

INTRODUCTION

Mary Budinger

$\mathcal{I}$ remember waking up cold and oddly wet. The sheets in my bed were drenched with my sweat. I sat up and swung my legs over the side of the bed to stand up. Then the pain registered. Pain in every joint as if I were a 90-year-old arthritic woman. I could barely walk to the bathroom. The lymph nodes in my neck were big and hard as marbles. The night before, life had been normal. As of that morning, it would never be the same.

I was 35 at the time. I was an Emmy-award winning television journalist. But instead of moving up the career ladder, life came to a crashing halt. Suddenly, I became something of a regular at the Mayo Clinic.

I really, really disliked everything medical. Always had. My mom told me when she took me as a toddler for regular doctors' visits, I would pass out when the nurse brought out the stainless steel tray with the needles on it. All my life, just walking into a hospital makes me nervous. But at age 35, I entered the medical establishment in a big way.

Mayo Clinic was an impressive place. Spacious waiting areas and all the specialists you might need under one nicely appointed roof. In a single day, you could see three or four different specialists; the clinic's scheduling abilities rivaled the eighth wonder of the world. First stop: the blood lab. "Eighty percent of the time we can tell what is wrong with you by the blood tests," the doctor said. I would come to learn that doctors often use a bell curve, but I was often at the far edges of the bell curve so what worked for most people, did not work for me.

A nurse walked toward me with three blood collecting vials big enough to roll a golf ball through. "Do you faint easily?" Jeez. Is the sky blue or the Pope Catholic? She had me lie down and, three hours later, the lead doctor on my case had the results. I will never forget the way the paper with the test results rolled off his desk and reached all the way to the floor. Who knew there were so many things they could measure from blood?

"I have patients in here for annual exams who have more wrong with them than you do," the doctor said. "Except that your SED rate and triglycerides are high, and you get a rash in the sun, you look pretty normal. Yet clearly, something is very wrong with you. It is amazing you didn't use a wheelchair to get in here today."

My fear was so intense now I could hear the ocean roaring in my ears. Being sick had always been relatively simple. It meant getting a prescription – usually for antibiotics – and all was well a few days later. This time was going to be different. I wasn't among the 80 percent whose disease could be given a name after looking at blood tests. Now it was time for lots more tests and rude invasions into body parts in hopes of finding an answer that obviously wouldn't be fixed with a simple course of pills.

The doctor told me other pathologists might disagree, and that he was not 100 percent sure, but it looked as if I had a rare, pre-cancerous lymph node condition called angioimmunoblastic lymphadenopathy with disproteinemia, or AILD for short. I wanted to applaud that anyone could actually pronounce that. There had been only about five cases of it in the Mayo system and all of those people died – either of cancer or pneumonia. The doctor explained that he would knock it down with prednisone – a powerful pain killing steroid – and an antibiotic because the steroid would 7lower my immune system. He told me I would develop a "watermelon face" and gain about 50 pounds – big time weight gain is a normal side effect of the steroid. I was five-foot-seven, weighed about 130 pounds. I couldn't imagine weighing 180. (He failed to mention the acne from hell, the incredible insomnia, and the short term memory loss.) Over time, I would be weaned off the steroids and then we all would hope the AILD had been conquered and that it would never return.

About 18 months later, when I had been off the steroids about 3 months, I woke up and it was all back – night sweats, swollen lymph nodes, and pain in every joint. More tests at Mayo, ranging from AIDS and Lyme to Parkinson's Disease and anything that involves the lymph nodes. They even put my case up on the monthly satellite feed where the various Mayo Clinics around the country discuss their "interesting" cases. They decided my case probably wasn't AILD after all, but Still's disease, the juvenile form of rheumatoid arthritis (RA). But maybe not – I didn't test positive for the RA factor – but then again not everyone does. The doctor explained all the drugs with which they would manage my disease on the assumption it was RA. Was there something I could do with diet or lifestyle? No, they said. What about the rash I developed after just a few minutes in the sun? Probably an allergy – but never mind that, there were bigger fish to fry.

I didn't want my disease "managed," I wanted it gone. The doctor patted me on the knee and said something to the effect that I was young and that they would probably find a cure in my lifetime.

I was to come to Mayo for gold shots once a week for several months. The doctor explained they didn't know why gold works, but they noticed in the 1950s that when they gave gold shots to tuberculosis patients who also had RA, the RA got better because the overactive immune system calmed down somewhat. But injecting microscopic bits of gold could be tough on the body. Some people were allergic to it, some developed blood disorders, some people even ended up on dialysis because of kidney damage.

By this time, I had spent a weekend at the University of Arizona medical school library – this was 1991, before Google was a twinkle in anyone's eye. I learned that gold shots were pretty far along the continuum of "disease management." The drugs that would come after that would be even worse. My body would turn into a demolition derby. A wheelchair was almost certainly in my future.

To go through life as a sick person didn't fit my self-image. I refused to accept it. I felt that some switches in my body had gotten flipped in the wrong direction and *somebody* must know how to flip them back. What I read in the medical library talked a lot about the effects of drugs and various therapies on RA, but not how to fix what went wrong. I had thought that at Mayo Clinic I would find the top guns of medicine. But they had no cure, just management of a disease they weren't positive I had.

I decided I needed different answers. There was this thing out there called Alternative Medicine. I didn't know what it was – didn't know the difference between a homeopath and a naturopath or if it was any good – but I was going to find out.

♦ ♦ ♦

Tennis is a great game. I can play it now. That's something people with RA can never do. It took me about eight years to get well; if I had known then what I know now, I think I could have done it in three.

What I had was something the Mayo docs didn't look for, didn't have on their radar yet – Leaky Gut Syndrome. The Standard American Diet (inflammatory vegetable oils, lots of sugar, lots of calories but not so much nutrition) can inflame the gut. That can turn your small intestines into a leaky sieve. Undigested food and whatnot gets out of the gut into places it's not supposed to be. The immune system senses invaders and calls up the troops. The cascade of events gets uglier from there. I learned the hard way about autoimmune responses, not absorbing what you eat, infected synovial fluid, candida overgrowth, and that food allergies can affect your mind and as well as your body. It's the price I paid for not thinking that what I ate was important. It's kind of embarrassing to admit this now, but one of my favorite dinners in the single days of my 20s was potato chips and sour cream. Another was fish sticks. And a handful of cookies for breakfast – yummy and easy to eat on the run. Yet if you had asked me, I probably would have said yes, I eat a balanced diet. I didn't. Nor did I get away with it. Most of us don't one way or another.

I owe a world of thanks to Jana Riter, a colonic therapist who steered me in the right direction about diet. I asked her which one book had it pretty darn right when it came to food. She handed me Sally Fallon's *Nourishing Traditions*. It took me almost a year to read it. I had found a treasure chest of secrets about food – the truth, the whole truth, and not a word of it bought and paid for by food manufacturers. Today as I write this, I have been to the farmers' market and am making stock. (I used to think the stock pot was for pasta.) Nutrient-rich stock was the first real food I learned to make from scratch. Thank you Sally Fallon Morell and the Weston A. Price Foundation. Food is the best medicine.

To get where I am today, I made a boatload of changes. On one hand, it was hard for me to do that because I was so clueless. Growing up, it was my job to wash the dishes, not help with the making of dinner. I remember every Sunday night my family would watch TV and eat a bucket of fried chicken that Dad had picked up. Living the single life as a TV news person, I wasn't home much to cook. Food was merely a pit stop and often it was fast food.

On the other hand, it was easy for me to make big changes because I was heavily motivated. Eating the right food was better at relieving pain than the prednisone had been – and there are no side effects to food. My personal care products and household cleaners got an overhaul too – I found non-toxic versions and I put filters on the water line to remove chlorine and fluoride.

For many people, it is tough to change the relationship with food. A lot of what is in the supermarket and in the fast food places is formulated to make people want to eat more of it. We are drowning in calories yet we are malnourished. How many of us know how to make meals from scratch or think we have time to do that? Working with a nutritionist was my first stop after leaving Mayo because I knew I had a problem with food – the pain level went up like clockwork every time I ate. The nutritionist realized that I was allergic to just about everything I ate regularly. She gave me a list of about 20 foods to eat for the next six to twelve months, and none of them had sugar in any way, shape, or form. I even switched to a toothpaste without sugar. The withdrawal symptoms were extreme for several days; I can only imagine the agony people must go through trying to withdraw from narcotics. Both act on the pleasure centers of the brain.

During that year of food elimination, I read a lot about juicing which taught me the importance of vitamins, minerals, and enzymes in raw food.

I figured my gas tank must have been on empty since I never ate vegetables. What if the rash I got after just a few moments in the sun was because I was lacking beta carotene? The doctors said the rash wasn't lupus but they didn't know what it was. Hm'm'm. When the time arrived that I could handle the sugar from carrots, I began to juice. A month later, I lay in the sun for ten minutes on each side. No rash. Problem solved. Food is medicine.

It can be hard to change our relationship with our environment because we really don't want to believe that there are carcinogens in our bathroom products, for example. I mean, the government is looking out for us consumers; *they* wouldn't let that on the market, would they? Actually, yes *they* do. We need to get our heads out of the sand. This "epidemic" of chronic disease in America isn't going away until we have a more honest dialogue about what we eat and what is in our environment.

◆ ◆ ◆

My husband had a mild heart attack a couple years ago. He was rushed into the cath lab and, with no prior discussion about options, came out with three stents in one of his arteries. Two hours later, he was served a hospital lunch that included caffeinated ice tea and a refined white flour biscuit accompanied by a vegetable oil spread. And we wonder why diseases of diet are spiraling out of control.

I had never had much reason to read up on stents before this event. Several studies read like the one published January 15, 2009 in the *New England Journal of Medicine:* people with clogged heart arteries are being overtreated with stents. Fewer deaths, heart attacks, and repeat procedures occur when doctors implant fewer stents. Don't you think the hospital might have talked to us about the possibility of stents and asked us what we wanted to do? But hey, insurance paid the bill, so all is well, right?

When you are frightened for your life, you tend to let "experts" wearing lab jackets make decisions for you. That's called the power of the white coat. We were bullied by the power of the white coat in the hospital just as so many breast cancer patients are bullied into immediately starting a severe regimen of chemotherapy. But we didn't take the statins and the blood thinners that were prescribed. We thanked the doctors for their service and headed for Dr. Grout's office to start a course of chelation.

◆ ◆ ◆

Dr. Martha Grout and I met several years ago. She was a level-headed voice in a meeting sprouting a wide swath of proposals. She struck me as unusually down to earth, as doctors go. She wears Birkenstocks and tee shirts. We had lunch and I briefly explained the odyssey that had taken me from reporting the daily news to writing about medicine. To this day, neither one of us can remember exactly what she said, but my jaw dropped to the floor. In several sentences, she pretty much summed up the gist of what I had learned since that morning I woke up drenched in sweat with a raging case of inflammation.

We have a much longer list of diseases than we did a hundred years ago, yet we seem to have a much smaller ability to stick any of them on people. I've seen many people, some even on oxygen because they have such diminished lung capacity, who do not know what is wrong with them. They have seen a lot of doctors, taken a lot of tests, and still no one can figure out what is causing their problems.

Our bodies are like a chain of links. Every day we are bombarded with many stressors that tug at those links. At some point, one of the links breaks and we fall sick. Which link breaks often depends upon the genetic deck of cards we've been dealt. My mother and her mother both had a great deal of arthritis so it's no wonder my problems befell my joints.

What I have seen tells me the label isn't so important. The fix is the important part, and the fix is often pretty similar for an amazing number of different diagnosed diseases. When you look down from the 20,000 foot level at illness in America today, many of us are getting sick for the same reasons and many of us can get well by doing a number of the same things. In Dr. Grout's view of the world, patients don't "complain." Patients feel and experience symptoms that create a road map of dysfunction that she uses to figure out how to customize the fix. She has meticulously assembled the ability to provide a broad array of healing "fixes," blending the conventional with the alternative and the functional, in a non-toxic environment. She practices green medicine.

Dr. Grout's view of the world also means that you educate your patients – a content-rich website, patient education materials, lectures, and now her first book. They don't make doctors like this every day.

Section I

The Three Pillars:

FOOD
CHEMICALS
ELECTROMAGNETIC ENERGY

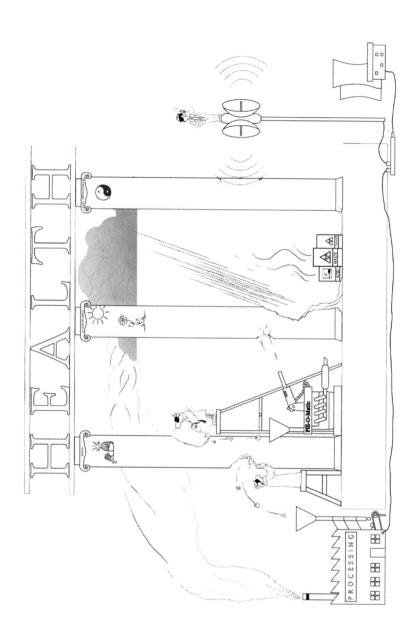

A toxic soup of heavy metals, EMF pollution, chemicals, and the body's own toxins produced by disease, is turning long-familiar microorganisms into super stars of destruction. Combined with junk food and a chemical-laden environment, they all add up to the perfect storm where perhaps a few types of biotoxins are produced in us in unprecedented rates.[1]

There is a trio of elements that is key to understanding chronic disease: **food, chemicals, and electromagnetic fields.** Understanding the impact they have on disease and healing makes all the difference in medicine in the 21st century.

Food can give good or bad information to the body. Some chemicals are essential, such as glutathione and glucose, but some chemicals are toxic, such as man-made plastics which can interfere with the endocrine system. The body's inner communication system is all about signaling with frequencies, but man-made devices generate unnatural frequencies that can interfere with the body's signaling.

Food, chemicals, and electromagnetic fields are like coins – they have a good side and a bad side. The bad side of the coin generates an intense stress that is driving the rates of chronic disease to epidemic proportions.

So let's go there first because understanding these three pillars of health and disease will go a long way toward explaining what went wrong and why so many people are sick.

---

[1] Mary Budinger. A "Perfect Storm" Accelerates the Chronic Disease Epidemic – Report from the LIA Conference of 2009. *Explore! For the Professional.* September, 2009

Food – Genetics, Addiction, and Politics

Your genes do not determine how your medical history will unfold. The environment – the way you eat, how much you exercise, how you deal with stress, your body's interaction with environmental toxins (chemicals and EMF) – will cause some gene mutations to express themselves. Or not.

Food is information to your genes. Each mouthful gives your genes, and the 60 trillion or so cells in your body, good information or junk information, depending upon what you choose to eat.

The "EPIC" study[1] published in 2009, for example, studied 23,000 people's adherence to four simple behaviors:

- not smoking
- exercising 3.5 hours a week
- eating a diet of fruits, vegetables, beans, whole grains, nuts, seeds, and limited meat
- maintaining a healthy weight, meaning a Body Mass Index of less than 30

In those adhering to these behaviors, 93% of diabetes, 81% of heart attacks, 50% of strokes, and 36% of all cancers were prevented.

A number of studies report similar findings that preventive lifestyle is the best medicine.[2] Food matters – a lot. Our eating habits and environment influence the fundamental causes of and biological mechanisms leading to disease:

- Changes in gene expression, which modulate inflammation (chronic inflammation drives most chronic diseases)
- Oxidative stress (free radicals kill micro-organisms, but in excess do damage to our own DNA)

- Metabolic dysfunction (can't excrete waste from cells because of hydrogenated oils, can't absorb nutrients because of leaky gut, can't utilize thyroid, can't, can't, can't...).

That, in a nutshell, is how we stop being well and start being sick.

Until relatively recently, food was not widely manufactured. People consumed meat that was grass fed, not processed hot dogs and deli meats made with chemical preservatives that are associated with a 42% higher risk of heart disease and a 19% higher risk of type 2 diabetes. Eggs came from chickens that scratched for bugs outside, not from factories where thousands of caged birds are fed soy and arsenic.[3, 4] There was no such thing as high fructose corn syrup, MSG, aspartame, BHT, propylene glycol, synthetic food colorings, genetically modified organisms, or chemicals made to trick the taste buds into thinking they were tasting real food. People ate animal fats (lard, butter) and unprocessed coconut oil, not oily vegetable fats high in inflammatory omega 6s, and not partially hydrogenated trans fats or the more recently manufactured and equally harmful interesterified fats. Parents gave their children a daily spoonful of cod liver oil (high in vitamins A and D). People drank their milk fresh and raw, and they made bread without bromide. But all that changed, and very quickly, within one generation.

We were taught to use "heart healthy" vegetable oils (corn, soybean, safflower, cottonseed, and sunflower) that helped fuel the rise in heart disease. Advertisements told us that aluminum-laced soy milk made from genetically modified beans was a smart purchase. We were told that toxic synthetic sugars were better than the real thing. We were scolded that eggs were bad, so we turned to starchy bagels and sugary breakfast cereals. We came to crave fast foods for their taste and convenience... We were marketed to death.

To peek into how the United States became the least healthy country in the industrialized world (in terms of life expectancy and obesity rates), is to find out how to get beyond this predicament.

Food Changed in a Generation

$\mathscr{C}$ancer, heart disease, and diabetes – the top three diseases we die of – are largely environmental. That means they are pretty much avoidable because they are a result of what we eat and the toxins in the environment around us. Man-made trans fats, for example, were estimated to kill 30,000 people a year.[5] That is 10 times more than the death total from 9/11.

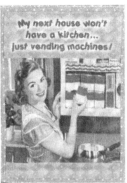

Our food began to change drastically in the 1950s because American productivity was humming after the war. Convenience was the new fashion – why bother to make soups from scratch when you could just open a can? White breads, white sugar – white anything – was thought to be much more stylish than your mother's old familiar brown version. Aluminum trays of frozen TV dinners were all the rage. Fresh food from the local farm was becoming a relic of the past.

The 1970s saw a period of high inflation when retail food prices rose an average of nearly nine percent a year. The public screamed. President Richard Nixon told his Secretary of Agriculture, Earl Butz, to do whatever it took to lower the price of food. New government policies sprang up to subsidize crops and create the system of monocultures – raising just one crop on a huge amount of acreage. As Michael Pollen, author of *The Omnivore's Dilemma*, describes it:

> [We] Americans only spend 9.5 percent of our income on food today. That's less than anybody in the history of civilization, and we have Earl Butz to thank. In the last thirty years, we have had this kind of agriculture industrial complex, which by some measures has worked quite well. It's kept the price of food low; it's kept the food industry healthy; it's given us a lot of power overseas—we're big food exporters—but what we're getting in touch with, I think, is that the by-products of that system, or the unintended consequences and costs, are catching up—every thing from obesity to diabetes.

3

> Because that was a system that specifically encouraged the consumption of cheap corn sweeteners, high fructose corn syrup, hydrogenated oils from soy, processed foods of all kinds, a lot of cheap meat. So, there's been a public health impact that's dramatic. That is what's bankrupting the health care system: the fact that half of us suffer from chronic diseases linked to the diet. ...Nutrition science is approximately where surgery was in the year 1650.[6]

Nutrition decisions based largely on studies funded by the processed food industries gave birth to the first USDA-sponsored Food Pyramid in 1992. The foods we were advised to eat the most of were the processed carbohydrates – six to eleven daily servings of bread, cereal, rice, and pasta.

Nutrition "experts" went with the flow and spread the message. The high-carb fad sold a lot of pasta and bread making machines and a lot of cookbooks extolling the starchy and glutinous carbs. It was a disaster for blood sugar levels.

Today, everyone has gotten the message that those starchy carbs are the "bad" carbs that spike insulin levels, and vegetables are the "good" carbs. The industry moved on to the next disastrous fad – low fat. With so much political pressure from the food processing industry, sound nutritional advice squeaks out only in drips and dabs.

America Is a Hay Belly Nation

Ever wonder why hay bales are kept in barns instead of outside exposed to the elements? Because when it rains, the nutrients wash out of the hay. When the cattle eat this hay, their bodies signal them to eat more of it than usual in an effort to get a full quota of nutrients. Their bellies get really big – what farmers call hay bellies. It is a sign of poor quality food.

Same thing happens with people. When we eat food, our body is looking for nutrients. When the food is nutrient-poor, the body signals us to keep eating because it is still looking for its quota of nutrients.

The desire to eat junk food is a vicious cycle – the more you eat it the more your body craves it because junk food distorts your hormonal profile, stimulating your appetite and causing you to crave unhealthy foods, while making you feel unsatisfied when you eat only healthy ones.

What we are about to tell you goes against the Great American Marketing Machine. The food producing industry goes to great lengths to ensure that you don't hear this. The cancer industry would have fewer clients. The pharmaceutical industry would sell fewer drugs. The vegetable oil makers would lose sales. The soy sellers and the food additive companies would struggle to survive.

Truth be told, how to eat right is not a major mystery. In one sentence it is this: *eat food as nature made it, not as man has processed it.*

Eating good fats (butter, grass fed meats, cod liver oil, nuts, unrefined coconut and olive oil) is the prescription for providing energy, making strong cell membranes, making hormones, and eating in moderation. Without fat at the table, your body has trouble absorbing the vitamins and minerals from the veggies on your plate. Without fat, you don't feel full so you don't stop eating. Eating hamburger from cows or buffaloes raised organically on grass is a good quality fat; a fast food hamburger from a cow fed hormones, steroids, genetically modified corn and then positioned between two refined pieces of bread, slathered in hydrogenated vegetable oils masquerading as mayonnaise and high fructose corn syrup masquerading as a catsup, is not. Eating truly unprocessed coconut oil may even help you lose weight. Eating a salad with the typical manufactured salad dressing made of vegetable oils will likely pack on the pounds. Green leafy salads were not even part of the American diet prior to the 1930s; lettuce doesn't pack that much nutritional punch. The idea of salads was largely the creation of the vegetable oil industry to sell more product in the form of salad dressing. Real food is a whole egg of the farmer's market variety, not a pasteurized egg-white only liquid in a carton.

Glucose (sugar) is essential to life because the body uses it to perform all its functions. But we do not have to eat sugar for our bodies to make glucose. Our ancestors ate fruits and grains that were not refined or processed. In other words, their sugars and carbs came with the vitamins, minerals, enzymes, and minerals needed for metabolism. When B vitamins are absent for example, the breakdown of carbohydrates cannot take place. Yet modern refining usually removes most of the B vitamins.

With obesity and other food-related diseases rampant in America, why is it so hard to get back to basics? Because food – how we think about it, how much money we spend on it – is a daily dance of politics, economics, habit, and addiction.

Politics Invaded Your Kitchen

Thanks to lobbying in Washington, Congress subsidizes the very foods that we're supposed to eat less of. The effects of huge government subsidies to huge agribusinesses make high fructose corn syrup, corn oil for frying, and cheap fast food burgers:

Federal Subsidies for Food Production, 1995-2005

- Meat and diary – 73.8%
- Grains – 13.23%
- Sugar, oil, starch, alcohol – 10.69%
- Vegetables, fruits – 0.37%

Source: Physicians Committee for Responsible Medicine
Accessed at http://www.pcrm.org/magazine/gm07autumn/health_pork.html

---

Fruit and vegetable farmers receive less than one percent of the government subsidies. You might remember the scene in the Oscar-nominated film *Food Inc.,* that revealed some dark sides of the industrial food system. In the documentary, a lower-income family wants to eat healthy and buy vegetables, but cannot afford them so they spend what little money they have on the cheaper fast food fare.

Columnist Nicholas Kristof, writing in the *New York Times*, December 2008, stated:

It is time to rethink the very notion of a Department of Agriculture [USDA] ... The problem isn't farmers. It's the farm lobby – hijacked by industrial operators – and a bipartisan tradition of kowtowing to it. The farm lobby uses that perch to inflict unhealthy food on American children in school-lunch programs, exacerbating our national crisis with diabetes and obesity.[7]

New York Times columnist David Leonhardt dug through data from the Bureau of Labor Statistics and found that over the last 30 years, fresh fruits and veggies became 40 percent more expensive, while soda got 30 percent cheaper:

The average 18-year-old today is 15 pounds heavier than the average 18-year-old in the late 1970s. Adults have put on even more weight during that period.[8] The average woman in her 60s is 20 pounds heavier than the average 60-something woman in the late 1970s. The average man in his 60s is 25 pounds heavier. When you look at the chart, you start to understand why.

Who Controls Our Food?

*M*ost economic sectors have concentration ratios hovering around 40%, meaning that the top four firms in the industry control 40% of the market. Agriculture far exceeds those ratios.[9]

Never before have the safety and sustainability of our food supply depended upon the decisions of so few people. The USDA and the Department of Justice held public workshops throughout 2010 to address issues of concentration and antitrust violations in agriculture.

According to the Organic Consumers Association:

- 80 percent of non-organic beef in the U.S. is slaughtered by four companies.
- 75 percent of non-organic pre-cut salad mixes are processed by two companies.
- 30 percent of non-organic milk is processed by one company.

Concentration narrows consumer choice and presents barriers to accessing locally-grown, organic, sustainable, and family farm-identified food. This puts the food supply at risk. Remember the E. coli outbreak of 2006 that took bagged spinach off the shelves? And the 2010 salmonella outbreak, caused by contaminated eggs? Concentration breeds food-borne diseases that spread quickly over a large area – there were confirmed cases of E. coli O157:H7 from bagged spinach in 26 states. The E. coli O157:H7 bacterium is a newly emerged pathogen, thanks to the rise of huge feedlots. When commercial feedlot cattle poop, pathogens can travel via groundwater to nearby organic vegetable fields, allowing even the organic vegetables to share the contamination.

Feedlot concentration breeds something else: stressed animals. The cells of all living things communicate by means of what is called "cellular signaling." A cell under stress reads somewhat different signals than a healthy cell, and therefore sends out different signals. One school of thought says that meat from animals raised under stressful conditions with hormones and steroids inevitably imparts those stress signals to those of us who eat the meat.[10,11]

Feeding Your Stomach by Doping Your Brain

What has been driving us to overeat?

Harvard-trained doctor and former FDA Commissioner David Kessler went dumpster-diving behind popular chain restaurants to see what Americans are really eating. He found a trio of ingredients guaranteed to keep us coming back for more – salt, fats, and sugar. (Note – most restaurant food uses vegetable oils which are inflammatory.)

Initially, he says, the food industry discovered that adding these ingredients increased product shelf life. But the salt/fat/sugar trio also makes food addictively compelling. It stimulates neurons that trigger the brain's reward system and release dopamine, a feel-good chemical that motivates our behavior to have more of what makes us feel good.

8

Combined in the right way, Kessler said, those three elements act upon our brains like an addictive drug.

"Much of the scientific research around overeating has been physiology – what's going on in our body," he wrote in his book, *The End of Overeating: Taking Control of the Insatiable American Appetite*. "The real question is what's going on in our brain."

Kessler gives an example of a popular appetizer:

> What's in Buffalo wings? You start with the fatty part of the chicken. Many times it's fried in the manufacturing plant first. It's fried again in the restaurant. That red sauce? Sugar and fat. That creamy sauce? Fat and salt. So what are we eating? Fat on fat on fat on sugar on fat and salt.

Instead of satisfying hunger, the salt/fat/sugar combination will stimulate the brain to crave more, and the food industry manipulates this neurological response, designing foods to induce people to eat more than they should or even want, Kessler found. He sees parallels between the tobacco and food industries in that both are manipulating consumer behavior to sell products that can harm health:

> The food the industry is selling is much more powerful than we realized. The challenge is how do we explain to America what's going on – how do we break through and help people understand how their brains have been captured?[12]

After just one meal of junk food, tissue becomes inflamed, just as it does when infected. Blood vessels constrict. Free radicals that cause cell damage are generated. The body's stress response raises blood pressure. The sudden surge and subsequent drop in insulin leaves people feeling hungry again soon after eating, despite having had plenty of calories. Junk food sets up a vicious cycle – the more you eat it, the more your body craves it because junk food distorts your hormonal profile, stimulating your appetite and causing you to crave unhealthy foods, while making you feel unsatisfied when you eat only healthy food.[13]

9

For countless millions of Americans living now, the generic fast-food flavor is one of the indelible smells and tastes of childhood, a comfort food that bathes the brain in feel-good chemicals. Today's generation of kids may come to think of processed food the way ex-smokers and ex-drinkers think of their former addictions – forever a temptation that needs to be kept at arm's length.

Your Blood On Pizza and Fries

The Weston A. Price Foundation (WAPF) extensively studies what traditional societies ate – before outsiders brought sacks of sugar and flour – and promotes that dietary wisdom. WAPF conducted a novel study comparing the blood of people who eat a WAPF diet to that of people who eat today's standard American diet. The most easily monitored tissue that shows changes in response to nutritional status is the blood. Fascinating results.

The picture below on the left is the blood of a 30-year-old woman who has been eating according to WAPF guidelines for eight years. Note the mostly round red blood cells of relatively uniform size, without any debris in the plasma, which is characteristic of normal healthy blood, with the blood initially showing no activation of clotting or plasma debris.

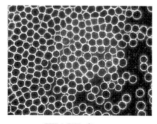 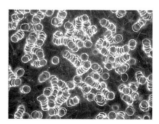

WAPF diet   **Standard American diet**
Reprinted with permission of Sally Fallon Morell
See the complete study at the Weston A. Price Foundation

The picture on the right is the blood of a different 30-year-old woman who eats the standard American diet. Note how the red blood cells stick together and are aggregated into loose "rouleaux" (rolls or stacks of coins) and the presence of the clotting protein, fibrin, in a network. Fibrin is seen here as white fibers that look much like a disorganized spider web. This photo shows viscous (thick, sticky) blood with activated clotting factors.

The woman who eats the WAPF diet eats like this: 90 percent of meat eaten is from pastured animals, one quart of raw milk per week, twelve eggs per week, cod liver oil daily (source of vitamins A and D), six tablespoons of saturated fat daily, fermented foods three times per week, preparation of 100 percent of grains and nuts by soaking or sourdough; and no alcohol consumption. The WAPF diet does not contain any processed foods including soy milk or pasteurized milk with denatured components that may act to promote inflammation in the body. There are no trans fats and no genetically modified organisms in natural unprocessed organic foods.

We showed just one comparison here; the study compared people of various ages. The older the person was on the standard diet, the worse the comparison looked.

Note that the WAPF diet is not vegetarian. In the words of one of the doctors allied with the Foundation:

> Let me tell you, the first cancer patient who comes in with a rumen [first of
> 4 digestive compartments in a cow], I'm putting them on a vegetarian diet,
> I don't care what blood type they are. If they have very long intestines and
> a rumen with bacteria to ferment cellulose, I'd put them on a vegetarian diet.
> –Dr. Thomas Cowen

Industry Muscle

Industrialized food manufacturing is big business. When threatened, it acts to protect sales as any business would.

As the nation gets sicker, more people are beginning to argue there are moral as well as financial considerations to cheap food with unhealthy additives. The current soda wars are a classic case.

Sweetened beverage consumption accounts for 50 percent of the sugar intake in the U.S. diet. PepsiCo is the second largest food company in the world. Here's an excerpt of a 2010 interview PepsiCo CEO Indra Nooyi gave to *Fortune* magazine:

Q – "You've said that Pepsi should be part of the solution, not the cause, of obesity. How are you and PepsiCo planning to go about that?"

A – "If all consumers exercised, did what they had to do, the problem of obesity wouldn't exist. ... If I look at our portfolio, I think you can classify them into three groups: 'fun-for-you foods' like Pepsi, Doritos, Lays, and Mountain Dew, 'better-for-you' products like Diet Pepsi, PepsiMax, Baked Lays, Sobi Life Water, Propel, all of these products, and 'good-for-you' products like Quaker, Tropicana, Naked Juice, Gatorade."[14]

People strenuously disagree. Many see that "Fun-for-you" is just PR spin "Bad-for-you." The majority of the states have a sales tax on soda now; it used to be that soda was exempt like most groceries. Efforts are building to impose a "sin tax" on soda akin to the high taxes on cigarettes. Professor Kelly Brownell at the Rudd Center on Food Policy and Obesity believes consumers need a financial dis-incentive to buy sweetened drinks:

You can educate people all day long, but you can never compete with the amount of marketing money that the industry spends to educate people to consume these beverages.[15]

In the first quarter of 2010, the American Beverage Association (ABA) exponentially upped its lobbying expenditures 3,785 percent over the last quarter of 2009. According to the Center for Responsive Politics, the ABA went from spending just $140,000 to spending $5.4 million.[16]

Gail Woodward-Lopez with the Center for Weight and Health at U.C. Berkeley states that "sweetened beverages should be consumed a maximum of once per week, but definitely it should not be a part of your daily intake."[17]

That's the last thing companies like PepsiCo want consumers and lawmakers to hear. And they built a war chest to get out their message.

Veiled Third Party Endorsements

The American Dietetic Association (ADA) has been working on a long-range plan to determine who can dispense information about nutrition. Typically, dietitians plan menus for hospitals, schools, and prisons with the goal of holding food costs to a minimum. The organization has attempted to pass laws in just about every state designating ADA-certified dieticians as the *only* legal entity allowed to set nutritional standards. (The effort came to Arizona in the form of House Bill 2406; it was killed in April 1990.)

This organization lists among its corporate sponsors soft drink giants Coca-Cola and PepsiCo, cereal manufacturers General Mills and Kellogg's, candy maker Mars, and Unilever, the multinational corporation that owns many of the world's consumer products brands in foods and beverages.[18]

Would it be a conflict of interest to have an organization with that parade of corporate sponsors be the same organization that endorses nutrition standards? You betcha. But it would be a great way for big food manufacturers to get what in the public relations business is called a third party endorsement that sodas and candy and processed junk foods are part of a "balanced" diet.

And it's not just the American Dietetic Association. The American Academy of Pediatric Dentistry accepted $1 million from Coca-Cola to "promote improved dental health for children."[19] The American Academy of Family Physicians made headlines in 2009 when it accepted $500,000 from Coca-Cola "to develop consumer education content related to beverages and sweeteners."[20] In November 2006, the *New York Times* front page questioned the American Diabetes Association's ethics. The organization took $23 million in 2005 from drug and food companies, especially food companies whose primary business is selling products high in calories and synthetic sugars.

13

Medical-professional organizations and health charities are among the biggest recipients of industry funding, according to Center for Science in the Public Interest (CSPI). In 2003, CSPI published a report, "Lifting the Veil of Secrecy," a review of corporate sponsorship. CSPI wrote:

> Nonprofit organizations... are usually considered to be objective and serving the public interest. In recent decades, though, a new factor has crept, often secretly, onto the scene. Corporations, with their own motivations, have learned that they can influence public opinion and public policy more effectively by working through seemingly independent organizations... Their power to persuade is significantly enhanced when they can get an apparently independent nonprofit organization to advocate on their behalf.[21]

And then there's the problem with industry money tainting medical journals, studies, and guidelines. For example, eight of the nine doctors who formed a committee in 2001 to advise the government on cholesterol guidelines for the public were making money from the companies that make cholesterol-lowering drugs.[22] No wonder the public thinks dietary cholesterol is bad, causes heart disease, and must be drugged out of existence.

Marketing masquerades as information. Advocacy groups like CSPI, Weston A. Price Foundation, Farm Aid, Organic Consumers Association, and Cornucopia Institute try to counter the marketing with knowledge and non-industry sponsored studies. They are grossly outspent by the industrial food companies like Monsanto, Kraft Foods, Proctor & Gamble, etc. It's a war with consumers as the target – buyer beware.

The Center for Science in the Public Interest (CSPI) put McDonald's on notice in 2010: Stop the predatory practice of using toys to sell unhealthy foods to kids or we'll sue you.

Consumers Have Real Power with Education

After a chocolate-flavored toddler drink hit the market in February 2010, the mommy blogosphere began to rail about it. Four months later, CBS News was reporting that:

> With childhood obesity rates soaring, a new chocolate-flavored toddler formula has sparked outrage from parents and nutritionists and has forced the manufacturer to pull it from the market.[23]

That clearly demonstrates the power of consumers to shape the marketplace.

Let's look at a can of Enfagrow's "Gentlease Next Step" toddler drink and see what the label tells us is in it: "Corn syrup solids, partially hydrolyzed nonfat milk and whey protein concentrate solids (soy), vegetable oil (palm olein, soy, coconut, and high oleic sunflower oils), and less than 2% Mortierella alpina oil…" according to the label we saw in May, 2010. The biggest ingredient is listed first, so corn syrup solids are the largest part of the formula. Why isn't the mommy blogosphere up in arms about feeding toddlers corn syrup solids, chocolate flavored or not? Corn syrup, soy, and vegetable oils are cheap, but they are not good food for human beings, especially little ones with developing bodies and brains. If you want to raise a generation of children with a taste for a sugary, oily diet that opens the door to obesity, diabetes, cancer, and heart disease – this kind of recipe is just the thing.

In November 2010, San Francisco became the first U.S. city to ban restaurants from offering a free toy or prize with meals that exceed 600 calories, 650 mgs of sodium, and fat levels exceeding 35% of total calories. All meals (except breakfast) must also contain a half-cup of vegetables and fruit.

A spokeswoman for McDonald's said, "Parents tell us it's their right and responsibility – not the government's – to make their own decisions and to choose what's right for their children."

On one side of the debate are people who feel that this was an over-reach by the "nanny state." Government should stay out of it. But on the other side is a grown army of people who believe a kind of moral line has been crossed in the pursuit of business and profits.

"Our children are sick," said San Francisco Supervisor Eric Mar who sponsored the measure. "Rates of obesity in San Francisco are disturbingly high, especially among children of color. This is a challenge to the restaurant industry to think about children's health first."*

*Baertlein, L. Law curbs McDonal's Happy Meal toys *Reuters*. November 3. 2010

A fascinating essay in pictures about what people eat around the world was done by photographer Peter Menzel and author-journalist Faith D'Alusio. They chronicled visits to families in 24 countries. Each family was asked to purchase a typical week's groceries. In American kitchens you see cases of soda and lots of packaged foods. Elsewhere in the world, you see sacks of vegetables, eggs, and foods the average American can't even name. This photographic tour through many different kitchens worldwide makes it crystal clear that what families eat is a combination of what they have available, and what they make available.

In America, parents likely have more choices of what to feed children than any other nation on earth. If Johnny will only eat pizza and fries, it's because he learned that from the adults around him who were swayed by mass media telling them that junk food is kid food. Children will eat healthy food – if that is what they are given.

A REAL EXPERIENCE

One of my patients told me she was babysitting her grandsons one day and they all went to the mall. My patient stopped at the juice bar and got some freshly squeezed vegetable juice. "I didn't even think to ask the kids if they wanted any because at ages 4 and 6, they were already into soda," she said. "As soon as I got my drink, the boys put their hands up toward me and asked for some of what I had. I gave them my drink and to my surprise, they drank it all down. Of course! Children learn by example. I ordered seconds. Yet their mother was adamant that they didn't like vegetables; I shouldn't even try. I wasn't trying it and it was so easy. If these children lived with me, I would use the juicer I have at home and use the organic veggies I get at the farmers markets."

Public Leadership

It is curious to note that campaigns against trans fats, sodas, and salt were not launched by any federal governmental agency charged with overseeing public health. One would expect the Food and Drug Administration (FDA) or the National Institutes of Health (NIH) to become involved in the healthy nutrition of our population. Rather, these campaigns were launched by several cities and states.

The FDA, the American Academy of Pediatrics, the American Dietetic Association and others have not wanted to cross swords with the powers that be who make the foods concocted from cheap corn-based sugars, refined salt, and heavily subsidized vegetable oil fats. Indeed, the federal government announced in 2010 its intention to step up its promotion of genetically modified food despite the fact the American Academy of Environmental Medicine called for a moratorium on GM food the year before. The CDC in 2010 released that 1 in 3 Americans will be obese by 2050.

So who is the face of change? Who is working to correct the legacy of former Secretary of Agriculture Earl Butz? One of the most prominent faces isn't even American:

> My name's Jamie Oliver. I'm 34 years old. I'm from Essex in England ... I'm a chef. I don't have expensive equipment or medicine. I use information, education... America is one of the most unhealthy countries in the world... Diet-related disease is the biggest killer in the United States... Your child will live a life 10 years [shorter] than you because of the landscape of food that we fill around them.[24]

When Jamie Oliver reformed the meals in the UK, the result was reduced absenteeism and improved test scores. Oliver told the *Guardian*:

> We could see that asthmatic kids weren't having to use the school inhalers so often, for example. We could see that [the healthy lunches] made them calmer and therefore able to learn.

The *Guardian* reporter also observed that:

> [In the U.S., Oliver] appeared on the Late Show, and was forced to listen to host David Letterman predict he would fail in his crusade to transform people's health. Letterman insisted diet pills were the only way to lose weight in the US.[25]

Diet pills have proven to be ineffective and sometimes dangerous. Fen-phen was withdrawn years ago for killing at least 120 people. Meridia, one of the few diet drugs on the market, was given heart attack and stroke warnings from the FDA. Who can forget Alli and Xenical which, by blocking the body's absorption of fat, caused "oily bowels" and "anal leakage" yet produced no more weight loss than a placebo – and the FDA just added a "severe liver injury" warning. The only weight-loss product that works fairly consistently and safely is homeopathic hCG, but because it is a natural product, the drug companies do not promote it.

Obesity has become a national security issue in the U. S. because one in four of our 17- to 24-age group is too overweight to serve in the military. Ironically, the school lunch program was started in the 1940s to prevent the widespread malnutrition common in the Great Depression that kept many young men from serving during World War II.

How is it possible to change the mind-set of a nation? The idea that food brings us information has to be brought into our consciousness. Then, and only then, do we have the opportunity and the capability to make an informed decision about what information we allow our bodies to process.

It is not always easy to look beyond the PR spin, the marketing disguised as official pronouncements, the TV commercials, and the addictive effect of processed salt/oily fat/sugar. But which alternative might you pick: How about giving up your limbs or eyes for diabetes? How about sidelining your career because you came down with a debilitating autoimmune disease? How about getting around in a wheelchair after a stroke? How about a prognosis of less than ten years [or six weeks] to live after a series of brutal chemo treatments for cancer? How about never having post-retirement years because you dropped dead of a heart attack?

For the first time in two centuries, the current generation of children in America may have shorter life expectancies than their parents:

> Obesity is such that this generation of children could be the first basically in the history of the United States to live less healthful and shorter lives than their parents. We're in the quiet before the storm. It's like what happens if suddenly a massive number of young children started chain smoking. At first you wouldn't see much public health impact. But years later it would translate into emphysema, heart disease and cancer. There is an unprecedented increase in prevalence of obesity at younger and younger ages without much obvious public health impact.
>
> —Dr. David S. Ludwig
> Director of the Obesity Program at Children's Hospital Boston
> and one of the authors of a landmark report in the
> *New England Journal of Medicine*[26, 27]

Little by little, parents are coming to see that they can leave their children with an awful legacy of addiction to processed food.

They also are realizing they have a choice to turn back the clock to a time when food did not push kids down the slippery slope toward chronic diseases. Meal preparation took a little more time, food was more local, there were fewer chemicals and additives, and each generation had a reasonable expectation that they could create a better life for their children.

Food is a constant stream of information to our genes. What will you choose to feed your genes today?

RESOURCES

Want to learn more about food? We invite you to go to our website:
http://www.arizonaadvancedmedicine.com/articles.html

- Food 201 – Is Organic Really Better?
- Kid Food – What Is It?
- Jamie Oliver's Nutrition Revolution
- What's In Your Milk? by Samuel S. Epstein, M.D.
- Fish Oils and Oils, Fats and Trans Fats
- A Public Relations Campaign on Oils by Beatrice Trum Hunter
- Gluten Free
- Chef Rachel Q&A on Gluten Free
- Salmon and Red Meat
- Soda and Diet Soda - Obesity and Hyperactivity in a Can
- New York Health Department Ad Campaign Targets Sugary Drinks
- Sugar - A Sweet Invitation to Disease
- Sugar Affects Memory
- Aspartame (NutraSweet®) Addiction by Dr. H. J. Roberts
- Aspartame – History of Getting FDA Approval by Betty Martini
- The Scary Truth About Sugar by Dr. Carolyn Dean, M.D., N.D.
- MSG - Monosodium Glutamate
- Genetically Modified Food

- Genetically Modified Foods, A White Paper by the American Academy of Environmental Medicine, May 2009

---

[1]Ford ES, Bergmann MM, Kroger J, Schienkiewitz A, Weikert C, Boeing H. Healthy living is the best revenge: findings from the European Prospective Investigation Into Cancer and Nutrition-Potsdam study. *Arch Intern Med.* 2009 Aug 10;169(15):1355-1362.

[2]American College of Preventive Medicine. *Lifestyle Medicine--Evidence Review.* June 30, 2009. Available at: http://www.acpm.org/LifestyleMedicine.htm.

[3]Arsenic In Chicken Feed May Pose Health Risks To Humans. *Science Daily,* April 10, 2007

[4]Douglas Gansler. A Deadly Ingredient in a Chicken Dinner. *Washington Post,* June 26, 2009

[5]Nicholas Kristof. Killer Girl Scouts. *New York Times,* May 21, 2006

[6]Michael Pollan: Forget Nutrition Charts, Eat What Grandma Said Is Good for You. Excerpted from Harry Kreisler's *Political Awakenings: Conversations with History*, published by The New Press, 2010. Reprinted February 16, 2010, in *AlterNet.*

[7]Nicholas Kristof. Obama's 'Secretary of Food'? *New York Times,* December 10, 2008

[8]http://www.cdc.gov/nchs/data/ad/ad347.pdf

[9]Food and Water Watch. December 2009. Accessed at http://www.farmaid.org/atf/cf/%7B6ef41923-f003-4e0f-a4a6-ae0031db12fb%7D/ASK_FARM_AID-CORPORATE_CONCENTRATION-LARGE.GIF

[10]Yun AJ, Doux JD. Unhappy meal: How our need to detect stress may have shaped our preferences for taste. *Med Hypotheses.* 2007 Mar 19.

[11]Rostango MH. Can Stress in Farm Animals Increase Food Safety Risk? *Foodborn Pathogens and Disease* 6;7(2009). DOI: 10.1089=fpd.2009.0315.

[12]Lyndsay Layton, Crave Man: David Kessler Knew That Some Foods Are Hard to Resist; Now He Knows Why. *Washington Post,* April 27, 2009

[13]James H. O'Keefe, Neil M. Gheewala and Joan O. O'Keefe. Dietary Strategies for Improving Post-Prandial Glucose, Lipids, Inflammation, and Cardiovascular Health. *J Am Coll Cardiol,* 2008; 51:249-255, doi:10.1016/j.jacc.2007.10.016

[14]JP Mangalindan, PepsiCo CEO: If All Consumers Exercised .. Obesity Would Not Exist. *Fortune,* April 27, 2010

[15]National Public Radio's *All Things Considered.* Soda In America: Taxes and a Debate Over Health. May 4, 2010

[16]http://www.opensecrets.org/news/2010/04/special-interests-continue-federal-lobbying-blitz.html

[17]National Public Radio's *All Things Considered.* Soda In America: Taxes and a Debate Over Health. May 4, 2010

[18]ADA 2009 Annual Report, Page 4

[19]Press release of March 3, 2003: Partnership to Promote Pediatric Dental Health

[20]AAFP press release of October 6, 2009: Coca-Cola Grant Launches AAFP Consumer Alliance Program

[21]Center for Science in the Public Interest. Lifting the Veil of Secrecy: Corporate Support for Health and Environmental Professional Associations, Charities, and Industry Front Groups. 2003. Introduction.

[22]Cholesterol Guidelines Become a Morality Play, *USA Today,* October 16, 2004

[23]http://www.cbsnews.com/stories/2010/06/11/health/main6572476.shtml

[24]http://www.ted.com/talks/lang/eng/jamie_oliver.html

[25]Rachel Williams, Jamie Oliver's school dinners shown to have improved academic results. *The Guardian.* March 29, 2010

[26]S. Jay Olshansky, PhD, Douglas J. Passaro, MD, et al; A Potential Decline in Life Expectancy in the United States in the 21st Century. *New England Journal of Medicine,* March 17, 2005

[27]Ludwig DS. Childhood Obesity – the Shape of Things to Come. *NEJM* 357;23 (Dec 6, 2007).

Chemicals

The cold, remote wilderness of the High Arctic, up near the North Pole, conjures up thoughts of some of the most pristine landscape in the world. Mankind hasn't set foot there much. But birds have and they tell a dirty story. Recently, scientists looked at seabird poop and found a toxic cocktail high in cadmium and mercury, plus lead, manganese, and aluminum. The Arctic is polluted because the world in which we live has become polluted. From plankton to polar bears, the Arctic is the recipient of contaminants whose sources travel from thousands of miles away on currents of water and air.[1, 2]

Heavy metals such as lead, mercury, cadmium, manganese, aluminum, thallium, antimony, and arsenic lodge in human bodies. Heavy metals are natural components of the earth's crust. As trace elements, some metals – copper, selenium, zinc – are essential to human health. However, at higher concentrations, even they can be poisonous.

Heavy metals in water are odorless, tasteless and colorless. As levels rise in our environment, they also rise within our bodies. They enter with our food, water, the air we breathe, and by skin contact. They slowly accumulate in the kidneys, liver, pancreas, bones, central nervous system and brain where they contribute to chronic diseases, learning disorders, cancer, dementia, and premature aging. They are subtle, silent, stalking killers. What makes them particularly dangerous is:

- Their tendency to bioaccumulate – we absorb and store them faster than we can metabolize or excrete them from the body. For example, we have perhaps 1,000 times more lead in our bones than people did 500 years ago, thanks to increasing contamination.[3,4,5]
- Their tendency to act as a catalyst for chronic disease. Heavy metals poison us by disrupting our cellular enzymes which run

23

on nutritional minerals such as magnesium, zinc, and selenium. Toxic metals kick out the nutrients and bind to their receptor sites (take their place), causing diffuse symptoms by affecting nerves, hormones, digestion, and immune function. Instead of calcium being present in an enzyme reaction, for example, lead or cadmium may be there in its place. Toxic metals can't fulfill the same role as the nutritional minerals, and so their presence becomes critically disruptive to enzyme activity.

- Their tendency to cause hyperactive, aggressive behavior.[6]
- Their tendency to be more dangerous in combination with each other[7] than singularly. Mercury and lead together have about 1,000 fold increase in toxicity as compared with either one separately.[8]
- They participate in the creation of biofilms[9] like those that surround the spirochete Borrelia burgdorferi, the bug that causes Lyme disease. Biofilm makes Lyme invisible to the immune system and able to dodge a barrage of antibiotics.[10]

Mercury exposure is an everyday occurrence for all of us, no matter where we live. And mercury levels are rising. When mercury is on board, the ability to handle infections is significantly impacted. Mercury damages 20,000 or so enzymes in the human body.[11]

"As long as compartmentalized toxic metals are present in the body, microorganisms have a fortress that cannot be conquered by antibiotics, Enderlein remedies, ozone therapy, UV light therapy and others," says Dr. Dietrich Klinghardt who specializes in persistent chronic disease. Heavy metals make it harder for our body's detoxification system to keep us cleaned out and they feed the bugs within us. This is why so many people today have chronic, low level infections.[12] People go to the doctor to find out what is wrong and can't get an answer because medical schools didn't teach heavy metal toxicity.

The damage done by heavy metals is not limited to just the body. Concentrations can disrupt neural pathways in the brain and deplete neurotransmitters. Disorganization of thoughts, problems with planning, and short-term memory disturbances can be a chronic issue.

Lead comes first to mind when we think of environmental toxins that suppress IQ – dumb down the human brain. In fact, lead may have been responsible in great part for the fall of the Roman Empire. In the late phase of the empire, it was considered a privilege of the reigning aristocracy to drink out of lead cups. Wine and food were sweetened with a honey extract boiled in lead pots. Many of the water lines in the city of Rome were made of lead pipes. Some historians believe the infamous neurological deficiencies of the Roman emperors were due to lead intoxication.[13]

Global Economies, Global Air Pollution

The electric power industry is the largest toxic polluter in the United States. Producing electricity from coal and oil releases a wide range of pollutants into the environment. In addition to toxic air pollution from power plant smokestacks, large volumes of toxic chemicals are produced at coal- and oil-fired power plants and included in millions of tons of solid and liquid wastes that are typically disposed of at or near the power plants that generate these wastes.[14]

Many of America's coal-fired power plants lack widely available pollution controls for the highly toxic metal mercury, and mercury emissions recently increased at more than half of the country's 50 largest mercury-emitting power plants, according to a 2010 report by the nonpartisan Environmental Integrity Project.[15]

In addition to what the U.S. generates, there is "transboundary air pollution." Coal burning in China emits 25 percent of global mercury, for example. High levels of mercury from China and India have been detected on both coasts of the United States. Research found that one-fifth of the mercury entering Oregon's Williamette River comes from abroad, mostly from China. Mercury is especially suited for long distance travel because at the smokestack in China it is in elemental form and insoluble. However, by the time it reaches the U.S. west coast, it has transformed into a reactive gaseous material that dissolves in Oregon's wet climate – falling onto the Williamette River's watershed and slowly building up toxic levels of mercury in the local wildlife. In California, for example, some researchers believe at least one-third of California's fine particulate pollution – known as aerosol – originates from Asia. These pollutants threaten California's progress on meeting stricter Clean Air Act requirements. In May 2006, University of California-Davis researchers claimed that almost all the particulate matter over Lake Tahoe was from China. The great irony is that these pollutants are mainly due to the burgeoning demand of U.S. and EU consumers for cheap Chinese goods – which is driving the Chinese economic development.[16]

Air pollution is getting credit for causing heart disease and strokes. According to findings from one of the largest studies ever to examine the issue, women living in the most polluted cities had the highest heart disease and stroke risks, while women living in the cleanest cities like Tucson, Arizona had the lowest. Fine particulate air pollution – caused primarily by vehicle exhausts, coal-fired power plants, and other industrial sources – is the problem.[17] Heavy metal toxicity can cause the blood pH to become acidic. The body buffers this acidity by extracting calcium from the bones. The calcium tends to accumulate in the soft tissue of the arteries causing hardening of the arteries.

When a fetus is exposed to urban air pollution in the womb, chemicals in that air interfere with brain development, resulting in lowered intelligence. Studies involving more than 400 pregnant women in New York City and Krakow, Poland, found that 5-year-olds exposed in the womb to above-average levels of polycyclic aromatic hydrocarbons, or PAHs, score lower on IQ tests. PAHs, created by the burning of fossil fuels, are ubiquitous in urban environments.[18] The pair of studies "adds to the growing literature implicating exposures to environmental toxicants with stunting of children's intellectual abilities and increased risk for attention deficit hyperactivity disorder and conduct disorders," said Bruce Lanphear, professor of children's environmental health at British Columbia's Simon Fraser University. "At some point, we will cease blaming parents and teachers for children's failure to learn or thrive in academics and focus our attention on reducing their exposure to widespread neurotoxicants."[19]

In my opinion, the greatest error which I have committed has been not allowing sufficient weight to the direct action of the environments, i.e., food, climate, etc., independently of natural selection.

CHARLES DARWIN, 1888

Man-Made Chemicals

Mankind loves colors. For centuries, people colored their clothing with dyes made of natural substances like mollusks, wood, and indigo plants. The color purple holds a special place in history, however.

In 1856, a young English chemist named William Perkin made the first synthetic dye. A combination of aniline and potassium dichromate ($K_2Cr_2O_7$) rinsed with alcohol produced a beautiful purple known as mauve. It was a huge hit with the French textile industry. Perkins retired a rich man at age 35, having founded the first industry based on synthetic, man-made chemicals.[20]

The chemical age that came to transform life as we know it started after World War I when new discoveries and new techniques revolutionized industry and led to an era of explosive production of synthetic chemicals.

When the Japanese attacked Pearl Harbor, the United States was in a bind. It had depended on natural rubber from trees in Southeast Asia. Necessity was the mother of invention; American ingenuity created synthetic rubber from petroleum. That accelerated the development of polymer engineering (think plastic materials made from petroleum). Polymers and plastics comprise the majority of the chemicals in our environment. They are used in cars, computers, planes, houses, eyeglasses, paints, bags, appliances, medical devices, carpets, tools, clothing, boats, batteries, pipes, and more. It would be hard to imagine a world without plastics. But they hand us all kinds of environmental problems because plastics never break down, and they deposit chemicals in our bodies that gum up the works.

As the decades went by, synthetic chemical technology gave us fertilizers, oleochemicals (oils, fats, and waxes), explosives, pharmaceuticals, semiconductors, fragrances, and flavors. For example: to use real strawberries to make a fast-food milkshake is inconvenient because berries mold easily. Food manufacturers can use a synthetic chemical that tastes like strawberries and not have to worry about losing money to moldy berries. For better or for worse, the chemical industry is central to the modern world economy.

Today, there are some 80,000 synthetic chemicals on the market in the United States; about 10,000 of them are used in food processing, packaging, wrapping, and storage. These chemicals are largely unregulated, and only about 200 have been studied for safety. Many are carcinogenic – able to cause cancer. For example, a 2001 pilot study looking at residential toxin exposure detected the presence of 33 different carcinogens implicated in breast cancer in house dust, and 24 different compounds in the air.[21]

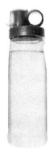

Bisphenol A (BPA) is the chemical that makes polycarbonate plastic drinking bottles clear and virtually shatterproof. But it is an endocrine disrupter – it mimics the body's own hormones. A 2009 review of available studies concluded that "perinatal BPA exposure acts to exert persistent effects on body weight and adiposity." In other words, if you are exposed to BPA as a fetus, you are predisposed to be a fat person. (Rubin 2009). A National Institutes of Health panel found "some concern" about BPA's effects on fetal and infant brain development. Canada banned BPA in baby bottles.

American law is reactionary, not precautionary. In other words, chemicals essentially are innocent until someone – usually an environmental activist group – goes to court and proves them guilty of harm. The burden for protecting children and adults falls on families, not industry or government.

The Cancer Connection

𝒪n 2010, the President's Cancer Panel issued a surprisingly candid report about our chemical world. The Panel said it was "particularly concerned to find that the true burden of environmentally induced cancer has been grossly underestimated," and that "grievous harm from carcinogens "has not been addressed adequately by the National Cancer Program."[22] Among the pollutants the Panel pointed out as causing cancer:

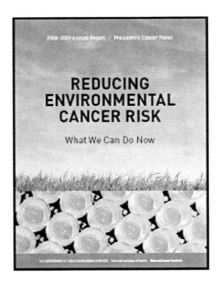

- Medical imaging – Americans now are estimated to receive nearly half of their total radiation exposure from medical imaging and other medical sources, compared with only 15 percent in the early 1980s.
- Pharmaceuticals – We are drinking each other's drugs. Drugs of all types enter the water supply when they are excreted or improperly disposed of and they have become a considerable source of contamination.
- Pesticides – The entire U.S. population is exposed on a daily basis to numerous agricultural chemicals, some of which also are used in residential and commercial landscaping. Many of

these chemicals have known or suspected carcinogenic or endocrine-disrupting properties. Pesticides (insecticides, herbicides, and fungicides) approved for use by the EPA contain nearly 900 active ingredients, many of which are toxic. Many of the solvents, fillers, and other chemicals listed as inert ingredients on pesticide labels also are toxic, but are not required to be tested for their potential to cause chronic diseases such as cancer. Chemicals used for household pest control can become a component of carpet dust, posing a risk to children when they play on the floor.

- Military sources – Nearly 900 Superfund sites are abandoned military facilities or facilities that produced materials and products for or otherwise supported military needs. Some of these sites and the areas surrounding them became heavily contaminated due to improper storage and disposal of known or suspected carcinogens including solvents, machining oils, metalworking fluids, and metals.

- Chlorine by-products – Disinfection of public water supplies has dramatically reduced the incidence of waterborne illnesses and related mortality in the United States, but research indicates that long-term exposure to disinfection by-products such as trihalomethanes may increase cancer risk.

- Manufacturing – Numerous chemicals used in manufacturing remain in or on the product as residues, while others are integral components of the products themselves. (Think lead in purses from China and melamine in baby formula.)

- Lifestyle – Modern conveniences such as dry-cleaning fluid, cell phones, and tanning booths are toxic.

It is predicted now that 1 in 3 women and 1 in 2 men will develop cancer in their lifetime.

"There are far too many known and suspected cancer-causing chemicals in products people, young and old, use every day of their lives," said Kenneth A. Cook, president and co-founder of the advocacy organization Environmental Working Group (EWG). "Many of these chemicals are believed to be time bombs, altering the genetic-level switching mechanisms that lead to cancerous cellular growth in later life."[23]

The Panel pointed out that "The requisite knowledge and technologies exist to develop alternatives to many currently used chemical agents known or believed to cause or promote cancer." The Panel called for a new national strategy that focuses on such threats in the environment and workplaces. Finding the political will to do that is another matter.

The Obesity Connection

In 2006, scientists at the Harvard School of Public Health reported that the prevalence of obesity in infants under 6 months had risen 73 percent since 1980. Babies aren't eating fast food burgers and fries, so what's up with that? As Sharon Begley explained in *Newsweek*, the answer lies in early-life exposure to traces of chemicals in the environment:

> Evidence has been steadily accumulating that certain hormone-mimicking pollutants, ubiquitous in the food chain, have two previously unsuspected effects. They act on genes in the developing fetus and newborn to turn more precursor cells into fat cells, which stay with you for life. And they may alter metabolic rate, so that the body hoards calories rather than burning them, like a physiological Scrooge. 'The evidence now emerging says that being overweight is not just the result of personal choices about what you eat, combined with inactivity,' says Retha Newbold of the National Institute of Environmental Health Sciences (NIEHS) in North Carolina, part of the National Institutes of Health (NIH). 'Exposure to environmental chemicals during development may be contributing to the obesity epidemic.' They are not the cause of extra pounds in every person who is overweight – for older adults, who were less likely to be exposed to so many of the compounds before birth, the standard explanations of genetics and lifestyle probably suffice – but environmental chemicals may well account for a good part of the current epidemic, especially in those under 50. And at the individual level, exposure to the compounds during a critical period of development

31

may explain one of the most frustrating aspects of weight gain: you eat no more than your slim friends, and exercise no less, yet are still unable to shed pounds."[24]

Estrogen-mimicking chemicals are everywhere: Vinyl flooring; detergents; shampoo; deodorants; perfumes; hair spray; moisturizers; garden hoses; inflatable toys; pesticides; fertilizers processed carbs (bread, pasta, cereal) trigger excess insulin, which builds fat and stimulates feminizing estrogen.

For example, bisphenol A (BPA), the chemical found in plastic water bottles, in the lining of cans, and some cash register receipts, prompts some cells to become fat cells.

The fact that chemicals could cause obesity was a radical theory when it was first proposed in 2002 by Paula Baillie-Hamilton, a doctor at Stirling University in Scotland.[25] But now these chemicals that make us fat actually have their own label: obesogens. Obesogens are natural estrogenic-hormones found in soy products, hormones administered to animals, plastics in some food and drink packaging, ingredients added to processed foods, and pesticides sprayed on produce. They act in a variety of ways: by mimicking human hormones such as estrogen, by misprogramming stem cells to become fat cells and, researchers think, by altering the function of genes.

Toxins can do great damage, and the body, in its wisdom, looks for a safe place to park them to keep them out of the bloodstream and away from the organs. One of the body's responses to toxins is to encapsulate them in fat cells. Think of putting something dangerous in a safe deposit box. Nature makes these fat cells tough to remove so the body is not endangered. This belly fat – medical books call it adiposity – does further damage because it is more biologically active than other kinds of fat, meaning it produces more hormones and chemical messengers that cause chronic inflammation throughout the body.

So the epidemics of obesity and chronic disease cannot be blamed just on the addictive quality of fast food and sodas, or the excess calories and out-of-control insulin levels triggered by processed foods. A good portion of the blame also goes to chemicals, particularly estrogen-mimicking chemicals. Whether you're a man or a woman, too much estrogen makes you fat, slow, tired, and diseased.

Many diseases, including pervasive and chronic ones such as autism and autoimmune diseases, will respond to treatment that includes helping the body eliminate toxins.

The Law & Order Connection

British Professor Derek Bryce-Smith put forth a thesis in 1974 that violent criminals who commit crimes involving loss of control are hyperactive people with a high heavy metal body burden, particularly lead. He concluded that "… offenders of this type would be better treated with penicillamine [a chelating agent] than prison."[26] His suggestion that society should adopt a more 'humane approach' of tackling the medical issues that predispose a person to criminal behavior went unheeded.

But he kept at it. Twelve years later he wrote:

> Changed brain chemistry can alter behaviour, and changed behaviour can alter brain chemistry: the interaction is two way. It therefore follows that behaviour, cognition, social interactions, and other expressions of brain function are subject not only to the social environment but also to certain aspects of the chemical environment. The relevant chemical factors include (a) neurotoxic pollutants in general, of which lead is evidently now the most serious in its impact, (b) certain common nutrient deficiencies, particularly of zinc, and (c) neurotoxins of voluntary abuse, of which ethanol is still probably producing the most widespread social damage.[27]

By 1995, methods to analyze such things were more precise. Dr. Neil I. Ward got permission to obtain hair and blood samples from a group of incarcerated men, aged 16-19 years, and he compared them with a control group.[28] He was particularly interested in 28 of those young men whose crime involved violence. Hair samples provide a "diary" of long-term exposure and tend more to show whole-body accumulation of toxins, whereas blood samples tell a more transient story concerning recent absorption of nutrients before they have been stored or excreted. Looking at the 28 violent offenders, Dr. Ward found their hair analyses had about four times as much lead and aluminum, and twice as much cadmium. He also found remarkable deficits in certain essential trace metals – chromium, selenium and zinc. The blood samples told pretty much the same story.[29]

Did the post WWII chemical age spawn several generations of 'toxic metal kids' roaming the streets?

America's crime rates have been falling since the early 1990s. New York and Los Angeles, once the twin capitals of violent crime, have calmed down significantly, as have Phoenix and most other big cities. In 2009, violent crime fell an impressive 5.5 percent nationwide, despite the economic downturn. Criminologists debate why: the crack war petered out, new community policing tactics worked, the economy had improved for a long spell. But many felt that didn't fully explain it and looked beyond the criminal justice system for answers. Professor Bryce-Smith's hypothesis was gaining traction. As reported in *The Week*:

> One intriguing hypothesis about why Americans were so prone to violence in the 1980s was that many young people were suffering the effects of lead poisoning. The link between lead poisoning and aggressive or impulsive behavior is well established. And peaks in children's exposure to the toxic metal, first due to lead paint and then to leaded gasoline, were followed roughly 20 years later by two of the 20th century's worst crime eras. Under this theory, the phasing out of lead paint and leaded gasoline explains the reduction in crime.[30]

Neurotoxic metals, absorbed in the brain due to poor diet and deficiencies in vitamins and minerals, can disturb normal brain development and neurotransmitter function. Some hypothesize that environmental pollution interacts with poverty, poor diet, alcohol or drug use, and social stress to put some individuals at risk for subclinical toxicity, leading to a loss of impulse control and increased violent crime.[31]

Magnesium, for example, protects us from aluminum. Zinc, amino acids, calcium, iron, vitamin C, and vitamin E protect us from lead.

The Autism and ADHD Connection

One out of every six children in the U.S. has been diagnosed with a developmental disability;[32] most often that diagnosis is for autism, ADHD, or bipolar disorder.

Evidence strongly suggests that thimerosal (the mercury-based preservative used in multi-dose vials of vaccines) may be responsible in some part for the exponential growth of autism, attention deficit disorder, speech delays, and other childhood neurological disorders now epidemic in the United States. In the early 1990s, public health officials dramatically increased the number of thimerosal-containing vaccinations. In a 1991 memo, Dr. Maurice Hilleman, one of the fathers of Merck's vaccination programs, warned that 6-month-old children administered the shots on schedule would suffer mercury exposures 87 times the government safety standards. He recommended that thimerosal be discontinued. Merck ignored Hilleman's warning. Autism rates began rising dramatically in children who were administered the new vaccine regimens.[33]

Also, thimerosal tends to settle in the vial. It stands to reason that if it was not shaken up before being drawn, whoever got the tenth and final dose would get an enormously high concentration of mercury.

The key issue has turned out to be whether or not you were dealt the genes to be a "good excreter" of mercury. Can your body get it out? One of the first hair-sample studies was done by Amy Holmes, M.D. She found strikingly lower levels of mercury in the hair of children with autism than in the hair of neurotypical children. Typical children excreted lots of mercury after they were vaccinated. Autistic children excreted almost none. That means children with autism cannot excrete mercury from their systems; the mercury builds to toxic levels.[34]

Mercury is still included in a few vaccines including the seasonal flu shot and the swine flu shot.

Although mercury got all the media attention, some vaccines contain aluminum and MSG, and they are also neurotoxins. Vaccines containing high concentrations of aluminum were added to the child immunization schedule when several vaccines containing mercury were removed. Two-month-old babies now receive 1,225 mcg of aluminum from their vaccines – 50 times higher than safety levels.[35]

> Aluminum is not perceived, I believe, by the public as a dangerous metal. Therefore, we are in a much more comfortable wicket in terms of defending its presence in vaccines.
>
> Dr. John Clements
> World Health Organization vaccine advisor, May 2000 [36]

People ask if vaccines cause autism. The answer: yes and no. No, because there are children who have never been vaccinated who have become autistic. Yes, because the neurotoxins in the vaccines add to an already heavy load of environmental pollution. The CDC and Environmental Working Group has tested umbilical cord blood and found more than 200 chemicals in newborns' blood – mercury, lead, fire retardants, pesticides, plastics, Teflon – a virtual toxic stew of modern day life. Vaccines appear to have been the proverbial straw that breaks the camel's back for some children.

Heavy metal toxicities such as lead and cadmium have also been associated with attention deficit hyperactivity disorder.[37] Autism and ADHD differ in how the children react to their world – one mostly withdrawn, the other mostly hyperactive. But both manifestations share much of the same origins and both require heavy metal detoxification as a fundamental element of treatment.

Autistic children commonly suffer from yeast overgrowth which, according to the National Autism Association, may be eliminated in the long-term only by removing the heavy metal burden from the body.[38]

Author Dr. Mary Ann Block suggests that what we call "diseases" are actually symptoms, rather than psychiatric disorders requiring medication. "If you've got heavy metal toxicity, then you don't have autism, you have the symptoms caused by heavy metal toxicity."[39]

Dr. Fred Baughman, an author and outspoken critic of the use of drugs for children with hyperactive disorders, points out that the ADHD diagnosis does not exist in other countries and didn't exist anywhere two generations ago. "They have taken entirely normal children and made patients out of them by diagnosing them with fictional chemical imbalances of the brain. It's a total fraud."[40]

In other words, there is more profit in prescribing drugs than performing a heavy-metal detox.

> Industrial chemicals are responsible for a silent pandemic that has caused impaired brain development in millions of children worldwide. Fetal and early childhood exposures to industrial chemicals in the environment can damage the developing brain and can lead to neurodevelopmental disorders – autism, attention deficit disorder, and mental retardation. About half of the 202 chemicals known to be toxic to the brain are among the chemicals most commonly used.
> —P. Grandjean, P. Landrigan
> "Developmental Neurotoxicity of
> Industrial Chemicals –Silent Pandemic"
> *The Lancet*, November, 2006

Chemicals In the Bathroom

The U.S. government doesn't regulate cosmetics and body care products for safety, long-term health impacts, or environmental damage. There are many harmful synthetic chemicals and petroleum-based ingredients including lead in lipstick, arsenic in eye shadow, mercury in mascara, coal tar in shampoos, and mineral oil in lotions.

Many cosmetics are made from petroleum. They are toxic. As Ronnie Cummins, founder and director of the Organic Consumers Association (OCA) put it in June, 2010:

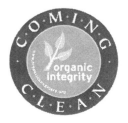

There's an oil spill leaking from U.S. bathrooms that's roughly the same size as the BP disaster in the Gulf of Mexico. It's coming from the petrochemical-based cosmetics we're rubbing into our hair and skin and rinsing down the drain ... All of these products can be replaced with petrochemical-free, certified organic alternatives that work just as well.[41]

Ingredients that use petroleum have no business being in products labeled "organic" but, as Cummins points out, it is a fairly common practice.

Brands that carry the USDA certified Organic Body Care and Cosmetics should be free of toxic elements made from or with petroleum, but there is a lot of cheating going on in the marketplace. Efforts are underway for better self-regulation of the industry. OCA is one of the leaders. It launched a "Coming Clean Campaign" to encourage retailers to take action to address widespread organic labeling fraud in their health and beauty care aisles. In June 2010, Whole Foods Market became the first retail chain to adopt an organic integrity policy for health & beauty products sold in their stores. By June, 2011, all organic claims on personal care products sold at Whole Foods are to be backed up by third-party certification to USDA organic standards.

Who is cheating and who is not? The OCA website tells you and constantly updates their database.

www.organicconsumers.org/bodycare/cc-endorsers.cfm

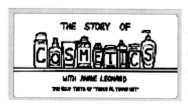

You'll find that many brand name cosmetic companies that donate to breast cancer awareness use toxic chemicals. It happens so much, it has been given the term "pink washing."

Check out one of our favorite videos, *The Story of Cosmetics* at www.safecosmetics.com. Teenagers will enjoy this one too. You will never look at the word "natural" on the label again and think it means "safe."

By some estimates, women use 12 cosmetic products each day and absorb five pounds of cosmetic chemicals a year. The evidence of damage to human health is mounting:

- More and more girls are experiencing "early onset puberty" meaning they reach puberty earlier, growing breasts by ages seven and eight.[42] Researchers are beginning to examine the link between cosmetics ingredients that mimic the effect of estrogen and premature puberty. Young bodies interpret the extra estrogen as the call to develop breasts and sexual traits, despite the fact they are still children.

- Girls younger than 10 with early onset puberty show a high rate of exposure to endocrine disruptors found in nail polishes and other cosmetics.[43] Phthalates, triclosan, musks and parabens are also known to alter the hormone system.[44]

- Exposure to phthalates, endocrine disrupting chemicals found in perfumes, nail polish and other cosmetics, is linked to childhood obesity.[45]

- Fragrances can be particularly nasty synthetic chemical concoctions and what goes into a fragrance need not be listed on labels because the law considers them trade secrets. Many fragrances contain hormone-disrupting chemicals which have been linked to increased risk of cancer, especially breast and prostate cancers; reproductive toxicity and effects on the developing fetus; and predisposition to metabolic disease such as thyroid problems or obesity. Fragrance is now considered among the top five allergens.[46]

- The polishes, acrylics and other products used in nail salons contain some twenty chemicals flagged as having "potential symptoms and health effects" by the EPA. Nail salon workers exposed to solvents without proper ventilation face an increased risk for miscarriages and birth defects similar to fetal alcohol syndrome. "Most kinds of house paint are less toxic than what you find in nail polish," says Cora Roelofs, Sc.D., an assistant professor at the University of Massachusetts.[47]

Environmental Working Group (EWG) has a wonderful resource called "Skin Deep," an online cosmetics safety database which they established in 2004. It provides safety ratings for more than 62,000 products on the market and receives about one million hits per month. You find it at www.cosmeticsdatabase.com. Jane Houlihan, vice president for research at EWG:

> When you get online and use it, you'll find more than 500 products that contain ingredients that are banned in other countries. You'll find a hundred products that contain ingredients that the industry itself has said are unsafe in cosmetics. And you'll find that 99 percent of the products you find in our database contain at least one ingredient, and many times dozens of ingredients, that haven't been assessed for safety by the FDA, by the cosmetics industry itself, or any other publicly accountable institution.[48]

Other very handy sources of information include:

- Not So Sexy (2010) – the perfume industry's 3,100 stock chemical ingredients are used to concoct a complex cocktail of natural essences and synthetic chemicals, often toxic petrochemicals. www.ewg.org/notsosexy
- A Little Prettier (2008) – cosmetic companies deny health problems related to phthalates, but are they secretly reformulating? A follow up to the prior Not Too Pretty report. www.safecosmetics.org
- Teen Cosmetic Study (2008) – Laboratory tests reveal adolescent girls across America are contaminated with

chemicals commonly used in cosmetics and body care products. www.ewg.org/reports/teens

- Beauty Secrets (2000) – Nail polish contains the plasticizer dibutyl phthalate (DBP) and the CDC found the compound in everyone they sampled. DBP causes a number of birth defects in lab animals, primarily to male offspring. An environmental release of just 10 pounds of DBP must be reported to environmental authorities under the Superfund law. The cosmetics industry, in contrast, puts hundreds of thousands of pounds of DBP into nail polish each year, with no requirements for safety testing or reporting. www.ewg.org/reports/beautysecrets

Chemicals in the House

On May, 2009, Canadian activists Rick Smith and Bruce Lourie published the book, *Slow Death by Rubber Duck: The Secret Danger of Everyday Things*. It got noticed, if for nothing else, because the cover attacks one of the icons of children's fun in the bath tub – the rubber ducky.

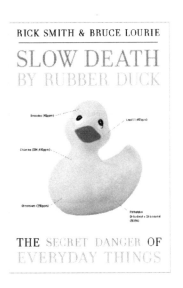

But alas, the duck perfectly symbolizes the new and surprising kind of pollution that threatens our health and environment. Most rubber ducks aren't rubber; they are vinyl and full of toxic phthalates.

Smith and Lourie voluntarily ate, drank, breathed, and absorbed commonly encountered toxins, then measured samples of their blood and urine for intake levels. Experiments involved such seemingly benign activities as sitting on upholstery (flame retardants) and using microwave popcorn bags (Teflon), soft plastic (bisphenol A), shampoo (phthalates), and anti-bacterial soap (triclosan). In most cases, with even brief exposure, their levels of toxicity rose significantly.

The *Wall Street Journal* gave their book a negative review. The authors wrote back:

> The *Wall St. Journal* insults the intelligence of concerned parents and scientists who know it is dangerous for children's health to use products such as baby bottles and sippy cups made from plastic containing BPA ... The *Wall St. Journal* is putting powerful vested interests above children's safety on toxic chemical issues. Its editorial rejects the basic purpose of scientific research saying 'Environmentalists hope that if researchers run more tests, they'll come up with more links...Thus, they ask for tests unto eternity.' In fact, it was the lack of studies that prompted us to use ourselves as lab rats. Our families would have certainly preferred it if studies had been conducted in modern laboratories, instead of us pioneering them in our homes.[49]

The take-home message is that we don't have the luxury to wait for governments to impose limits on chemicals.

And mainstream environmental groups may not be what you think. Christine MacDonald's 2008 book, *Green Inc.*, exposed cozy relationships many groups have with corporate donors who, as she sees it, turn green groups into the handmaidens of corporate benefactors.

A couple years later, journalist Johann Hari picked up where MacDonald left off. His 2010 article in *The Nation* magazine suggests that addiction to corporate cash has changed these groups at their core.

> [As Christine MacDonald reported] many of the green organizations meant to be leading the fight are busy shoveling up hard cash from the world's worst polluters – and burying science-based environmentalism in return. Sometimes the corruption is subtle; sometimes it is blatant. . . . The Sierra Club was approached in 2008 by the makers of Clorox bleach, who said that if the Club endorsed their new range of "green" household cleaners, they would give it a percentage of the sales. The Club's Corporate Accountability

Committee said the deal created a blatant conflict of interest – but took it anyway. Executive director Carl Pope defended the move in an e-mail to members, in which he claimed that the organization had carried out a serious analysis of the cleaners to see if they were "truly superior." But it hadn't.[50]

The argument for taking corporate dollars is basically that such alliances are the way to steer environmental policies within the business community.[51]

Groups who have not taken corporate money, like Greenpeace, say that is a lot of baloney from those who are not willing to do the hard work:

> Greenpeace has maintained our financial independence, refusing money from corporations. A few years ago, Greenpeace and our allies decided to stop deforestation in the Amazon by "convincing" the major industries driving the problem to cease and desist ... Greenpeace activists throughout the United States and Europe nudged Nike and Timberland to cancel their contracts with leather [companies] causing deforestation. A few cancelled contracts later, the major ranching companies agreed with Greenpeace Brazil to a moratorium on any ranching that causes deforestation.[52]

Our Top 10 List for Cleaning Up Our Own Corner of the World

Here are 10 things we have found possible to do in our lives to mitigate the impact environmental chemicals have on our health:

1. You can't do much directly about China's air pollution, but you can remove mercury fillings and get fluoride-free toothpaste. Removing amalgam fillings is usually an out-of-pocket expense because the powers-that-be do not want the enormous liability that would come from acknowledging the harm of having put this neurotoxin in the mouth. In addition to poisoning enzyme reactions and potentiating the effects of pesticides and aluminum, mercury negatively affects the heart. Heart disease is the number one killer – we need to do all we can to reduce the incidence of heart attacks, strokes, and hypertension. Fluoride has never

been proven to prevent cavities; there is no reason to put a poison in our mouths that attacks our bones and thyroid. Much of the fluoride added to municipal water supplies across the United States is imported from China, and is contaminated with other heavy metals.[53] A credible resource on the subject is the Fluoride Action Network (fluoridealert.org).

2. Invest in a water filtration system. Claims and counterclaims abound with different systems, but anything you can do is a big help. Our bodies are about 70 percent water, so get it as clean as you can. The closer you are to the water treatment plant, the more chlorine you will have in the household water you use for drinking and showering. You want to remove chlorine and its by-products. The first step is to use a carbon filter. Getting the fluoride out takes a different filter because it is a smaller molecule; there are multi-part filtration systems that include a fluoride filter. Reverse osmosis water is "clean," but it is often an acid pH and all the minerals have been removed from it – not to mention it takes about nine gallons of water to make one gallon of RO. Alkalinized water systems have some merit.

Invest in a re-usable BPA-free water bottle so you can carry your own water. That way you don't toss plastic bottles into the trash, and you are not at the mercy of the bottled water companies who often charge a lot for a natural resource.

3. Eat nutrient-dense, organic food. Get less pesticides; get more nutrition. And we don't mean go buy organic pretzels and cookies. Buy organic vegetables, and organic meats and dairy – grass fed if you can afford it. If you're eating non-organic celery today, you may be ingesting 67 pesticides with it (EWG). Fruits and vegetables are one of your biggest exposure risks to chemicals and pesticides.

"To the extent you can afford to do so, [parents] should simply buy organic, because there have been some very good studies that shows people who eat mostly organic food reduce 95 percent of pesticides [in their body] in two weeks," said Dr. Philip Landrigan, chairman of the department of preventive medicine at Mount Sinai School of Medicine in New York. "A kid's brain goes through extraordinary development, and if pesticides get into the brain, it can cause damage."[54]

Vegetarians argue that eating fish, meat, and dairy increases the risk of heavy metal contamination. But that argument overlooks that fruits, vegetables, legumes, nuts and seeds are easily contaminated by heavy metals in top soil and air. Meat contains amino acids, natural chelators, and vitamin B12 (after about seven years of B12 deficiency, irreversible brain damage can result). Eat butter, olive oil, and coconut oil – not man-made, processed vegetable oils which are inflammatory.

While you are at it, ditch the soda, the "energy" drinks, the flavored waters, the mocha lattes. There's lots of money in this for the multi-national companies, but there is no redeeming value in this stuff for you. You don't need the caffeine, the sugar, the high fructose corn syrup, the aspartame, the Splenda®, the benzene, the phosphoric acid, etc. Your bones will thank you, your liver will thank you, your brain will thank you – what more could you ask? Oh, wait, there is one thing more. You'll love the money you save.

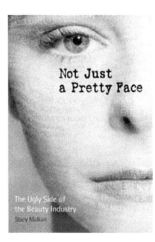

Not Just a Pretty Face

The Ugly Side of the Beauty Industry
Stacy Malkan

4. Clean up the cosmetics and household products. You will spend a little more buying organic cosmetics, but you can save big on the household products. One of the best germ killers and degreasers is distilled white vinegar. It's cheap, and it doesn't create superbugs as triclosan can. Its natural acidity kills germs. We recommend the Heinz brand – it is made from corn; other brands of distilled white vinegar are made from petroleum products. (And it doesn't matter if it is genetically modified corn; you're not eating it.)

Butyl cellosolve is the principal ingredient in many household cleaners; the Material Safety Data Sheet says acute conditions include irritation of eyes, skin, lungs, headaches, dizziness, nausea, diarrhea; chronic conditions include damage to liver, kidney, and skin. You can avoid this toxic chemical and many others by reading labels.

You can get cleaning products without ammonia (poisonous), pine oil (irritant), glycol ethers (used in countertop cleaners; can cause liver and kidney damage, as well as nervous disorders), formaldehyde (used as a preservative; a suspected carcinogen, inhalation extremely destructive to mucous membrane tissue), paradichlorobenzene (used in toilet bowl cleaners; causes cancer in laboratory animals), parabens (an inexpensive preservative used in liquid soaps and cosmetics; found in breast cancer tissue), and mineral acids (such as muriatic acid used in pools or phosphoric or hydrochloric acids which clean well but are toxic).

5. Read up on formaldehyde. It is classified as a known carcinogen and has been linked to cancers of the throat, blood, and lymphatic system. It irritates the nasal and respiratory passages. Formaldehyde is a common chemical found in everything from plywood to nail polish, car exhaust and cigarette smoke. It's part of the "new car" smell. It is in room air fresheners to deaden your sense of smell. It bestows permanent-press qualities to clothing and draperies. It is put into glues and adhesives, and used as a preservative in some paints and coating products. And yes, it's the same stuff morticians use to embalm people and the toxin that made those Katrina trailers infamous. The Campaign for Safe Cosmetics found formaldehyde in bath products. When you buy particle board furniture, you can block the off-gassing of formaldehyde by brushing the exposed ends with a sealer (easy to use).

6. Read labels. If you can't pronounce the ingredients, question if you should buy the item. For example: a popular sales tool is to play on the fear of germs. Thus antimicrobials are popular in hand soaps, dish soaps, etc., but we overuse them, just as we did antibiotics, and we are breeding resistant super-bugs. Look for the small print on a variety of everyday products: Colgate Total® toothpastes, Clearasil Pimple Treatment Cream®, and Right Guard Sport Deodorant® all contain triclosan, according to EWG.

Need a handout on triclosan to take to your children's school so they switch to something better? **Beyond Pesticides.org** has one.

EWG surveyed 3,300 parents in 2007 asking what products they use and compared the ingredients to lists of chemicals known to cause allergies, hormone disruption, damage to the nervous system, and cancer. The study found 89% of products labeled "recommended by a doctor" actually contain what EWG considers dangerous chemicals.[55]

Phthalates most commonly show up on labels as DEP (diethyl phthalate) and MEP (monoethyl phthalate).

7. Get wise to electrosmog. Two years ago when we walked into the cell phone store and asked about the SARs rating (Specific Absorption Rate), the sales staff pretended not to know what we were talking about – talking about radiation emissions implied liability. But now the city of San Francisco requires the SARs rating to be displayed on each cell phone sold. The SARs rating is far from perfect, but it's a great start on building awareness that cell phones expose us to dangerous radiation. We have encased ourselves in a net of electronic signals 24/7 and those pulsating signals don't vibrate on at the same frequency as the energy signals our cells use to repair and regenerate our bodies.

8. Avoid medical and security imaging – PET scans, CT scans, annual mammograms, airport X-ray scanners. Radiation causes cancer. We Americans get the most medical radiation in the world. The average American's dose has grown sixfold over the last couple of decades. The risk of cancer is growing because people in everyday situations are getting imaging tests far too often. The use of CT scans – "super X-rays" that give fast, extremely detailed images – has soared in use over the last decade, often replacing tests that don't require radiation, such as ultrasound and MRI, or magnetic resonance imaging.[56] Doctors don't keep track of radiation given their patients – they order a test, not a dose. Now airports are installing X-ray scanners at security checkpoints. You don't feel the

radiation, so you don't think about it. But do think about it. Ask the doctor if there is another option. Choose thermography over mammography (it's a better screening test anyway). And choose the manual pat-down at the airport.

9. Beware of too much medicine. Legal medications like painkillers and sedatives send as many Americans to emergency rooms each year as hardcore street drugs. Vioxx killed some 60,000 people. Drugs to treat mental disorders, and statins, are the largest selling drugs in America, but they are notoriously ineffective long term and come with some very nasty side effects. Pharmacies filled almost 4 billion prescriptions in 2009. Drugs don't solve biological dysfunction; they generally poison a system so the body cannot produce certain symptoms of dysfunction.

In 2003, Gary Null and Dr. Carolyn Dean looked at all the peer-reviewed statistics available at the time and found that the American medical system is the leading cause of death and injury in the United States. Their landmark paper "Death by Medicine" documented unnecessary procedures and drugs used in hospitals.

In 2006, the Institute of Medicine concluded that at least 1.5 million Americans are sickened, injured or killed each year by errors in prescribing, dispensing and taking medications. Mistakes in giving drugs are so prevalent in hospitals that, on average, a patient will be subjected to a medication error each day he or she occupies a hospital bed. "Everyone in the health-care system knows this is a major problem, but there's been very little action, and it's generally remained on the back burner," panel member Charles B. Inlander said.[57]

Did we mention that hospital-acquired infections, MRSA, killed 48,000 Americans in 2006?[58]

10. Ditch the perfume, scented candles, scented laundry soaps and softeners, air fresheners, car fresheners, and fake fire place logs. They are loaded with synthetic chemicals that add greatly to indoor air pollution.

Education and Choices

The next time you are in a public place, look around. Notice how many people are overweight, walking painfully. Notice how the kids have changed – more allergies and asthma, more developmental disabilities, more overweight, and growing up faster biologically. Notice the news stories about the rising rates of infertility, diabetes, and cancers. Along with poor nutrition, too many chemicals in our environment – especially estrogen mimickers and heavy metals – have changed our society drastically.

We all have the ability to lessen our body burden of chemical toxicity. We can learn how to reduce our intake of pesticides, hormone-mimicking chemicals, and the like. We can lessen the heavy metals already stowed in our bodies by doing a heavy metal detox.

Removing Heavy Metals

Several different chelating agents are used to pull heavy metals out of the body. EDTA, ethylenediaminetetraacetic acid, is one. EDTA features four carboxylic acid and two amine groups that can all bind to metals. It attracts the metals, attaches to them, and pulls them out of the body, mainly through the kidneys into the urine. EDTA is not broken down in the body; it goes in and comes out as EDTA. DMPS, dimercapto propane sulfonate, is used preferentially for elevated body burden of mercury, since it binds more tightly to mercury than EDTA. On the other hand, EDTA binds lead better than DMPS. DMSA, dimercapto succinic acid, is an oral sulfur-containing chelating agent which also has a high binding coefficient for mercury. It is approved by the FDA for removing lead and mercury from the brains of children with lead or mercury poisoning.

Chelating agents have a half-life of several hours. Their effectiveness comes from consecutive administration of consistent dosages, not from the magnitude of the dose.

Removal of heavy metals is preferably done with intravenous (IV) therapy. The IV method is more effective because it gives higher levels of the chelating agent. EDTA, for example, is poorly absorbed by the GI tract. The IV actually delivers EDTA to the cells. Each chelation IV takes 30-40 minutes. Heavy metal removal is a slow process; plan on a series of sessions with on-going oral chelation.

In an ideal world, you undergo both IV and oral because the oral provides a continuous low level of chelating agents in the intestinal tract and in the blood, to continue to pull out heavy metals in between the IV treatments. The IV once a week gives you the big push.

Your blood work should be monitored regularly to make sure kidney and liver functions are stable and hopefully improving. Urine should be tested weekly to make sure there is no protein, another measure of kidney health. Every three to six months, measure the excretion of heavy metals into the stool and urine. Science is not yet able to measure how much is stored in the body without grinding the body up – which seems like a poor option. We can, however, measure how much is coming out of the body and compare that data with how much comes out of most people's bodies under similar conditions. Over a relatively short period of time, the body makes every effort to clear the metals from the blood, with lead going preferentially to bone, arsenic and cadmium to soft tissues, aluminum and mercury to fatty tissues and brain.

Chelation therapy tackles a fundamental and common cause of the chronic inflammation that underlies a lot of chronic illnesses.

RESOURCES

The web site EnvironmentalHealthNews.org has daily updates on environment and health.

Environmental Working Group www.ewg.org

U. S. Dept. Health and Human Services Household Products Database

http://householdproducts.nlm.nih.gov/index.htm

Campaign for Safe Cosmetics

Breast Cancer Fund

Center for Environmental Health

Moms Rising

Washington Toxics Coalition

---

[1] Arctic Pollution: How Much Is Too Much? *Northern Perspectives*, Volume 18, Number 3, September-October 1990. Published by the Canadian Arctic Resources Committee.

[2] Jane George. Arctic bird poop loaded with environmental poisons, biologists say. *CanWest News Service.* June 15, 2010

[3] Dr. Robert J. Rowen. Oral Chelation – Hoax or Heart Protector? *Second Opinion Newsletter*

[4] Press Release: Scientific Pioneer Clair C. Patterson Dies. California Institute of Technology. December 6, 1995 http://media.caltech.edu/press_releases/11683

[5] Hirao Y, Patterson CC. Lead aerosol pollution in the High Sierra overrides natural mechanism which exclude lead from a food chain. *Science.* 1974 May 31; 184(140): 989-92.

[6] D.Bryce-Smith and H.Waldron. Lead, Behaviour and Criminality. *The Ecologist.* 1974,4,347-358,353

[7] http://www.atsdr.cdc.gov/interactionprofiles/index.asp

[8] Schubert J, Riley EJ, Tyler SA. Combined effects in toxicology. A rapid systematic testing procedure: cadmium, mercury, and lead. *Toxicol Environ Health*, 1978;4(5/6):763-776

[9] Dahle UR, Sunde PT et al. Treponemes and endodontic infections. *Endodontic Topics,* 2003, 6, 160–170.

[10] Mary Budinger. Pasteur's Legacy Feeds the Epidemics of Lyme and Autism. *Townsend Letter*, November, 2008

[11] Ibid

[12] Dietrich Klinghardt, MD, PhD. Heavy Metals and Chronic Diseases. Klinghardt Academy for the Healing Arts

[13] Milton Lesser. Lead and Lead Poisoning from Antiquity to Modern Times. *Ohio Journal of Science*, 88 (3): 78-84, 1988

[14] Clean Air Task Force. "Laid to Waste: The Dirty Secret of Combustion Waste from America's Power Plants", March 2000

[15] Dirty Kilowatts – America's Top 50 Power Plant Mercury Polluters. Environmental Integrity Project. March 2010

[16] A China Environmental Health Project Fact Sheet. Transboundary Air Pollution – Will China Choke On Its Success? The Wilson Center. February 2, 2007

[17] Saylnn Boyles. Air Pollution Linked to Heart Deaths – Risk May Be Higher Than Previous Studies Suggest. *WebMD*, Jan 31, 2007

[18] Edwards SC, Jedrychowski W, et al. Prenatal Exposure to Airborne Polycyclic Aromatic Hydrocarbons and Children's Intelligence at Age 5 in a Prospective Cohort Study in Poland. *Environ Health Perspect*, April 20, 2010

[19] Marla Cone, Emily Elert. Urban air pollutants may damage IQs before baby's first breath, scientists say. *Environmental Health News*. July 26, 2010

[20] John Olmstead, G Williams. *Chemistry, the Molecular Science*. Second Edition, 1997, p 396

[21] Ruthann A. Rudel, Julia G. Brody, et al. Identification of Selected Hormonally Active Agents and Animal Mammary Carcinogens in Commercial and Residential Air and Dust Samples. *Air & Waste Manage. Assoc.* 51:499-513. 2001

[22] Reducing Environmental Cancer Risk – What We Can Do Now. 2008–2009 Annual Report, President's Cancer Panel. April, 2010

[23] Lindsey Layton. U.S. facing 'grievous harm' from chemicals in air, food, water, panel says. *Washington Post*, May 7, 2010

[24] Sharon Begley. Born to be Big - Early exposure to common chemicals may be programming kids to be fat. *Newsweek*, September 11, 2008

[25] Paula F. Baillie-Hamilton. Chemical Toxins: A Hypothesis to Explain the Global Obesity Epidemic. *The Journal of Alternative and Complementary Medicine*. April 2002, 8(2): 185-192. doi:10.1089/107555302317371479.

[26] D.Bryce-Smith and H.Waldron. Lead, Behaviour and Criminality. *The Ecologist*. 1974,4,347-358,353

[27] D. Bryce-Smith. Environmental Chemical Influences on Behaviour and Mentation. *Chem. Soc. Rev.* 15, 93-123 (1986).

[28] N. Ward. Heavy Metal status of Incarcerated Young Offenders and Control Individuals, 10th Conference on Heavy Metals in the Environment, Hamburg Symposium 1995, 277-280; CEP Consultants, Edinburgh, 1996

[29] Nicholas Kollerstrom PhD. Violent Crime, Hyperactivity and Mental Balance – A review of Neil Ward's work. *The Nutrition Practitioner*. Summer 2006

[30] The Mystery of Falling Crime Rates. *The Week*, July 16, 2010, page 13

[31] Roger D. Masters, B Hone, A Doshi. Environmental Pollution, Neurotoxicity, and Criminal Violence. *Brain Biochemistry, Neurotoxicity, and Criminal Violence*. September 3, 2007

[32] Monitoring Developmental Disabilities. CDC http://www.cdc.gov/ncbddd/dd/ddsurv.htm

[33] Robert F. Kennedy, Jr. Autism, mercury, and politics. *Boston Globe*. July 1, 2005

[34] Amy Holmes, MD. My Son, the King of Metals. Excerpted for the Autism Research Institute from the book, *Recovering Autistic Children*

[35] Neil Miller. *Aluminum in Vaccines – a Neurological Gamble*, Thinktwice Global Vaccine Institute. 2009

[36] Ibid

[37] Tuthill RW. Hair lead levels related to children's classroom attention-deficit behaviour. *Arch Environ Health*, 1996;51:214–20.

[38] Ed Arranga. Autism Overview. The National Autism Association

[39] Dr. Mary Ann Block. *No More ADHD, No More Ritalin*. The Block System. August 2001

[40] Neurologist Dr. Fred Baughman talks about the fraud of ADHD and the poisoning of U.S. children. *Natural News* interview with Mike Adams. August 30, 2006

[41] Ronnie Cummins. The Oil Spill in the Bathroom. *Huffington Post*. June 16, 2010

[42] Denise Grady. First Signs of Puberty Seen in Younger Girls. *New York Times*, August 9, 2010

[43] Douglas Quenqua. Graduating From Lip Smackers. *New York Times*, April 28, 2010

[44] Environmental Working Group. Teen Girls' Body Burden of Hormone-Altering Cosmetics Chemicals: Cosmetics chemicals of concern.

[45] Mary S. Wolff, Philip J. Landrigan. Mount Sinai Center for Children's Environmental Health and Disease Prevention Research

[46] Environmental Working Group. Scented Secrets. February 12, 2007

[47] Virginia Sole-Smith. The High Price of Beauty. *The Nation*, October 8, 2007

[48] Interview with Amy Goodman of *Democracy Now*, July 21, 2010

[49] http://slowdeathbyrubberduck.com

[50] Johann Hari. The Wrong Kind of Green. *The Nation*. March 22, 2010 edition

[51] Mark Pawlosky. Green, Inc. author says big environmental groups have sold out to big business. *The Grist*. October 3, 2008

[52] Special on-line forum. Conservation Groups and Corporate Cash: An Exchange. *The Nation*. March 10, 2010

[53] http://www2.fluoridealert.org/Alert/United-States/Maryland/Chinese-fluoride-is-a-homeland-security-matter

[54] Danielle Dellorto. 'Dirty dozen' produce carries more pesticide residue, group says. *CNN*, June 1, 2010

[55] EWG Study: Dangerous Chemicals In Common Baby Products. October 31, 2007

[56] Americans Get the Most Radiation From Medical Scans. *Associated Press*. June 14, 2010

[57] Marc Kaufman. Medication Errors Harming Millions, Report Says. *The Washington Post*, July 26, 2006

[58] Hospital-Acquired Infections, MRSA, Killed 48,000 Americans In One Year. *Medical News Today*, February 23, 2010

Additional note:

In 1895, less than two decades after production of synthetic dyes had begun in Germany, it was reported that one of every ten industrial dye factory workers had bladder cancer. Exposure to carcinogenic aromatic amines were taking their toll. By 1930, the high risk of bladder cancer among those who worked regularly with such dyes was clear enough that Germany and Switzerland officially agreed to pay dye workers who developed such cancer, making this one of the first formally compensable occupational illnesses.

[Michaels, David. When Science Isn't Enough: Wilhelm Hueper, Robert A. M. Case, and the Limits of Scientific Evidence in Preventing Occupational Bladder Cancer. *Int J Occup Environ Health* 1995 July ; 1(30: 278-288.]

Electromagnetic Energy

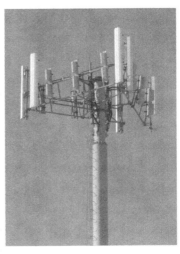

℘homas Edison switched on his first light bulb about 130 years ago. Since then, the world has become enveloped in an invisible net of radio and television signals, military networks, cell phone towers, WiFi, baby monitors, etc. Add to that the deluge of AC energy used to run electrical appliances in the house – refrigerators, printers, hair-dryers, electric clocks by our bedside, dimming light switches, and more. Electrosmog, pollution through electromagnetic energy, is relatively new in human experience.

A human being is a complex organization of electrical fields. The body is about 70 percent water with a high mineral content making it highly electrically conductive. We have some 60 trillion cells, and between the nucleus and the membrane of each cell is a measurable electrical field. Brain cells, nerve cells, bone cells, all vibrate at different rates in order to communicate with one another. Cells know when to divide by vibrating. When you look at an EKG, for example, you see the electrical functioning of your heart. Although Western medicine has been focused on chemistry for last century, electricity is what drives our biology.[1]

Electromagnetic fields (EMFs) produced by modern technologies are artificial intrusions with unnatural intensities, signaling characteristics, pulsing patterns, and wave forms. They can misdirect cells in myriad ways.[2] "If you put a radio near a source of EMFs you will get interference," says Olle Johansson, Associate Professor of Neuroscience at the Karolinska Institute in Sweden. "The human brain has an electric field so if you put sources of EMFs nearby, it is not surprising that you get interference, interaction with systems and damage to cells and molecules."[3]

Not So Good Vibrations

When astronauts first traveled to space, they came home sick. They had been separated from gravity and from the Schumann Wave – the earth's natural frequency, a constant vibration to which our bodies are attuned. When later space flights installed a Schumann Wave generator, astronauts came home in good shape. The steady rhythm of the Schumann Wave regulates our biological clock, our sleep/dream patterns, our patterns of arousal, and hormonal balance. Our optimal brain wave pattern duplicates the Schumann Wave. Human beings do best when they resonate with this frequency, which is what we have done since time began.[4]

SCHUMANN WAVE

A frequency of energy created by the amount of times lightning strikes the earth every second of every day. The Schumann Wave is a steady frequency of energy that measures 7.83 Hz, and beats 7 to 10 times per second.

Man-made frequencies exert a constant pressure on the cells to shift their natural vibration. Our DNA is affected because these unnatural fields carry enough energy to break the chemical bonds that hold DNA together. EMFs also slow our brain waves and affect our long term mental clarity, according to Eric Braverman, M.D., an expert in the brain's global impact on illness and health.[5]

The term **electrosmog** here refers to:

- Electrically charged wires or appliances that exert a magnetic pull on our cells, entraining them into alternate potentially less healthy vibrations.

- Frequencies from wireless communication networks which penetrate the body.
- "Dirty electricity," which is very-low-frequency voltage signals (1-100 kHz), by-products of modern energy-efficient appliances, halogen lamps, computers, wireless routers, plasma TVs, dimmer switches, etc. What all of these devices have in common is that they tamp down the electricity they use. This manipulation of current creates a wildly fluctuating electromagnetic field. Say you bought an "Energy Star" refrigerator. You plug it in. It receives 110 volts, but it ramps down to use less and the unused excess is directed away from the appliance toward you and back onto the electrical lines. "Dirty electricity" increases your risk of melanoma, thyroid cancer, and uterine cancer.[6]

ELECTROSMOG, EMF

EMF = Electromagnetic field, a field of energy created by electrically charged objects.

EMFs occur naturally in storms, in the Earth's magnetic field, etc. The development of man-made electricity and rapid technological progress over the past century have multiplied their sources and diversified their characteristics. EMFs are an invisible form of air pollution.

Electricity powering our homes exposes us to magnetic fields as the current flows to power appliances and lights. Ever-present electric fields are produced by the wiring in the walls, floors and ceilings, and wiring to appliances, etc. If you are sleeping with your head against a wall that has a refrigerator on the other side, for example, every time the refrigerator goes on in the middle of the night, you are bathed in its unnatural electromagnetic field.

Nighttime exposure is the worst. It is at night that your body regenerates, organs detoxify, and cancer-fighting melatonin is produced. Dr. George Carlo, the researcher who first blew the whistle on cell phone hazards, explained that when there is a constant pulsing signal like what you get from "Energy Star" appliances and WiFi networks, human cellular receptors are fooled into entraining to the frequency of that pulsing signal. DNA within the cell has to decide whether the vibration is friend or foreign. If foreign, the cell thinks it is under attack and closes its "doors" which means nutrients do not get in, and toxins do not get out. The medical term is oxidative stress. At night it is essential that the cell membrane be permeable. Think about those 60 trillion cells in your body. Because the cells are not releasing toxins, you get free radical buildup and DNA repair is disrupted. Cellular communication is also impacted, causing confusion within the cells as to how and when to divide. This is the path for the development of tumors associated with cell phone usage.[7]

RF (radio frequency) signals + chemical toxins = damage. It has been shown that mammalian brains are affected negatively by mobile phones, causing increased permeability of the blood-brain barrier and leakage of albumin from the capillaries into the surrounding tissues.[8]

When pathogens are grown in a Petri dish and bathed in electro-magnetic energy, it was found they reproduce ten times faster than normal. It is theorized this is because the pathogens feel threatened and rapid reproduction is a survival strategy. This could explain why, in part, we see disease states manifesting in younger people and becoming more virulent.[9]

When Science Meets Politics

The Russians first noticed during World War II that radar operators often came down with symptoms we now call electrical hypersensitivity syndrome. When television was introduced in Australia in 1956, researchers there documented a rapid increase in cancers among people who lived near transmission towers.

In 1960, neuroscientist Allan Frey "heard" the persistent low-level hum of radar at GE's Advanced Electronics Center at Cornell University. The "hearing," however, didn't happen via normal sound waves perceived through the ear. It occurred somewhere in the brain itself, as electromagnetic waves interacted with the brain's cells, which generate tiny electrical fields. This told scientists that by pulsing a radio signal, it is possible to have the signal interact with the brain and nervous system. This idea came to be known as the Frey effect, and it caused an uproar in the neuroscience community. Frey had stumbled upon the fact that microwaves open up the blood-brain barrier. He was pressured to stop further investigation. (Since then, no meaningful research into the effect of microwaves on the blood-brain barrier has been pursued in the United States.)[10,11]

> Cell phones radiate microwaves, as do microwave ovens. If cell phones had been called "microwave phones" when they came on the market, would you have bought one?

When cell phones went on the market in the 1980s, federal regulators did not require proof they were safe. The telecommunications industry came to see storm clouds on the horizon and hired Dr. George Carlo, a first-rate public health scientist, to study the product. Six years and some $23 million later, Dr. Carlo and his team reported the unexpected – there are definite human health risks:

- cell phones caused leakage in the blood brain barrier
- radiation from wireless phone antennae causes genetic damage in human blood
- there was a doubling of risk for a certain type of cancer

The industry did not renew his research funds and began to discredit him.

Meanwhile, industry lobbyists were at work. The Telecommunications Act of 1996 was a boon to the telecom companies. It specifically prohibits citizens and municipalities from stopping the placement of a cell tower due to health concerns. You can go to your city council and argue whether or not a tower looks pretty enough, but you can not argue that cell towers should not be allowed because they make people sick. The worrisome studies kept coming.

In 2007, the Bioinitiative Working Group released a 650-page report citing more than 2,000 studies that detail the toxic effects of electrosmog ranging from DNA damage and immune system dysfunction to brain cancers and childhood cancers like leukemia. "Every single study of brain tumors that looks at 10 or more years of use shows an increased risk of brain cancer," said Cindy Sage, M.A., co-editor of the report.[12]

In the wake of that report, the European Environmental Agency (EEA) called for immediate action to reduce exposure to radiation from WiFi, mobile phones and their masts (cell towers). The agency suggested that delay could lead to a health crisis similar to those caused by asbestos, smoking and lead in gasoline:[13]

> The case studies of public hazards analysed in the *Late Lessons* publication show that harmful exposures can be widespread before there is both "convincing" evidence of harm from long-term exposures, and biological understanding of how that harm is caused.
>
> ...There are many examples of the failure to use the precautionary principle in the past, which have resulted in serious and often irreversible damage to health and environments.[14]

But in America, the agencies were quiet, waiting for the Interphone Study that came out in 2010. *Microwave News* put it this way:

> There's an old saying that a camel is a horse designed by a committee. Welcome to Interphone.
>
> The good news is that the Interphone paper has finally been made public after a four-year stalemate within the 13-country research team. But it comes at a price. A series of compromises over how to interpret the results of the largest and most expensive study of cell phones and brain tumors ever attempted has left the paper with no clear conclusions other than more research is needed.
>
> At the very least, the risks are greater than many believed only a few years ago. In a series of interviews, a number of the members of the Interphone project told *Microwave News* that they now see the risk among long-term users as being larger than when the study began. Some think the risk warrants serious attention.[15]

The Interphone Study began with cases – people with brain tumors – and controls – people with no cancer – and asked them to remember how much they had used mobile phones in previous years.

At the Bioelectromagnetics Society annual meeting shortly thereafter, Lloyd Morgan, B.Sc., Senior Fellow of Environmental Health Trust, demonstrated that the risk of brain tumors from cell phone use is in fact much higher than the Interphone Study acknowledged: "What we have discovered indicates there is going to be one hell of a brain tumor pandemic unless people are warned and encouraged to change current cell phone use behaviors."[16]

We are all being affected by personal cell phone usage, and also as by-standers subject to second-hand radiation from nearby cell phone users, cell phone antennae, and wireless networks. This is why the concept of second-hand smoke is being applied to wireless technology and cell phones in particular, and why cell phones are sometimes called the cigarettes of the 21st century – toxic, addictive, and heavily defended by an army of industry lobbyists.

"Electromagnetic pollution may be the most significant form of pollution human activity has produced in this century, all the more dangerous because it is invisible and insensible."

—Andrew Weil, M.D.
author of *Spontaneous Healing and 8 Weeks to Optimum Health*

People Began to Say No

In 2003 the teachers at La Quinta, California middle school complained that they, the staff, and the students had more cancers than would be expected. They demanded an EMF investigation. Sam Milham, M.D., an experienced epidemiologist, studied high-frequency voltage transients now called "dirty electricity." In some classrooms he found the surges of transient pollution so high, they exceeded his meter's ability to gauge them. In 2008 he reported in the *American Journal of Industrial Medicine* that cumulative exposure to transients in the school increased the likelihood a teacher would develop cancer by 64%. The teachers' chances of developing melanoma, thyroid cancer, and uterine cancer were as much as 13 times higher than the average.[17]

Dr. Milham's findings served as the first public alert in the U.S. about the health link between occupational exposure to electromagnetic fields and human disease. This helped explain why office workers, like the school

61

teachers, have high cancer incidence rates. It also explains why indoor workers had higher malignant melanoma rates, and why melanoma occurs on parts of the body never exposed to sunlight.

> "The 'War on Cancer' has been a failure because people have missed the major carcinogen." —Dr. Sam Milham

In September 2007, the German Government issued a warning to citizens to avoid using WiFi in the workplace or at home, suggesting cabled connections instead. In late 2007, the French National Library removed all WiFi systems in Paris due to health complaints from staff. The Austrian Medical Association is lobbying against the deployment of WiFi in schools.[18] Lakehead University in Ontario, Canada has limited its use of WiFi and relies on a comprehensive fiber-optic computer network throughout the campus. University policy states:

> There will be no WiFi connectivity provided in those areas of the University already served by hard wire connectivity until such time as the potential health effects have been scientifically rebutted or there are adequate protective measures that can be taken.[19]

Various doctors began to speak out. Three neurosurgeons went on Larry King Live in May, 2008 saying they observed widespread dangers from cell phones and that they personally never put it next to their head – they use earpieces or the speakerphone feature. A couple months later, Dr. Ronald B. Herberman, who headed up the prominent University of Pittsburgh Cancer Institute, issued an unprecedented warning to his faculty and staff: Limit cell phone use because of the possible risk of cancer.[20] He testified to Congress in September, 2008, that the Interphone Study and industry-sponsored studies often discarded data from studies that involved heavy cell phone usage:

> Some recent studies in Nordic countries, where phones have been used the longest, find that persons who have used cell phones for at least a decade have 30% to more than 200% more brain tumors than do those without such use, and only on the side of the head where the user holds his or her phone. To put these numbers in context, this is at least as high an increase

as the added risk of breast cancer that women face from long-term use of hormone replacement therapy [HRT].[21]

In 2009, a collaborative of non-industry funded scientists published "15 Reasons for Concern" about cell phones: including:

- Independent studies show that for every year of cell phone use, the risk of brain cancer increased by 8%, and that after 10 or more years of digital cell phone use, there was a 280% increased risk of brain cancer.
- Electromagnetic fields cause DNA damage.
- Cell phone radiation has been shown to cause the blood-brain barrier (BBB) to leak; the BBB protects the brain from many molecules that are toxic to the brain.
- Cell phone radiation decreases sperm counts and reduces sperm motility.

Despite heavy lobbying from industry, the city of San Francisco voted in 2010 to require all retailers to display the SAR number, the amount of radiation each cell phone emits. ElectromagneticHealth.org called it "a watershed moment for health advocates in the U.S. and families who have or have had members with brain tumors."

EMF Hypersensitivity and Diabetes Type 3

Could dirty electricity raise elevated blood sugar levels among diabetics and prediabetics who are especially sensitive to EMFs? Dr. Magda Havas, Associate Professor of Environmental and Resource Studies at Trent University in Canada, has seen and documented it. Her research represents a paradigm shift in the way we think about diabetes.

She found that blood sugar levels went up when subjects were on a treadmill or in a doctor's office where there is dirty electricity; blood sugar levels went down when subjects walked outside. She calls EMF-induced higher plasma glucose Type 3 Diabetes:

Type 1 diabetics require less insulin in an electromagnetically clean environment and blood sugar levels for Type 2 diabetics increase with increasing exposure to dirty electricity ... Type 3 diabetics may be better able to regulate their blood sugar with less medication, and those diagnosed as borderline or pre-diabetic may remain non diabetic longer by reducing their exposure to electromagnetic energy.

What we describe here is a totally different type in the sense it has an environmental trigger ... We recognize that there is, as yet, no accepted definition of Type 3 diabetes and that our definition may be in conflict with others that have been suggested.[22]

She tells us that for those who are hypersensitive to EMF, blood sugar measurements need to be done in an electromagnetically clean environment (medical offices are typically in buildings with dirty electricity, homes often have wireless networks and portable phones) to prevent misdiagnosis and to accurately determine the severity of the disease.

Riskier for Children

When Dr. Ronald B. Herberman issued his warning to staff and testified before Congress,[23] he included the illustration below which shows how much higher the absorption rates are in a child's brain than in an adult's. Electromagnetic radiation penetrates almost straight through the entire brain of a 5-year-old child.

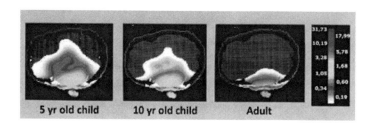

This is a modification of the iconic illustration made in 1996 by Om Gandhi, Professor and Chairman of Department of Electrical Engineering at the University of Utah, Salt Lake City.[24] Dr. Herberman worked with Gandi to turn the illustration into a three-dimensional model that estimates the absorption of electromagnetic radiation.

Scientists feel children are more susceptible to harmful effects of cell phones because:

- Pre-teen children have a smaller head and brain size, the skull bones are thinner, and the percentage of water volume is greater (water conducts electricity).
- Children's brains and central nervous system are still developing so they are more sensitive to exposures.
- Today's children have started to use cell phones at a younger age, therefore their lifetime exposure to cell phone RFs will be greater. Those who started using cell phones before the age of 20 may be five times more likely to develop a glioma, a type of brain tumor, according to Swedish independent researcher, Lennart Hardell.[25]

The UCLA School of Public Health collaborated with University of Aarhus in Denmark to study 13,000 children born in 1997 and 1998. They found children who were exposed to cell phones – either in the womb by their mother's cell phone use or as youngsters themselves – had more behavioral problems at the age of seven than non-cell phone users. Researchers found inattention, hyperactivity, and problems with peers.[26]

Recently, France and Germany dismantled wireless networks in schools and public libraries. Israel has banned the placement of cellular antennae on residences. Russian officials have advised against cell phone use for children under the age 18.

The French government announced in 2009 plans for the most comprehensive action to date taken by any government worldwide: ban advertising of cell phones to children under 12, ban manufacturing of phones specifically designed for children ages six and younger, put more restrictive limits for radiation from the phones, and make it compulsory for handsets to be sold with earphones. Lyon, France's second largest city, launched an advertising campaign before Christmas 2008 aimed at dissuading people from buying mobile phones for children as presents, with the slogan "Let's keep them healthy, away from mobile phones!"[27]

Is brain cancer on the rise among young Americans? Depends on who interprets the stats. At the September 2008 congressional hearing on cell phone safety called by Rep. Dennis Kucinich, Robert Hoover of the National Cancer Institute said government statistics show no increase from 1987 to 2005 – end of story. But Dr. Ronald Herberman testified that as he looked at the same government statistics, he was struck by the fact that the incidence of brain cancer has been increasing over the last ten years, particularly among 20-29 year-olds.

America Lagging Behind?

The American Federal Communications Commission established radiation standards for cell phones in 1996, 13 years after cell phones went on the market. The agency adopted limits recommended by industry that were established to protect against high-dose thermal effects. So they allow a 20-fold higher exposure to the head (1.6 W/kg) compared to the rest of the body (0.08 W/kg) for both adults and children.

At the beginning of the Cold War in the 1950s, radio frequency (RF) standards were set, primarily by the Air Force. It was an era of air raid drills and fear of Soviet missile launches. Decisions were based on the nation's urgent security needs of the day. At that time, the thinking was focused only on the hazardous biological effect from short-term, acute RF exposures of sufficient power to raise body temperatures in excess of one degree centigrade. This is called the "thermal-effects-only" viewpoint and it contradicted Russian and other Eastern European research that claimed to have found a whole range of biological interactions at power levels far below that which was needed to cause tissue heating. That is called the "non-thermal theory" of RF.[28]

Can you have human health problems from non-thermal RF – in other words, from something other than heating? Yes. Though difficult to measure definitively, when a cell phone is being used (making phone calls, searching the internet, downloading music) the non-thermal effects extend about three to six feet. Non-thermal effects from cell towers can affect people thousands of feet away from the originating signal. Often, multiple antennae are all transmitting simultaneously so your home or office is being impacted at the same time from different directions.[29]

From David Carpenter, M.D., co-editor of the *BioInitiative Report*:

The fields associated with electricity are commonly called "extremely low frequency" fields (ELF), while those used in communication and microwave ovens are called "radiofrequency" (RF) fields. Studies of people have shown that both ELF and RF exposures result in an increased risk of cancer, and that this occurs at intensities that are too low to cause tissue heating. Unfortunately, all of our exposure standards are based on the false assumption that there are no hazardous effects at intensities that do not cause tissue heating ... We need to educate decision-makers that 'business as usual' is unacceptable.

Yet in the United States, it is still business as usual; the science seems to get little official attention.

In 2006, the New York based publication *Microwave News* examined the 85 papers on microwave effects on DNA that were published in peer-reviewed journals since 1990.

They found that of the 42 papers which reported no effect, 32 of them were funded by either the U.S. Air Force or industry. Of the 43 yes-effects papers, only 3 were funded by Air Force or industry. The source of funding appears to have a strong influence on the outcome of research. The published results, however, with an approximately equal mix of positive and negative studies, support the mobile phone industry's viewpoint that "the science is inconclusive" and "more data is needed."[30]

As the public relations spin masters describe it, this is the technique of paralysis by analysis.

Cordless Phones

Cordless phones are EMF monsters. The base is the problem, not the handset. The base can exert radio frequencies that extend between one quarter and one half mile, depending on the strength of the phone. This means that even if you do not have a cordless phone, your neighbor's phone can impact you – and every other cordless phone within range of your house. Because as these waves pass through your windows (not through walls), they tend to concentrate in rooms with natural lighting. This is why it is said we are bombarded with more than a 1,000 times more electromagnetic energy now than ever before in the history of mankind.

Most cordless phones emit pulsing microwave radiation from their base station even when the phone is not being used.

Make sure your cordless phone base station is not in your bedroom or close to where you sit a lot. You can put a metal bucket over the base of a cordless phone at night or just unplug it. Better yet, replace it with a hard wired phone and use two 25 foot spiral cords attached them together with a coupler to give you a 50 foot tether for mobility.

Cell Phones

*H*olding the cell phone against your head ensures that you will absorb most of the microwave energy. A speakerphone is better because it puts more distance between the emissions and your head. Using a headset designed with an air-filled, wireless tube also reduces exposure. You can choose to limit your calls to a couple minutes. Use less than 500 minutes a month. Texting is better than talking (in terms of avoiding cell phone damage) because all the data is transmitted in a fraction of a second.

When your cell phone has fewer bars, it ramps up and uses more power; therefore, it is more dangerous to make calls from outlying areas.

Inside a vehicle, the RF frequencies bounce off the inside of the vehicle and bombard you. You increase your exposure when you use a cell phone in an enclosed area such as a car, train, airplane, or metal building.

Don't let your teenager sleep with a cell phone under the pillow. And turn off all wireless devices in the house at night.

Cell phone radiation is transmitted by the antenna and the circuit elements inside the handset. The antenna and the circuit elements send out the electromagnetic wave (RF radiation) to transmit the signal. EMF radiation emitted by a cell phone antenna is not very directional – similar amounts of radiation are transmitted outward, towards the base station, and inward, towards the ear/head of a cell phone user.

A worldwide-recognized, basic unit for the description of thermal effects of a cell phone is referred to as the specific absorption rate (SAR), which is given in watt per kilogram (W/kg). The higher the "SAR rating," the more thermal energy a phone gives off.

To play it safe, you can buy a cell phone with a SAR number of .08 or less – that would be half or less of what the U.S. allows. However:

- The SAR value compares just the thermal (heating) effect of different phones and does not give information about the non-thermal biological effect of that phone.
- SAR values are reported to the FCC by the manufacturer and there is little or no ongoing, independent monitoring of the SAR values submitted.
- Holding the phone in a slightly different way can actually render the worst SAR value phone better than the best SAR value phone.
- SAR values have been created based on simulations of exposure in a plexiglass head filled with fluid, not a human head, and many scientists consider them to be inaccurate and irrelevant at determining actual biological effects. The FCC, the industry, and the academic community all acknowledge that SAR measurements have significant precision problems.
- Some non-thermal, biological effects, such as blood brain barrier permeability, have been shown to be worse at lower SAR values compared to higher SAR values.

As Camilla Rees, founder of ElectromagneticHealth.org put it: "Physical distance of the phone from your brain, and less usage of the cell phone overall, more so than simply choosing a phone with a lower SAR value, is probably a far better insurance policy."

Wireless devices transmit a constant signal whether in use or not. IPhones and Blackberries are different than other cell phones; each device acts as antenna relay station, even when turned off – thus more exposure to you.

How many antennae and towers are near you? Check it out at
www.antennasearch.org

It varies from model to model, but in general when a cell phone is being used in a full-strength signal area, the signal can have a potential impact on anyone within approximately three to six feet of the cell phone.

Every time you use your cell phone, it is necessary for a nearby cell tower antenna to transmit and receive your signal. Therefore, anyone within the neighborhood of the cell tower will be impacted by your action. Each cell tower's signals eventually hit the ground. If your home is at that spot, the bombardment from the tower is usually many times greater than the bombardment from a wireless system you might have in your home office.

Reducing the Electrosmog

It is always good to know that you can have a BauBiologist check your home (www.wehliving.org), and find out exactly how badly you are being bombarded by neighborhood cell towers and where the wiring and such in your house are most intrusive. Parents who have autistic children and those with Lyme disease who have followed the BauBiologist's recommendations have reported significant improvement in their autistic children's behavior.

There are many devices on the market that claim to protect from electrosmog, but claims and counter-claims about their effectiveness abound. Also, this is often a case of you get what you pay for. Here are some of the options:

- Paint the interior walls of your house with shielding paint.
- Put a shielding film on windows and sliding glass doors. You can also use RF shielded material that can line drapes – most of these look like a silvery space blanket.
- Install a kill switch in the bedrooms to turn off electricity at night that runs through the walls. If a refrigerator or TV backs up to a wall that is also a bedroom wall, put RF shielding material behind it.
- Don't use your laptop computer directly in your lap.
- Use a cell phone protector. Buyer beware here. Skip past claims that a protector will "stop damage to your blood cells." You want a protector that has been measured with a meter for its shielding abilities.

Cell phones emit microwave energy – the stuff of thermal effects and the source of most of the publicity. Some cell phone protectors offer some protection from this. There are no cell phone protectors for the non-thermal effects. Something to shield from both does not exist that we know of at this time.

Absent prudent safety standards from government and manufacturers (adding a protective filter would add perhaps $5 to the cost of a laptop), protection is up to you.

As momentum builds, we may see the day when – by incentives or mandates – much of our wireless communications will be conducted on a fiber optic system. That would pretty much give us the technology we want, without the unnecessary risks.

Good Vibrations

Clint Ober decided to create a new life for himself after he almost died from a medical condition. He quit his cable TV executive life to get closer to nature. He found himself sitting on a park bench in Arizona in 1998 noticing that everyone walking by was wearing shoes with synthetic soles that impede their connection to the earth. He got an idea.

He researched EMF studies. He saw that effects from exposure found in some human studies were "inconclusive" because the same effects could not be reproduced in animal studies. Ober went where no one else had gone before. He theorized that animals don't wear shoes or sleep in beds so they are naturally grounded by the earth, unlike people today. He understood that the earth's natural grounding effect might protect people from EMFs the way it protects electrical systems from interference. Researchers laughed; Ober persisted and he did studies.

Simple ground contact, Ober observed, provides a neutralizing charge to the body and naturally protects the nervous system and the endogenous fields of the body from extraneous electrical interference. He expanded this to include the neutralization of free radicals produced within the body. Free radicals are produced by the body to destroy pathogens. But outside forces cause us to produce too many free radicals. Ground contact, he postulated, allows the earth's free electrons to neutralize excess free radicals.

Throughout most of evolution, humans walked barefoot and slept on the ground. The Earth is full of electrons. When a person's bare skin touches the earth, Ober says, electrons enter the body and work like antioxidants, disarming the free radicals that age us.

Dr. Maurice Ghaley, an anesthesiologist, set out to prove Ober wrong. Instead, he found that grounding the human body to the earth during sleep reduces nighttime levels of cortisol and re-synchronizes cortisol hormone secretion more in alignment with the natural 24-hour circadian rhythm profile:[31]

> Exposure to sunlight produces vitamin D in the body. It's needed for health. Exposure to the ground provides an electrical 'nutrient' in the form of electrons. Think of these electrons as vitamin G – G for ground. Just like vitamin D, you need vitamin G for your health as well.[32]

And like vitamin D, "earthing" is free. Well, mostly. There are gadgets you can buy to ground your bed to the earth. "Earthing ranks right up there with the discovery of penicillin," said Ann Louise Gittleman, author of several natural medicine books.

In our excitement to develop new technologies, we rushed past the natural and good vibrations of the ground beneath our feet. How ironic – a retired cable TV executive hands us a low tech idea for protection from the ever-increasing high-tech EMF net around us.

RESOURCES

Report: "Cell Phone Radiation: Science Review on Cancer Risks and Children's Health" by Environmental Working Group (ewg.org/cellphoneradiation/fullreport)

Look up the SAR rating on your phone at Environmental Working Group (ewg.org/cellphoneradiation/Get-a-Safer-Phone)

Learn how to "Create a Sleeping Sanctuary" at wehliving.org/sleeping_sanctuary.pdf

Emrpolicy.org is a good all-around source of the latest news and resources.

ElectromagneticHealth.org also offers free audio interviews with some of the world's leading experts in the field of EMF. They also post videos of industry discussions.

Electrosensitivesociety.com provides information and resources for those who are especially sensitive to EMF.

Dirtyelectricity.ca is a great source of information in "dirty electricity."

BOOKS

Dirty Electricity – Electrification and Diseases of Civilization
  by Dr. Sam Milham, 2010

Disconnect – The Truth About Cell Phone Radiation, What the Industry Has Done to Hide It and How to Protect Your Family
  by Debra Davis, 2010

Earthing
  by Clinton Ober, Dr. Stephen Sinatra, Martin Zucker, 2010

Public Health SOS – The Shadow Side of the Wireless Evolution
  by Camilla Reese and Magda Havas, 2009

Electromagnetic Fields: A Consumer's Guide to the Issues and How to Protect Ourselves by B. Blake Levitt, 2007

Cell Phones: Invisible Hazards in the Wireless Age
  by Dr. George Carlo and Martin Scram, 2001

---

[1] Pliquett, U. Electricity and Biology. Electronics Conference, 2008. BEC 2008. *11th International Biennial Baltic*. DOI: 10.1109/BEC.2008.4657474
[2] B. Blake Levitt. *Electromagnetic Fields, A Consumer's Guide to the Issues and How to Protect Ourselves*. Backinprint.com, 2007
[3] Nic Fleming. Scientists serious about 'electricity sickness' claims. *The Telegraph*. January 24, 2005
[4] Miller RA, Miller I. The Schumann Resonances and Human Psychobiology. *Nexus Magazine*, Volume 10, Number 3 (April-May 2003). Downloaded from http:twm.co.nz/schumann.html
[5] Bioinitiative Working Group, 2007 http://www.bioinitiative.org/index.htm

[6] Dr. Samuel Milham. *Dirty Electricity.* 2002 http://electromagnetichealth.org/electromagnetic-health-blog/sammilham

[7] Mary Budinger. Lyme-Induced Autism Conference Focuses on Biofilm and Toxicity. *Public Health Alert,* July 2009

[8] Salford LD, Brun AE et al. Nerve cell damage in mammalian brain after exposure to microwaves from GSM mobile phones. *Environ Health Perspect.* 2003 June; 111(7): 881–883.

[9] Dr. Dietrich Klinghardt. Electromagnetic Radiation, Electromagnetic Fields, Pollution, Microwave Radiation, Cell Phone Cancer

[10] Alan H. Frey. Headaches from Cellular Telephones: Are They Real and What Are the Implications? *Environmental Health Perspectives,* Volume 106, Number 3, March 1998

[11] Christopher Ketcham. Warning: Your Cell Phone May Be Hazardous to Your Health. *GQ Magazine,* February, 2010

[12] Michael Segell. Is 'electrosmog' harming our health? Electrical pollution from cell phones and WiFi may be hazardous. *Prevention Magazine,* January, 2010

[13] Geoffrey Lean. EU watchdog calls for urgent action on Wi-Fi radiation. *The Independent,* September 16, 2007

[14] Radiation risk from everyday devices assessed. European Environmental Agency. September 17, 2007

[15] Interphone Points to Long-Term Brain Tumor Risks-Interpretation Under Dispute. *Microwave News,* May 18, 2010

[16] Press release: Risk of Brain Cancer from Cell Phone Use Underestimated by At Least 25% in Interphone Study, According to Scientific Presentation Today at the Bioelectromagnetics Society. ElectromagneticHealth.org. June 15, 2010

[17] Milham S, Morgan LL. A new electromagnetic field exposure metric: high frequency voltage transients associated with increased cancer incidence in teachers in a California school. *Am J Ind Med* 2008;51(8):579–86.

[18] http://wifiinschools.org.uk/4.html

[19] WiFi and Cellular Antennae Policy. Lakewood University. Effective November 10, 2009

[20] Cancer institute warns of cellphone risks. *USA Today,* July 25, 2008

[21] Statement of Ronald B. Herberman, MD, Tumors and Cell Phone Use-What the Science Says. Testimony to the Oversight and Government Reform Committee. September 25, 2008

[22] Magda Havas. Dirty Electricity Elevates Blood Sugar Among Electrically Sensitive Diabetics and May Explain Brittle Diabetes. *Electromagnetic Biology and Medicine,* 27: 135-146, 2008.

[23] http://www.docstoc.com/docs/14940856/Ronald-B-Herberman-MD-%E2%80%9CTumors-and-Cell-Phone-use

[24] Om P. Gandhi, G. Lazzi, and C. Furse. Electromagnetic Absorption in the Human Head and Neck for Cell Telephones at 835 an 1900 MHz. *IEEE Transactions on Microwave Theory and Techniques,* 1996. 44 (10):p 1884-1897

[25] Lennart Hardell, M Carlberg. Long-term use of cellular phones and brain tumours: increased risk associated with use for > or =10 years. *Occup Environ Med.* 2007 Sep;64(9):626-32. Epub 2007 Apr 4.

[26] Press release: Study questions safety of children's exposure to cell phones during prenatal and early childhood period. UCLA School of Public Health, May 21, 2008

[27] Geoffrey Lean. French government bans advertising of mobiles to children. *The Independent,* January 11, 2009

[28] Donald R. Maisch, PhD. The Procrustean Approach – Setting Exposure Standards for Telecommunications Frequency Electromagnetic Radiation. Thesis submitted to University of Wollongong, 2010

[29] Hyland GL, Physics and Biology of Mobile Telephony. *The Lancet* 2000; 356: 1833-36.

[30] L. Slesin, 'Radiation Research and The Cult of Negative Results', *Microwave News,* vol. 26, no. 4, July 2006.

[31] D Minkhoff. Best Cases in Biological Medicine, Series #6. *Explore!* Volume 13, Number 6, 2004

[32] Clint Ober, Dr. Stephen Sinatra, Martin Zucker. Earthing: The Most Important Health Discovery Ever? *Basic Health Publications;* April, 2010

Sickness is a Slow Descent

$\mathcal{E}$very day, our bodies are bombarded with food additives, chemicals, and a plethora of substances that degrade health.

No wonder eventually something breaks down, just like a car running on dirty fluids and filters, and the wrong kind of oil and gasoline.

You may not realize how much the world throws at your body every day. Let's take a look at a typical day in the life of Fred.

Fred wakes up, having slept on a mattress manufactured with flame retardants (polybrominated diphenyl ethers). Laboratory studies using animals have linked the chemicals to behavior changes that bear an uncanny similarity to attention deficit and hyperactivity disorders common in children. New research has found that flame retardants have an ability to mimic thyroid hormones; it is thought that by acting hormonally, the chemicals wreak havoc in laboratory animals, where exposures have been linked to hyperactivity, impaired learning, and decreased sperm counts.[1]

Fred brushes his teeth with fluoride, never noticing that his tube of toothpaste contains a warning from the FDA that he should not swallow the toothpaste and to call a poison center if he does. Modern studies link fluoride to arthritis, allergies, kidney and thyroid dysfunction, bone damage and cancer even at the low levels dentists claim is optimal to reduce tooth decay.[2] As he brushes his teeth, his silver amalgam (mercury) fillings release a little mercury vapor, as they do every time he chews. He is unaware that in 1991, the World Health Organization acknowledged that the predominant source of human exposure to mercury comes

75

from fillings. His dentist hasn't told him that study after study shows that mercury negatively affects the heart – he could be setting himself up for a heart attack.

Found on toothpaste products, as required by law:
WARNINGS: Keep out of reach of children under 6 years of age. If you accidentally swallow more than used for brushing, seek PROFESSIONAL HELP or contact a POISON CONTROL center immediately.

He showers in chlorinated water where he absorbs more chlorine through his skin than if he were to drink eight glasses of tap water. According to the U.S. Council of Environmental Quality, "Cancer risk among people using chlorinated water is as much as 93% higher than among those whose water does not contain chlorine." Joseph M. Price, M.D., warned that "Chlorine is the greatest crippler and killer of modern times. It is an insidious poison."[3]

Fred washes his hair, unaware that 93 percent of shampoos contain harmful impurities linked to cancer or other health problems, and that 76 percent of conditioners contain ingredients that are allergens. The sodium lauryl sulfate (SLS) and sodium laureth sulfate (SLES) found in many shampoos and conditioners and may cause hair loss and scalp irritation.[4]

He puts on clothes his wife washed with fabric softener that emits a "springtime fresh" smell. Fabric softeners contain chemicals like chloroform, benzyl acetate and pentane that are known to cause cancer and/or damage to lungs, brain, and nerves. About 95% of the chemicals used in fragrances are made from petroleum products.

For breakfast, Fred eats bacon and eggs. The bacon, like many processed meats, contains sodium nitrite to add red color. It is known to cause cancer. The eggs came from "factory chickens" which never saw the light of day and were fed a grain and soy-based chicken feed laced with hormones and antibiotics to prevent the growth of disease-causing bacteria. He never thinks that these antibiotics may have allowed these MRSA bacteria to flourish – the ones that cause his recurrent boils.

He washes breakfast down with coffee laced with a powdered "creamer" concoction of hydrogenated oils – inflammatory vegetable fats which cause heart disease, nutritional deficiencies, general deterioration of cellular health, and much more.

Fred is proud of his new car. As he inserts the key, he breathes in that new car smell. He doesn't think that what he is really filling his lungs with is a toxic brew of fumes from adhesives, sealers, carpeting, lubricating compounds, and phthalates (plastic softeners) with chemical names like ethyl benzene, xylene, formal-dehyde and toluene.

Later at the office, Fred reaches for a diet soda and a health bar from the vending machine. The soda contains aspartame, a chemical additive which is the source of more FDA complaints than any other food additive. In the body, it converts to formaldyhyde which has been shown to cause cancer in animals and is listed by the EPA as a probable human carcinogen. It is an excitotoxin which harms nerve cells, over-exciting them to the point of cell death. The "health" bar contains the excitotoxin MSG hidden in safe-sounding ingredients like yeast extract.

On a scale of 1 to 10, Fred's nutritional intake so far today is at about a 2. He is unaware of the "Triage Theory" that says natural selection favors short-term survival over the long-term, and that our short-term survival is achieved by prioritizing the allocation of scarce micronutrients. In other words, to stop us from falling over from a lack of iron, for example, iron is pulled from non-essential sources. So illnesses like heart disease, cancer, and Alzheimer's may be unintended consequences of mechanisms developed during evolution to protect against episodic vitamin/mineral shortages.

He goes to the restroom where there is a chemical air freshener. It contains benzene, a carcinogen that's been linked to leukemia – and xylene, a toxic petroleum byproduct that has been associated with headaches and cognitive impairment. He washes his hands in antibacterial soap containing triclosan which promotes the emergence of bacteria that are resistant to antibiotics. TV ads have made him afraid of germs; he is unaware that even the American Medical Association and the U.S. Centers for Disease Control and Prevention advise against non-clinical use of antibacterial soaps, which may lead to bacterial resistance and don't clean any better than ordinary soap.[5]

He returns to his office which emits formaldehyde from particle board cabinets and insulation between the walls. Formaldehyde is associated with respiratory inflammation, watery eyes, burning mucus membranes, cough, skin rash, and even cancer. This is the chemical made infamous by the trailers provided by the federal government to those whose homes had been destroyed in New Orleans by Hurricane Katrina in 2005.

In the afternoon, Fred has a dentist appointment for a root canal. Dr. George Meinig, author of *Root Canal Cover-Up*, could tell Fred how "Root-canal-filled teeth always remain infected no matter how good they might look or how good they might feel." When bacteria get into the tooth's bony socket, the bacteria also get into the blood supply of the jaw, allowing the bacteria to travel to another gland, organ and tissue and cause a new infection.

Every day Fred's body works at detoxifying these kinds of things. It uses glutathione, folic acid, methyl groups, sulfate groups, liver enzymes and all the cellular machinery whose functions are to detoxify. The detoxifying agents are actually nutrients that we take in with food – if we are eating a nutrient-dense diet. However, the Standard American Diet of pizza, fast food hamburgers, French fries and soda is not nutrient dense. The body runs chronically low on detoxifying agents. The body continues to try to detoxify but when it doesn't have the complete "medicine chest" with which to do that, dangerous free radicals are created. Free radicals damage cell walls and eventually the cell DNA. Now the stage is set for chronic disease and cancer.

If the detoxification systems are compromised, it is virtually impossible to restore normal metabolic function unless we first remove the toxins. The adequacy of these detoxification systems can be tested, using sound principles of functional medicine.

When President Richard Nixon launched his "war on cancer" some 40 years ago, a large body of scientific literature already existed that linked chemicals in the environment to cancer. There were also hypotheses, but little else, linking retroviruses to cancer. One would have expected that most of the $30 billion spent on the "war" would have looked at proving the chemical connection. Instead we failed to prove that retroviruses cause cancer, and the "war" is today widely deemed a failure. Chemicals saturate our environment.[6]

Most of the chronic illness we see today is due to our environment and our food.

Our diets have changed tremendously in the past 100 years. Why don't most physicians warn people of unhealthy eating? Perhaps because medical school does not teach the importance of good food. Why have diabetes and obesity become rampant on the allopathic watch? Medical school gave doctors perhaps a scant 8 hours of nutrition study. The curriculum is shaped in part by the pharmaceutical industry. Med schools essentially train doctors to prescribe drugs to suppress symptoms. In many instances, looking for the root cause and using non-pharmaceutical modalities to prompt healing is "outside the standard of care."

Is it any wonder that so many people wander from one doctor's office to another trying to find out what's wrong and how to fix it?

People will look to their 90-year-old grandparent who ate lots of "cholesterol inducing" red meat and butter and marvel at how fit that person is for 90. What they do not realize is that older person spent the first several decades of his or her life before WWII – before processed foods, pervasive chemicals, ubiquitous wireless networks, and before the couch potato lifestyle that so many of us have adopted. They were outside in the sun getting good-sized doses of vitamin D. Their red meat and dairy were largely without hormones and steroids and the dietary hazards of today's modern feedlot. This was an era before drugs were touted as the answer to every problem.

We are giving drugs to children more than ever before. American children take anti-psychotic medicines, for example, at about six times the rate of children in the United Kingdom.[7] Lipitor® comes in a chewable form.

Infants are born with an average of over 200 toxic chemicals in their blood.[8] So children come into the world with a significant body burden of toxicity. According to a 1999 National Academy of Sciences report, half of all pregnancies in the nation end in the loss of the baby or a child with a birth defect or chronic health problem that manifests by age three.[9]

It's no wonder.

And it's not just what is happening to our bodies today. It's what is happening to our genes that are passed down to our children and grandchildren and their children. Epigenetics is turning the science of inheritance on its head. Use your search engine to find a BBC documentary called *The Ghost in Your Genes*. It will amaze you.

---

[1] http://www.theglobeandmail.com/servlet/story/RTGAM.20060529.wxenvironment-flames30/BNStory/specialScienceandHealth

[2] Lawyer Paul Beeber, President, New York State Coalition Opposed to Fluoridation, Inc.

[3] Joseph M. Price. *Coronaries/Cholesterol/Chlorine*. Jove Book, Alta Enterprises, 1969.

[4] Environmental Working Group. Skin Deep. 2004 summarized at http://www.ewg.org/node/17855

[5] see www.epa.gov/oppad001

[6] National Health Freedom. Politically Motivated Disease Causation-the Biggest Epidemic of All, by Marcel Girodian. May 5, 2005 http://www.thenhf.com/articles_117.htm Accessed January 2007

[7] Associated Press. U.S. kids prescribed more anti-psychotic drugs, May 5, 2008

[8] Body Burden – the Pollution in Newborns II. Environmental Working Group

[9] National Research Council. Hormonally active agents in the environment. *National Academy Press*, Washington DC. 1999. Also see http://www.protectingourhealth.org/newscience/birthdefects/2004-0501birthdefectspreview.htm, accessed February 2007

Section II
An Alphabet of Good Health

"Man's rise and fall has been a measure of his ability
to learn and obey Nature's laws of life."
—Dr. Weston A. Price

In this section, you will find a number
of popular health topics listed alphabetically.

The chapter on Chronic Disease and Inflammation is a must read,
for no matter what condition you may be curious to learn about,
inflammation is the common thread that underlies
almost every problem we see today and
drives many chronic diseases
to epidemic proportions.

Allergies

Our body tries to protect us against environmental insults by means of a very well developed immune system. In some people the response is over-active and harmful instead of accurate and helpful. What causes hyperactivity in the immune system? Is it physical? Energetic? Psychological? All of the above?

The body has an innate wisdom by which it distinguishes self from non-self. This is the fundamental dichotomy of our human existence – the Yin and the Yang of Chinese medicine, the one and the zero of the computer, the "yes" and the "no."

In the realm of ordinary human existence, the infant at first has no idea which body parts belong to itself, and which to "other," meaning its mother. How does the infant figure it out? It begins in the gut.

The infant's intestinal tract must not only distinguish self from non-self, but also pathogens (infectious bacteria) from non-pathogens (food, helpful bacterial residents of the GI tract).[1]

Most of our immune system is initially contained within the gut, where it is called the GALT, or gut-associated lymphoid tissue. This GALT has no lymphatics coming into it from the rest of the body, so it receives its information solely from the contents of the intestines. This information comes in the form of food antigens and "normal" intestinal flora, the helpful bacteria which produce vitamins and serve as guards against organisms which could make us really ill. The infant's GALT is poorly developed for up to several months after birth. B lymphocytes are produced in the GALT. These B lymphocytes then migrate throughout the body, eventually returning to the GI tract in the form of secretory IgA producing cells which then serve as gatekeepers, telling the body which substances are healthy to absorb, and which need to be guarded against.

85

> GALT tissue can become massively inflamed and enlarged in cases of measles enterocolitis, a disease which has been described in autistic children.*
>
> * Wakefield A J, Murch S H et al. Ileal-lymphoid-nodular hyperplasia, non-specific colitis, and pervasive developmental disorder in children. *The Lancet* 351. Feb 28, 1998: 637-641

In the United States today, we do not see infants with the severe gastrointestinal infections which characteristically cause high infant mortality in other parts of the world. Instead, we see different problems. We see an increase of food allergies in our population, to the point where entire websites and self-help groups are growing up to help people deal with allergic manifestations because conventional allopathic physicians seem either unresponsive, unknowledgeable, or unbelieving.

The fact that the information-carrying B lymphocytes migrate throughout the body, before returning to the GI tract from whence they came, goes a long way toward explaining why food allergy or sensitivity can manifest in so many different ways in so many different organs of the body.

Allergies are NOT a Mystery

The period immediately after birth is critical to the development of both food tolerance and food allergy. Dietary antigens other than breast milk need to be introduced slowly and carefully, in order to avoid the development of severe food allergy (introduce vegetables and meats first, not wheat and cereals). Genetics also play a part. People with specific genotypes have increased incidence of food allergy and inflammatory bowel disease.[2]

Normal intestinal flora are essential to prevent the development of food allergy.[3] If the composition of the intestinal flora is altered, (by antibiotics for example), then susceptibility to food allergy is markedly increased, as is susceptibility to disease.[4]

So which comes first? The food allergy? The antibiotics? The frequent infections? It's a little like arguing whether the chicken came first or the egg. Genetic susceptibility, environmental exposure, destruction of the normal intestinal flora... these can all occur very early in life. The result is children who are not only susceptible to food allergy – which they often appear to "grow out of" – but also to many other manifestations of both allergic and inflammatory disease which they grow in to later in life.

Infants can manifest eczema – severe dermatitis, skin rash – which is generally treated with inflammation-suppressing steroid creams. Infants may manifest colic – inconsolable crying, often in the evenings – with no discernible cause, sometimes with excessive intestinal gas, but not always. They often develop near constant ear infections. These are generally treated with antibiotics, thus destroying the few remaining beneficial bacteria. Then these children go on to acquire tubes in the ear drums at a very early age to treat the chronic infections. By the time they reach the age of four or five, they are now old enough to manifest nasal allergy – called "allergic rhinitis" – and/or chronic tonsillitis and swelling of the adenoids, necessitating surgical removal of the tonsils.

At about this age, they start seeing the pediatric allergist, who diagnoses airborne allergy (grasses, pollens, dust, etc) and starts them on a long course of allergy shots and pharmaceutical medication to treat the stuffy nose, the plugged ears, the swollen glands and the chronic cough which generally accompany the allergy symptoms.

The child may be less fortunate and go on to develop reactive airway disease, or asthma, which is then further treated with steroid medication and antibiotics, as well as antihistamines, resulting in a further loss of function.

Children sometimes "outgrow" asthma, and have no further manifestations of disease until they reach their late 30s or early 40s. The allergies do not actually disappear. Instead, they continue to cause chronic inflammation and provoke the immune system to continued low level response. They may not manifest overtly because the child grows and weighs more, has taken lots of antibiotics and immune suppressant drugs (steroids), therefore it takes more allergen to provoke a visible response.

Allergy-Induced Inflammation Causes Disease

 $\mathcal{A}$ s middle age approaches, these folks may have a recurrence of their asthma, or they may be among those unfortunates who develop deeper manifestations of disease. They may develop arthritis, irritable bowel syndrome, inflammatory bowel disease, colitis, Crohn's disease, type 2 diabetes, metabolic syndrome, multiple sclerosis, or a whole host of other diseases which are based upon chronic inflammation. Even at this late date, if the food allergy is diagnosed and the offending food is removed, substantial recovery is possible.

In the end, the chronic inflammation can manifest as high blood pressure, stroke, heart attack, memory loss and even Alzheimer's disease or cancer. The greater the progression of dysfunction, the less are the chances of complete recovery. Even still, symptoms may diminish markedly, if the offending allergens are removed.

It is clear that allergic reaction begets inflammation which begets yet more predisposition to allergic and inflammatory reaction. Some people develop progressively worsening food sensitivities, and even begin to notice they have trouble when they walk down the detergent and soaps aisle in the grocery store. They may start to cough or wheeze when they smell strong perfumes. In the end, some of these unfortunate people develop a syndrome known as "multiple chemical sensitivity" – loss of tolerance to multiple foods, and eventually to all kinds of chemicals as well,[5] resulting pretty much in confinement to their own environmentally safe home.

In other parts of the world, severe gastrointestinal infections cause high infant mortality. But in America, we have children hospitalized with asthma, on chronic steroid medication, inhalers and antihistamines... children with dry skin, eczema, rashes... children with type 2 diabetes and weight gain... children with ADD, unable to sit still or focus.

A runny nose leads to sinusitis – inflammation of the sinuses. Many people get infections in the sinuses that are behind the cheekbones – the maxillary sinuses – because this area drains from the top, not the bottom.

It is efficient in animals which walk on all fours with their heads down, but not as efficient for upright beings who walk on two feet.

Many people find their chronic sinus infections improve when they deal with their chronic constipation. It is a well known fact in Chinese medicine that the lungs, the respiratory system, and large intestine are on the same energetic meridian. If there is blockage in one area, there is blockage in the other. Relieve the blockage in one, and you relieve the blockage in the other. The way to relieve the blockage in the colon is through improved nutrition, not eating the things you are allergic or sensitive to, increasing fiber in the diet (fruits and veggies), and cleaning out the colon with colonics.

A study published in 2010 compared the gut flora of Italian children with that of children from a village in western Africa. The African children ate a high-fiber, low-fat, vegetable-heavy diet that reflects what people ate at the dawn of agriculture, whereas the Italian kids had a typical Western diet, low in fiber but high in animal protein, sugar, starch, and fat. Researchers found that only the African children had bacterial strains of Prevotella, Xylanibacter, and Treponema, which are excellent at breaking down fibrous foods and producing short-chain fatty acids that provide added energy. Studies have also shown that those same fatty acids help protect the intestines from inflammation, which could explain why inflammatory bowel disease is almost unheard of in African communities that eat high-fiber diets. The increased diversity of microbes in the gut also makes the body more resistant to intestinal pathogens while tempering the immune system's response to harmless molecules, leading to fewer allergies, the researchers concluded.[6]

CASE STUDY

A 28-year-old man with annual severe allergies. At the first whiff of pollen, he would plug up and didn't breathe well again till the first frost. We tried allergy shots and food elimination. It gave some improvement, but nowhere near 100 percent improvement. One day he got to talking about when he first experienced his allergies. He remembered sitting on the cellar stairs when he was four years old, very worried about what was happening between his parents who were in the process of divorce. He remembered that he wanted very much to cry but he didn't. He plugged it up inside. It was springtime. Since that time, his nose would plug up at the first whiff of a flower. After he made that conscious connection to the four-year-old child, his allergy symptoms dissipated. He never had a problem with plugging up in the springtime again.

Identifying energetic blockages and bringing them to consciousness can release them. This can be done in many ways. Hypnosis can put you in touch with the time and place where you can contact the emotion that manifested physically. For some people, acupuncture triggers the release.

Sometimes the body stashes a trauma because it was too hard to deal with at the time. Then later, we may be fortunate enough to realize that the coping mechanism no longer serves us and it is time to be rid of it.

Treating for Allergies

The diagnosis of allergies is done by using antigens – diluted substances with which we test for reactions. You can be tested for:

- Foods of all kinds
- Airborne allergies – pollens, mold, dust
- Yeast and skin fungus
- Animal allergies – cat, dog, horse, bird, etc.
- Chemical allergies – cologne, newsprint, car exhaust, building materials, cleaning products – you name it
- Hormones – some people react badly to their own hormones
- Special requests – almost anything can be made into an antigen

For foods, eliminating the offending menu items for a period of time allows the gut to repair itself, and the B cells to diminish in number. This has proven to be a most effective treatment. Eventually the immune system settles down, and the food can often be tolerated in small doses periodically, although it may never be tolerated again in large amounts daily. Treatment can be given for accidental or unpreventable exposure.

It is impossible to avoid many other substances. It is possible to be desensitized with antigens which are very diluted solutions of the substances to which you react. Antigens operate on approximately the same principal as a homeopathic remedy. If a large amount of something makes you sick, a tiny amount of the same substance reverses the symptoms. The antigen is a small enough amount that the body can let go of the histamine response. Over time, you take progressively larger doses of the substance until the body no longer reacts.

Most antigens are commercially prepared with glycerin or phenol added as a preservative. However, both glycerin and phenol are quite capable of producing a significant allergic reaction in some people. Additionally, glycerin gives a burning sensation when given in shots. Few medical clinics are able to formulate their own preservative free antigens. The Environmental Health Center of Dallas is one; the Arizona Center for Advanced Medicine in Scottsdale is another; Manhattan Health Consultants in New York City is a third. Antigens for just about anything to which you are allergic can be made.

The process of making preservative free antigens is very precise and very sterile. Every substance is measured and placed in a special solution for five days to extract the allergenic material. For people who are allergic to newsprint, for example, we can grind newspaper in a blender with the special solution, and extract the printer's ink, bleaches, and other allergenic materials.

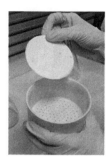 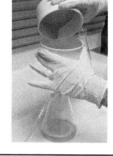 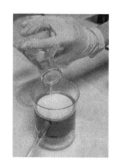

Each substance is put through 4 filters to remove particles and impurities.	Here we are working with liquefied oats. Suction pulls the liquid through each filter into a sterile beaker.	The forth and final filtration removes bacteria, and puts the concentrated solution into a sterile, one-time-use jar.

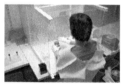 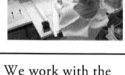 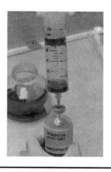 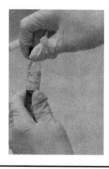

We work with the filtered concentrates in a sterile area with filtered airflow.	The concentrated mix is taken from the fourth filtration jar and put into a sterile injectable bottle.	A portion from each concentrate is set aside and double-checked regularly for any growth of contaminants.

Detailed records are made each time a concentrate is made. The finished concentrates are kept in a freezer which preserves them until they are used to make an individual diluted antigen for a patient.

Allergy treatment which gradually increases the dose of allergen over a period of time and then maintains the maximally tolerated dose for a period of 18-24 months appears to be effective in most people. Treatment can be given as allergy shots or drops which are taken sublingually (under the tongue). The sublingual route is nearly as effective as shots, and less painful for many people, especially children. The drops can be given at home, and the treatment requires only periodic follow-up visits, not weekly injections.

BOOKS

Is This Your Child? by Doris Rapp

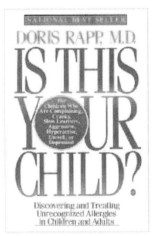

This best-selling book by Dr. Doris Rapp made her beloved by thousands of parents who were finally able to identify allergic substances that changed their child's behavior. The book tells how to pinpoint specifically the reason why some children and adults are unable to learn in certain rooms, outside the school, or at certain times after specific exposures at school, home or work. It clearly explains ways to verify your suspicions using fast, easy and relatively inexpensive as well as more expensive methods.

[1]MacDonald TT, Monteleone G. Immunity, Inflammation, and Allergy in the Gut. *Science* 307;5717:1920-25 (25 Mar, 2005)

[2]Hampe J, Cuthbert A et al. Association between insertion mutation in NOD2 gene and Crohn's disease in German and British populations. *The Lancet* 2001; 357:1925-1928.

[3]Bashir MEH, Louie S et al. Toll-Like Receptor 4 Signaling by Intestinal Microbes Influences Susceptibility to Food Allergy. *The Journal of Immunology*, 2004, 172: 6978-6987.

[4]Isolauri E, Rauteva S. Role of probiotics in food hypersensitivity. *Curr Opinion All Clin Immunol* 2(3):263-271 (June 2002).

[5]Miller CS. Toxicant-induced Loss of Tolerance – An Emerging Theory of Disease? *Env Health Perspectives* 105; suppl 2: 445-453 (Mar 1997).

[6]Carlotta De Filippo, Duccio Cavalieri, et al. Impact of diet in shaping gut microbiota revealed by a comparative study in children from Europe and rural Africa. *PNAS*, August 2, 2010, doi: 10.1073/pnas.1005963107

Asthma

Asthma is a chronic inflammatory disease of the airways and lungs. Its impact can be profound because it can interrupt sleep, limit physical activity, and disrupt family routines.

Cases of asthma are rising so fast it is now widely viewed as an epidemic. Asthma affects about 7% of the adult population, and up to 25% of children in big cities like Harlem, N.Y.[1,2] Asthma is on the rise among every age group all across the county.

Worldwide, the asthma incidence has increased by 45% since the 1970s. The increase is seen mainly in countries which are industrialized. This suggests that some factor in the lifestyle of industrialized nations is causative – although it is difficult to design ethical placebo-controlled double blind studies to prove exactly what might be the primary cause.

Quick Facts

- Asthma accounts for more hospitalizations in children than any other chronic illness.
- Asthma is the number one cause of school absenteeism
- American Lung Association finds that 130 of every 1000 students have asthma, which equates to about 3 children per classroom in the United States (2004)
- Asthma is seen in more boys than girls.
- Between 1980 and 1993, the numbers for asthma in children nearly doubled.

Signs & Symptoms

*A*sthma is a "syndrome" or disease characterized by:

- Airway obstruction
- An exaggerated narrowing of the small airways in response to irritating stimuli (called a bronchoconstrictor response)
- Inflammation of the airways resulting in production of thick sticky mucus which is difficult to cough out
- Recurring attacks, with wheezing or cough caused by factors which do not affect most of the population

Asthma's symptoms may range from mild shortness of breath to life-threatening airway obstruction. Most commonly, people wheeze when they exhale and experience an increased rate of respiration. Sometimes the wheezing can actually be heard by another person as a whistling sound when the asthmatic breathes out. Sometimes people have ronchi, rattling sounds caused by mucus in the larger airways.

Occasionally asthma sounds like a cough that just won't stop – no wheezing. If the asthmatic attack is extremely bad, you sometimes do not hear wheezing because the air flow is so low.

Patients are generally anxious during an acute asthma attack. The anxiety subsides as the attack diminishes. If wheezing diminishes but anxiety increases, this indicates worsening of an asthma attack, and strongly suggests need for immediate medical care.

What Type of Asthma Do You Have?

- Aspirin-induced asthma: Some people are extremely sensitive to aspirin and other salicylates, even those contained naturally in fruits and vegetables. These people may even wheeze when they take other Cox-2 inhibitors like ibuprofen.

- Childhood asthma: Generally brought on by food allergy, sometimes by infection. Twin studies show that about 60% of identical twins both have asthma. This suggests that there is a genetic susceptibility, but that there must also be some other environmental exposure which triggers the disease.
- Adult-onset asthma: May be associated with a recurrence of childhood asthma. Adults may also develop asthma without any prior symptoms in childhood. Frequently they have food or environmental chemical allergies which can be diagnosed and treated.
- Allergy-induced asthma: Allergies may express themselves in the nose as "allergic rhinitis" (chronically runny stuffy nose), or "allergic sinusitis" (chronic plugging of the sinuses associated with pain in the face and around the eyes). Allergies may present as itchy red eyes ("allergic conjunctivitis") or skin rash ("atopic dermatitis" or "eczema"). Allergies may also present with wheezing and airway obstruction, and now they are called "asthma".

The well-known *Cecil Textbook of Medicine* states that asthma is a "clinical syndrome of unknown etiology," meaning that conventional Western medicine does not know what causes asthma.[3] Approximately 60% of asthmatics have asthmatic parents, meaning that asthma has both genetic and environmental causes. There may be a predisposition, but there also needs to be some environmental insult to trigger the asthma.

Asthma is seen in association with allergies to foods or chemicals, pollens and molds, and cigarette smoke. It is seen in people who have allergies to chemicals in their workplace environments, particularly to molds or to formaldehyde and other volatile organic compounds (VOCs) used in new carpets and glues.

Smoke and environmental chemicals create free radicals. Research suggests asthma is caused in part by increased levels of free radicals. Vitamin E inhibits IgE responses to allergic stimuli in animals. "These findings may explain the beneficial effect of dietary vitamin E on the incidence of asthma," researchers wrote in *The Lancet*.[4]

Asthma is seen more frequently in households of smokers, and is found especially in children and grandchildren of smokers, if the smoking continued during pregnancy.[5]

Studies have linked asthma and allergies with the consumption of pasteurized milk. "Fewer and fewer people can tolerate commercial milk," states Sally Fallon Morell of the Weston A. Price Foundation. "Pasteurization distorts the delicate protein compounds in milk. The body recognizes these warped components as foreign and mounts an energy-sapping immune response." Many people who are allergic to pasteurized/homogenized milk are not allergic to raw milk.

Asthma may also develop after severe respiratory infection – those people whose colds always go to their chests. Infants infected with certain respiratory viruses (RSV, for example) develop wheezing and symptoms suggestive of asthma which may persist long after the respiratory infection has cleared. Foods, chemicals, pollens, molds, fungi, and certain viruses are well-known to cause wheezing, and may induce chronic asthma in susceptible patients.

Asthma can also be triggered by emotional upset, or by grief. The lungs, in Chinese medicine, are affected by grief. When the grief is dealt with, often the lung problem is improved.

Why does asthma hit children so hard? The National Academy of Sciences has found that, in general, children are more vulnerable than adults to toxic chemicals in the environment.[6] Pound for pound, children eat more food and drink more water and juices than adults, and thus they take in more pesticides and toxic chemicals relative to body weight. Children also have a more rapid respiratory rate and take in a greater volume of air per unit of body weight than adults. At the same time, children's organ systems are still developing and therefore are more vulnerable and less able to detoxify hazardous chemicals. According to researchers at the Mount Sinai School of Medicine in New York City, children's developing organs create "early windows of great vulnerability" during which exposure to toxins can cause great damage.[7] Exposure to chemical irritants can have significant effects on respiratory development.

Tests & Diagnosis Methods

*P*ulmonary function tests will show decreased maximal expiratory air flow (PEFR, peak expiratory flow rate), increased lung volume, decreased forced expiratory volume (FEV1, how much air can be exhaled in one second). Even after an attack has subsided, we may see continued changes in how rapidly a breath of air can be exhaled from the lungs (called MMEFR, maximal mid-expiratory flow rate). People with chronic asthma may not recover completely between attacks.

Nitric oxide is increased in exhaled air of asthmatics.

Arterial blood gases will show decreased oxygen, and may show decreased carbon dioxide if the attack is mild, and the person is simply working hard for their oxygen. When we see increased carbon dioxide, we know that the attack is very severe. As the person worsens, the oxygen decreases and the carbon dioxide increases.

Chest X-ray may be normal, if the person is healthy and the attack is not too severe. It may also show increased lung volume with flattened diaphragms, if the attack is severe. In that case, there may be significant air trapping behind swollen air passages – kind of like a one-way ball valve.

Routine blood work may show a high concentration of eosinophils, cells which are associated with allergic reactions. We may see high levels of IgE, an immunoglobulin directed against substances to which a patient is allergic.

Sputum coughed out from the lungs may be clear, or green, or yellow. Often we see long thin tubules of sputum, called "casts." This is debris from the lungs molded into the shape of the tubular air passages.

Treatment Options

Conventional Western medicine treats asthma with pharmaceutical medication and/or standard immunotherapy.

Time-tested alternative treatments are seldom mentioned in the allopathic literature:

- **Immunotherapy** – testing with preservative-free antigens in multiple dilutions to determine reactivity and then treating with progressively increasing strengths of antigen to help the body develop a tolerance to the substance.
- **Acupuncture** – tiny needles inserted into specific places on the body to change the flow of energy within the channel where the needle is placed. Specific locations will stop an acute asthma attack within a few minutes. Other locations are geared more at restoring proper lung function for the long term.
- **Intravenous magnesium** – because magnesium is a vasodilator and muscle relaxant, it can help to restore blood supply to muscles surrounding the bronchioles, or tiny air passages, and allow those muscles to relax and recover their proper function, thus relieving wheezing.[8]
- **Chelation** – to clear out heavy metals known to trigger chronic inflammation that can manifest in many ways.
- **Colonics** – to clean out the colon, reducing the inflammation in the intestinal tract and thereby reducing the level of inflammation throughout the body. Abnormal bacteria in the intestinal tract – frequently seen in children with multiple ear infections and multiple courses of antibiotics – is another cause of a chronic inflammatory state.

- **Anti-inflammatory diet** – to decrease the inflammatory levels of everyone in the household.
- **Homeopathic remedies** – certain remedies are specific to relieve wheezing. Different remedies are chosen, depending on whether the wheezing is accompanied by fever, yellow sputum, left-sided or right-sided chest pain, etc. Viruses like the Respiratory Syncitial Virus (RSV) can cause a chronic hyper-reactive state of the small airways of the lungs. These viruses may leave a signature in the body which can predispose the victim to react to any similar virus with similar symptoms. These signatures can be treated bioenergetically, using homeopathic remedies or other methods of manipulating the body's information systems, to allow healing of the respiratory system.

Sometimes, energetic blockages are the reason we have trouble breathing. We'll share a memorable case study with you:

CASE STUDY

A 23-year-old man often visited a house where there are 11 cats. He wheezed every time he walked in to that house. Acupuncture on his ears successfully relieved the symptoms. But he wanted to use hypnosis to get at the root cause so his symptoms would go away completely. The hypnosis session revealed a surprising energetic block. He saw himself as a young boy on his first zebra hunt in Africa. He'd become separated from his uncle, and was eaten by a lion. At this point in the session, he started to shake. Later in the session, he went back to the scene, but this time he saw himself looking down on events from above. He saw his uncle searching for him. He realized the awful part of it was not being eaten by the lion, but that his tribe would think he had run away and wasn't brave. In the hypnosis session, he saw his uncle look up at him and he was able to tell the uncle that he hadn't run away. Then the man walked along a path to see if there

101

were any obstructions [blockages to healing]. The man found the lion blocking his path. He jumped over the lion and the path was clear. Hypnosis session finished, now for the proof of the pudding... The young man came back to the house with cats many times after that and never had to use his inhaler again.

RESOURCES

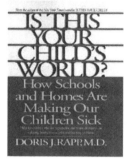

Is this Your Child's World? by Doris Rapp

[1] Asthma's Impact on Children and Adolescents, accessed 10/18/08 from http://www.cdc.gov/asthma/children.htm

[2] Richard Perez-Peña, Study Finds Asthma In 25% of Children In Central Harlem, Published in the *New York Times*, April 19, 2003.

[3] *Cecil Textbook of Medicine*, 23rd edition, pp 612-619. Accessed online through Merck Medicus at www.merckmedicus.com.

[4] Fogarty, Andrew MRCP, Dietary vitamin E, IgE concentrations, and atopy, *The Lancet* 2000; 356:1573-1574

[5] Li YF, Langholz B et al. Maternal and grandmaternal smoking patterns are associated with early childhood asthma. *Chest.* 2005 Apr;127(4):1232-41.

[6] National Research Council, National Academy of Sciences. 1993. Pesticides in the Diets of Infants and Children, Washington, DC: *National Academy Press*, 184-185.

[7] Landrigan, PJ, L Claudio, SB Markowitz, et al. 1999. Pesticides and inner-city children: exposures, risks, and prevention. *Environmental Health Perspectives* 107 (Suppl 3): 431-437.

[8] Rowe BH, Edmonds ML, et al. Evidence-based treatments for acute asthma. *Respir Care.* 2001 Dec;46(12):1380-90; discussion 1390-1.

Attention Deficit Disorder

The American Psychiatric Association gave official recognition to attention deficit disorder (ADD) in 1980. The drug Ritalin® became a household word. In 1997 with the epidemic standing somewhere around 500,000 to 700,000 nationwide, the American Psychiatric Association rewrote the diagnostic criteria by adding the term "hyperactivity" to the attention deficit attention deficit disorder. ADD became ADHD.[1] Mostly.

ADD differs from ADHD because there is an absence of hyperactivity. These children are withdrawn, they display what some might describe as the "lights on, but nobody home" type behavior. Usually, people say ADHD when talking about attention deficit disorders.

Three types of ADHD are diagnosed:[2]

- 80% = combined inattentive, hyperactive, and impulsive
- 10%-15% = predominantly inattentive
- 5% = predominantly hyperactive and impulsive

It is estimated that 7%[3] of children aged 4 to 17 are affected with ADHD. The Center for Disease Control estimated in 2004 that there were 4 million cases nationwide in children 17 and under. That is about 1 out of every 10 children in public schools.[4]

There is no physiological process of degeneration or disease that characterizes the disorder. The diagnosis of ADHD is most often made after a doctor or psychiatrist observes behavior and deems the patient has ADHD.

ADHD is characterized by the "inability to marshal and sustain attention, modulate activity level, and moderate impulsive actions."[5] This results in behavior which is markedly inappropriate to the child's age, and often gets them in serious trouble in school. These children are typically impulsive, often aggressive. They cannot seem to control their level of activity, and they spend three times as long as other children doing their homework. Even at that, they usually require the presence of a parent or other caregiver to enable them to finish their homework at all.

The diagnosis and treatment of ADHD has generated controversy. The DSM-IV (the American Psychiatric Association's Diagnostic and Statistical Manual of Mental Disorders), lists 14 symptoms; the diagnosis of ADHD can be made if a child is found to have eight of them:

1. often fidgets or squirms
2. has trouble staying in one's seat
3. is easily distracted
4. cannot wait one's turn
5. blurts out answers
6. has trouble following instructions
7. cannot sustain attention
8. shifts from one activity to another
9. does not play quietly
10. talks excessively
11. interrupts
12. cannot listen
13. loses things
14. does dangerous things

If you're thinking that sounds like you as a child and some adults you know today, you're not alone.

Stimulant Drugs

Drug therapy is the most common form of allopathic medical treatment for ADHD. Ritalin®, Concerta®, and Adderall® are popularly prescribed drugs. There is little doubt that stimulants help to control behavior in many cases. There is much doubt whether they improve scholastic performance.[6] And concerns about the drugs' side effects keep mounting.

Prescription drugs for ADHD are almost all stimulants and come with "black box" warnings, meaning they carry significant risk of serious or even life-threatening adverse effects. These drugs have been linked to cardio-vascular problems, sudden death, and violence. The more common side effects can be so devastating or unpleasant that many kids just don't want to take them.

Long term, drug therapy may turn out to have been a very costly short term fix.

There is evidence that the use of stimulants increases the risk of substance abuse in later life by over 50%.[7] There is substantial evidence that stimulant drugs increase the risk of hypertension, stroke and cardiovascular disease.[8] Many parents, and even some researchers, are questioning whether the use of stimulant drugs is warranted, given that other therapies are more effective in the long run.[9]

In April 2009, *USA Today* editorialized that we need more education, less drugs.[10] The paper reported that according to the government's leading, multiyear study of 579 children,[11] the effectiveness of the popular drugs for ADHD can dissipate after 14 months of use. By the six-and eight-year mark, across 30 measures of behavior and academics, children still given medication fared no better than their non-medicated counterparts, despite a 41% increase in the average total daily dose, failing to support continued medication treatment as salutary. The drugs can stunt growth. After three years, medicated children have grown almost an inch less than non-medicated ADHD kids. They also suffer from more muscle tics. The editors wrote:

> Response to what the study itself calls its "failure to find better outcomes associated with continued medication treatment" has been troubling. Psychiatrists who've publicly favored drug over non-drug therapy have downplayed the findings. And the website of Children and Adults with Attention Deficit/Hyperactivity Disorder, a leading ADHD advocacy and support group, buried mention of the study in a blog without noting any findings. Perhaps not coincidentally, 30% of CHADD's revenue is from drug companies. Such denial risks real harm. It's time for those with ADHD

children in their care to recalibrate their enthusiasm for long-term use of the drugs and to engage in some behavioral modification of their own.

School officials are prohibited from implying that medication is a requirement for school attendance but teachers, more than parents or doctors, refer children for an ADHD diagnosis. Drugs are the usual consequence. Yet most teachers surveyed are ignorant about many of the drugs' basic aspects, says a University of Wisconsin-Eau Claire study.[12]

California neurologist Dr. Fred Baughman, author of *The ADHD Fraud, How Psychiatry Makes "Patients" Out of Normal Children*, spearheads the arguments against the exploding ADHD diagnosis and increased drug treatment:

> The single, biggest heath care fraud in US history – the representation of attention deficit hyperactivity disorder (ADHD) to be an actual disease, and the drugging of millions of entirely normal American children, as "treatment," is spreading like a plague – still. Once children are labeled with ADHD, they are no longer treated as normal. Once methylphenidate hydrochloride, or any psychiatric drug, courses through their brain and body, they are, for the first time, physically, neurologically, and biologically abnormal.[13]

Some psychiatrists, including Peter Breggin, worry about the drug therapies too:

> ...we abuse our children with drugs rather than making the effort to find better ways to meet their needs. In the end, we are giving out children a very bad lesson – that drugs are the answer to emotional problems. We are encouraging a generation of youngsters to grow up relying on psychiatric drugs rather than on themselves and other human resources.[14]

Were Mark Twain writing *Huckleberry Finn* today, instead of reading about a couple of rambunctious and adventurous boys, we could be reading that Huck was told to take a pill, shut up, and sit still in class.

We need only look around us at the children today to see that something is clearly amiss.

The U.S. government admits that one in six children is born today with some kind of brain impairment.[15] By age three, an increasing number of children exhibit autism and other forms of toxicity-related illness such as asthma, diabetes, ADD, and depression.

Getting to the Root Cause

Root causes of the ADHD syndrome may be multiple, including brain processing abnormalities, problems with the entire listening/hearing system, food or environmental allergies, metabolic insufficiencies, or heavy metal toxicity, among other things.

Researchers at the University of California-Davis Center for Mind and Brain and M.I.N.D. Institute found that two brain areas fail to connect when children with attention deficit hyperactivity disorder attempt a task that measures attention.[16] The researchers measured electrical rhythms from the brains of volunteers. When part of the brain is emitting alpha rhythms, it is disengaged from the rest of the brain and not receiving or processing information optimally. "This is the first time that we have direct evidence that this connectivity is missing in ADHD," said researcher Ali Mazaheri in 2010.[17]

According to current models of how the brain allocates attention, signals from the frontal cortex should alert other parts of the brain, such as the visual processing area at the back of the head, to prepare to pay attention to something. That should be reflected in a drop in alpha wave activity in the visual area. However, children with ADHD showed no such drop in activity, indicating a disconnection between the center of the brain that allocates attention and the visual processing regions. "The brains of the children with ADHD apparently prepare to attend to upcoming stimuli differently than do typically developing children," Mazaheri concluded.

We know many cases of ADHD behavior have been cleared up by making a few extremely important changes in diet. Removing sugar has stopped some children from "bouncing off the walls." Removing specific foods to which they are sensitive has been the answer for others. Harvard and Columbia researchers stated that artificial food colorings are one reason for the surge in children's hyperactivity and attention problems. They asked, "Do children's foods really need to be colored with petroleum-based dyes like Red 40 and Yellow 5 when there are plenty of natural dyes available? Are food manufacturer's profits worth the tradeoff in our children's health?"[18]

In 2008, the American Academy of Pediatrics said the 2007 Southampton/McCann Study finally convinced them to reverse their long-standing position on food additives:[19]

> Thus, the overall findings of the study are clear and require that even we skeptics, who have long doubted parental claims of the effects of various foods on the behavior of their children, admit we might have been wrong.
>
> In real life, practitioners faced with hyperactive preschoolers have a reasonable option to offer parents. For the child without a medical, emotional, or environmental etiology of ADHD behaviors, a trial of a preservative-free, food coloring–free diet is a reasonable intervention.

Sometimes fish oils correct a fatty acid deficiency and restore normalcy. A 2005 Oxford study of 117 underachieving children found 40% of them made dramatic improvements in reading and spelling when given fish oil supplements high in omega-3 fatty acids.[20]

Australian researchers tracked a group of 1,799 children from their birth in 1989.[21] As young teens, some consumed relatively high amounts of fresh fruit and vegetables, whole grains, and fish. This diet pattern delivered more omega-3 fatty acids, folate (a B vitamin involved in brain health), and fiber. Others consumed a typical "Western" diet pattern – takeout foods, sweets, pastries, and processed, fried, or refined foods. This diet pattern delivered less omega-3s but more total fat, saturated fat, omega-6 fats, refined sugar, and sodium.

Out of the total of 1,799 teens, 91 boys and 24 girls had been diagnosed with ADHD by age 14. After adjusting the results to account for various known social and family influences on ADHD risk, the Aussie team found that the kids who ate the "Western" diet were more than twice as likely to have received an ADHD diagnosis. Omega-3 fatty acids are thought to hold benefits for mental health and optimal brain function.

So in some cases, ADHD can be vanquished by eating foods that build strong minds and learning how to eliminate those foods to which a child is allergic. That's the power of the refrigerator.

The Chicken or the Egg?

It's not always clear which came first – the processing problem or the metabolic insufficiency. For example: Children raised on commercial baby formulas (some are 50 percent corn syrup), likely have been metabolically challenged since their very beginning. They may have lost brain function because they took in more manganese than what is in breast milk. Manganese occurs at very low levels in breast milk, but it is added to infant formula made from cow's milk and occurs naturally at even higher levels in soy formula. It is dangerous for infants to consume more manganese than they would get from breast milk because infants have no capacity to excrete excess amounts until they are older. The effects of too much manganese include inattention, impulsivity, and hyperaggression.[22]

Soy baby formulas do not contain nearly as much protein as breast milk, depriving the developing brain of what it needs.

Researchers at Brown Medical School compared premature infants fed with breast milk to those fed formula and found breast fed babies clearly did better on tests of mental development by age 18 months. The more breast milk they consumed, the better they did on the tests. Ingredients in breast milk, particularly fatty acids, seem to help the brain develop properly. Additionally, breast milk builds a strong immune system.[23]

Some children are impacted by a high body burden of heavy metals, interfering with the normal developmental processes. Take lead, for example: children with higher exposures to lead are more easily distracted, less organized, and apt to be hyperactive, impulsive, aggressive, and easily frustrated. Sound familiar?

Governmental research reports the average American baby, at birth, has more than 200 chemicals in its body.[24] Even after nine months of growth in the womb, the infant's nervous, respiratory, reproductive, and immune systems are not yet fully developed. They are in a dynamic state of growth with cells multiplying and organ systems developing at a rapid rate. Pound for pound, children take in more air, food, and liquids than do adults. For example, carpets are typically made with toxic materials; children tend to make direct contact with carpet with their faces and hands as they play.

Neurotoxin experts Philippe Grandjean and Philip Landrigan reported in 2006 that the widespread use of pesticides, cleaning products, glues and other chemicals that contaminate our air, water, and homes are causing a "silent pandemic" of brain diseases in children. When children reach their "toxic overload" point, out-of-control behaviors can be the result. Medical schools do not train physicians in detoxification procedures, nor does medical school curriculum yet embrace the mounting evidence that environmental toxins cause breakdowns in body systems that cannot be corrected simply by adding a prescription drug – yet another toxic substance.

The Cincinnati Children's Hospital Medical Center study is the first to examine how genes, toxins and gender interact to shape ADHD. "Our analysis confirms a suspected link between prenatal tobacco exposure and ADHD, and it demonstrates that the greater the level of blood lead, the greater the risk of ADHD, says Bruce Lanphear, M.D., director of the Children's Environmental Health Center at Cincinnati Children's and corresponding author of the study. "These findings underscore the profound behavioral health impact of these prevalent exposures and highlight the need to strengthen public health efforts to reduce prenatal tobacco smoke exposure and childhood lead exposure." Investigators found approximately 270,000 cases of ADHD attributable to mothers smoking during pregnancy. Children exposed to tobacco before birth had a 2.5-fold higher risk of ADHD compared to children not so exposed to tobacco. The study is based on data gathered between 1999 and 2002 from a parent or guardian of 4,704 children.[25]

Food sensitivities and heavy metals create inflammation in the GI tract. If we have an inflamed gut, we are not able to efficiently process and absorb the nutrients in the food we eat. As some wise person once said: we are not what we eat, we are what we absorb.

It is important to have a strong body biochemistry and metabolism,[26] so that the brain processing can be corrected, and will hold fast even under stress.

Lyme Disease and ADHD

There is growing evidence that some children with ADHD symptoms actually have Lyme disease. Lyme's effect on the brain can appear as increasing anxiety, irritability, chronic depression, cognitive decline and memory loss, and much stronger ADHD tendencies.

Lyme Disease, like the similar disease syphilis, is called "The Great Imitator" since it can affect the entire body in a myriad of ways. It is often misdiagnosed as ADD, ADHD, rheumatoid arthritis, autism, depression, chronic fatigue, multiple sclerosis, and more. The co-infection Bartonella henselae has been associated with neuropsychiatric disease.

Most experts agree that the incidence of pediatric neurological dysfunctions, including autism and ADHD, has increased at least four to five times in the last decade. The vast majority of promising evidence connects many of these dysfunctions to the emerging inter-relationship of the neurological and immune systems.

Non-drug Approach

Comprehensive and holistic treatment for ADD and ADHD includes looking at brain processing, food sensitivities, environmental allergies, heavy metal and other toxicities, metabolism, and function of the intestinal (GI) tract, so we can determine the origin of the problems.

It is well known that people with ADHD,[27] depression,[28] head injury, and other forms of brain dysfunction[29] often have a slowing of the activity in the frontal lobes – that area of the brain in charge of executive function: planning ahead, decision-making, judgment, language, and other important cognitive functions. Sometimes an ADHD individual has been robbed of the ability to hear and process specific frequencies, because of chronic ear infections, severe allergies or lots of very loud concerts. The ear becomes unresponsive and must be stimulated, in order to be able to tune into the desired sound. Attention, focus, learning, and language abilities can all be improved by retraining the brain to listen[30,31] using different frequencies of sounds, so that whatever is available is working at maximum capacity. This kind of brain dysfunction can be treated without drugs.

Hemoencephalography (HEG) uses light to measure activity in the frontal lobes by measuring the oxygenation in the blood. Oxygenation of blood flowing to the frontal lobes can be increased through a computer-assisted biofeedback mechanism. This can improve all the functions dependent upon frontal lobe activity, bringing order from chaos in the brain of a child – or an adult – with ADHD.

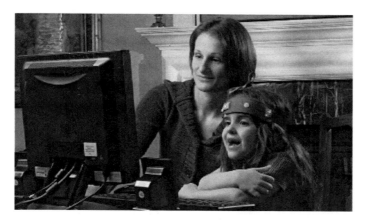

HEG neurofeedback is a technique using near infrared light to measure brain blood oxygen levels, and the information is used as feedback to the client. Users don a simple headband with no electrodes or gooey gel. Can be combined with audio/visual entrainment, sound therapy, neuromotor skills training, and cognitive training. © *BrainAdvantage, LLC 2009 Used by permission*

As oxygenation increases, neurons are able to make new connections. HEG is combined with exercises for auditory processing and vestibular function, cognitive development, and brainwave entrainment in a successful program called BrainAdvantage™. It is a unique program that encourages neural connections all over the brain and brainstem. It can be extremely effective in only 20 sessions. The program helps the brain re-establish broken pathways and make new ones. We've seen people whose brains could hardly function well enough to read a newspaper work through the various exercises and "get their brain back." The person who was trapped inside is able to come out.

The pieces of the puzzle necessitate a focus on nutrition. In some people, ADHD symptoms can be reversed by eliminating sugar, wheat, corn, and chemical additives from their diets. Parasitic infections are common with ADHD and good homeopathic remedies can correct the problem. Sleep deprivation is another piece of the puzzle that can be addressed through both behavioral and nutritional means, sometimes with specific supplements.

Some children have turned around just by removing specific foods to which they are sensitive and adding omega-3 fish oils to correct a fatty acid deficiency. Others get a big boost with chelation to remove metals which are silently warehoused in brain and bones and gum up the works.

By treating the origins of the dysfunction, and determining if Lyme disease is also a factor, we can avoid the need for dangerous stimulant medication. But most importantly, parents can restore their child's health naturally and bring forth the person who got lost when the body's functions got confused.

RESOURCES

BrainAdvantage (www.BrainAdvantage.com) – bringing more oxygen to the brain and developing new connections. This non-drug approach re-trains the brain to improve memory and focus, and to lessen ADHD, depression, and other disorders.

BOOKS

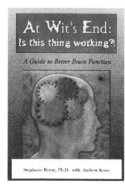

At Wit's End: Is this thing working?!

Stephanie Reese, Ph.D. with Andrew Reese

"*At Wit's End* is a scientific, yet easy to read, book that is essential reading for parents and practitioners alike. Dr Reese provides an authoritative look into how the brain and body work together and how that symbiotic relationship can be a recipe for health and happiness."–Randy D. Danielsen, Ph.D., PA-C Dean and Professor emeritus, Arizona School of Health Sciences, A.T. Still University, Mesa, Arizona

---

[1] Fred A. Baughman Jr., MD. *The ADHD Fraud, How Psychiatry Makes "Patients" Out of Normal Children* by Trafford Publishing, 2006

[2] Rappley, MD. Attention Deficit Hyperactivity Disorder. *N Engl J Med* 2005;352:165-73.

[3] http://www.cdc.gov/nchs/data/series/sr_10/sr10_231.pdf

[4] Mike Adams interview, "Neurologist Dr. Fred Baughman talks about the fraud of ADHD and the poisoning of U.S. children," August 2006, http://www.naturalnews.com/020227.html

[5] Rappley MD. Attention Deficit-Hyperactivity Disorder. *NEJM* 2005;352:165-73.

[6] Purdie, N., Hattie, J. and Carroll, A. (2002) 'A Review of the Research on Interventions for Attention-Deficit Hyperactivity Disorder: What Works Best?', Review of Educational Research 72(1): 61–99.

[7] Sales, A. (2000) 'Substance Abuse and Disability', Substance Abuse and Counseling. A Perspective. ERIC document reproduction service, no. 440352. Also Lambert N, Hartsough CS. Prospective study of tobacco smoking and substance dependence among samples of ADHD and non-ADHD subjects. *J Learn. Disabil.* 1998;31:533-544

[8] Nissen SE. ADHD drugs and cardiovascular risk. *NEJM* 354;14 (April 6, 2006).

[9] Doggett AM. ADHD and drug therapy: is it still a valid treatment? J *Child Health Care* 8;1:69-81.

[10] Ben O'Brien. *USA Today*. "Our view on helping hyperactive kids: New findings raise questions about use of ADHD drugs." Accessed April 13, 2009 at http://blogs.usatoday.com/oped/2009/04/our-view-on-helping-hyperactive-kids-new-findings-raise-que stions-about-use-of-adhd-drugs.html

[11] Molina B, Hinshaw S et al. MTA at 8 Years: Prospective Follow-up of Children Treated for Combined-Type ADHD in a Multisite Study. *Journal of Amer Academy of Child & Adolescent Psychiatry*: doi: 10.1097/CHI.0b013e31819c23d0 POST AUTHOR CORRECTIONS, 23 March 2009

[12] Snider VE, Busch, T. et al (2003). Teacher Knowledge of Stimulant Medication and ADHD. *Remedial and Special Education*, 24(1), 46-56

[13] Fred A. Baughman Jr. Presentation to the Parliamentary Assembly, Council of Europe, November 23, 2001, http://www.adhdfraud.com/frameit.asp?src=commentary.htm

[14] Breggin PR. Psychostimulants in treatment of children diagnosed with ADHD: Risks and mechanism of action, *International Journal of Risk and Safety in Medicine*,1999;12

[15] Canfield RL, et al. Intellectual impairment in children with blood lead concentrations below 10 mcg/dl, *New England Journal of Medicine*, 348:1517-26, 2003

[16] Ali Mazaheri, Ingrid L.C. Nieuwenhuis, Hanneke van Dijk, Ole Jensen. Prestimulus alpha and mu activity predicts failure to inhibit motor responses. *Human Brain Mapping*, 2009

[17] Press Release: Disconnect Between Brain Regions in ADHD. University of California-Davis. January 11, 2010

[18] Do artificial food colorings promote hyperactivity in children with hyperactive syndromes? A meta-analysis of double-blind, placebo-controlled trials, D.W. Schab et al., *Journal of Developmental and Behavioral Pediatrics* 25(6):423-434, December 2004

[19] ADHD and Food Additives Revisited. AAP Grand Rounds 2008;19;17. Accessed February 2008 at http://www.feingold.org/Research/PDFstudies/AAP08.pdf

[20] A.J. Richardson, P. Montgomery. The Oxford-Durham study: a randomized, control trial of dietary supplements with fatty acids in children with developmental; coordination disorder. *Pediatrics* 115(5):1360-6, May 2005

[21] Al Howard, M Robinson. ADHD Is Associated With a 'Western' Dietary Pattern in Adolescents. *J Atten Disord.* 2010 Jul 14. Also see http://www.ichr.uwa.edu.au/media/1185

[22] Former U.S. Public Health Service director Philip R. Lee, keynote speech February 2003 to the National Institute of Environmental Health Sciences

[23] Betty R. Vohr, et al. Beneficial Effects of Breast Milk in the Neonatal Intensive Care Unit on the Developmental Outcome of Extremely Low Birth Weight Infants at 18 Months of Age, *Pediatrics*, Jul 2006; 118: e115 - e123.
Also, Carla K. Johnson. Infants' brains developed better with breast milk, *The Boston Globe*, July 10, 2006

[24] Landrigan PJ, Sonawane B, Drollaer D. Early environmental origins of neurodegenerative disease in later life, *Environmental Health Perspectives*, 113;9:1230-33, 2005

[25] Cincinnati Children's Hospital Medical Center, news release of October 5, 2006: "Tobacco Smoke and Lead Exposure Linked to One-third of ADHD Cases." Full study published in *Environmental Health Perspectives*, September 19, 2006. Braun JM, Kahn RS et al. Exposures to Environmental Toxicants and Attention Deficit Hyperactivity Disorder in U.S. Children. *EHP* 114;12:Dec 2006.

[26] Ferguson SA, Berry KJ. Behavioral effects of prenatal folate deficiency in mice. *Birth Defects Res A Clin Mol Teratol.* 2005 pr;73(4):249-52.

[27] Castellanos FX, Lee PP, Sharp W, et al: Developmental trajectories of brain volume abnormalities in children and adolescents with attention deficit/ hyperactivity disorder. *JAMA* 2002;288:1740-1748.

[28] Dotson VM, Davatzikos C et al. Depressive symptoms and brain volumes in older adults: a longitudinal magnetic resonance imaging study. *J Psychiatry Neurosci.* 2009 Sep;34(5):367-75.

[29] Marcoux J, McArthur DA et al. Persistent metabolic crisis as measured by elevated cerebral microdialysis lactate-pyruvate ratio predicts chronic frontal lobe brain atrophy after traumatic brain injury. *Crit Care Med.* 2008 Oct;36(10):2871-7.

[30] Okamoto H, Stracke H et al. Frequency-specific modulation of population-level frequency tuning in human auditory cortex. *BMC Neurosci.* 2009 Jan 6;10:1.

[31] Leaver AM, Van Lare J et al. Brain activation during anticipation of sound sequences. *J Neurosci.* 2009 Feb 25;29(8):2477-85.

Autism

Autism is a complex syndrome based on physiological and biochemical disorders that have as a common endpoint the cognitive and emotional impairment we associate with autism.

—Jaquelyn McCandless, *Children with Starving Brains*

$\mathcal{A}$utism is a biomedical illness caused by an unfortunate combination of genetic susceptibility and exposure to more toxins than the system can handle, either before or after birth. The result is dysfunctional neural processing and significant social deficits.

Autism spectrum disorders, including Asperger's syndrome and pervasive developmental delay, are complicated illnesses. They are all characterized by delayed development in some aspect of our human existence. Autism and Asperger's syndrome characteristically involve repetitive behaviors that impair interpersonal relationships.

The incidence of autism-spectrum disorders has skyrocketed since the early 1980s, when large numbers of thimerosal-preserved vaccines came into common use, and when multiple vaccinations were given to children at about 15 months of age. That timing sparked a raging controversy, pitting parents against physicians against vaccine manufacturers against the government arguing whether the damage done to a generation of children should be blamed on mercury's use as a preservative.[1, 2]

That controversy still persists, but in 1999 it was agreed that thimerosal preservative should be removed from most vaccines. The vaccines continued to be sold until the thimerosal-containing stores were used. Finally by 2002 most vaccines no longer contained mercury.

In October 2009, two government studies raised the estimates of childhood autism from 1 in 150 to 1 in 91. In December 2009, the CDC officially pegged it at 1 in 110. Boys are four times more likely than girls to be diagnosed. Why? Studies suggest testosterone has an affinity for mercury. Research has shown that testosterone significantly potentiates mercury toxicity, whereas estrogen is protective.[3]

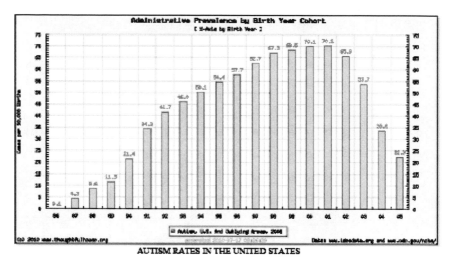

AUTISM RATES IN THE UNITED STATES

Used with permission of ThoughtfulHouse.org

If not always vaccines, what else?

Some children who are autistic have not been vaccinated. And autism existed well before the 1980s when the vaccination schedule increased, and the amount of mercury delivered skyrocketed.

Many factors can influence the development of an autistic child, including:

- intra-uterine or pre-natal maternal dietary deficiencies
- immunizations – too many, too soon
- infections
- deficiencies in the intestinal tract and immune system
- food or chemical allergies
- heavy metal and other toxicities

There does not seem to be one single factor which causes autism.

It has been proposed, but not proven, that if the mother has an infection, this can trigger either an inflammatory response in the fetus, or the development of antibodies to neural tissues, resulting in an autoimmune response in the fetal brain and body.

Amalgam fillings are the largest source of mercury in the body. There is considerable controversy about amalgam (or "silver") fillings as well – they are about 50% mercury – but there seems to be no doubt that mercury levels in the body are directly correlated with the number of amalgam fillings.[4] A mother with amalgam fillings will download mercury to her child both while the child is still in the womb, and also while breastfeeding. In 2008, Norway banned the used of mercury fillings; Germany, Sweden, and Denmark severely restrict the use of them. Were the American Dental Association to reverse its position that amalgams are safe, the potential liability claims could be spectacular.

Many parents like to remodel the house to accommodate a new baby. However, the process often introduces toxins in the environment. Carpet fibers and glues, for example, could be made with any of the 80,000 synthetic chemicals developed and released into the environment since World War II. Particle board furniture off-gasses formaldehyde. Paint releases VOCs for up to a year. Phthalates – a chemical added to soften plastic – are still used in children's chew toys. Children's bodies are ill-equipped to handle such a firestorm of exposure. Childhood is a period of critical organ development and fast growth. The brain growth spurt lasts all the way through age two, and once disruption occurs in the nervous system, it cannot be easily be repaired. A child's natural defense mechanisms are not yet fully developed, especially during the first few months, and they are less able to break down certain toxins and excrete them. And some children simply have better genes than others when it comes to detoxing chemicals.

Much corn now is a genetically modified food, and corn products are found in everything from baby formula to talcum powder. In the late 1930s, scientists were able to splice pesticides and antibiotic resistant bacteria into the DNA of crops. Convenient for the farmer perhaps, but what happens when that pesticide or unnatural bacterium inhabits an infant's gut? Most autistic children have intestinal malfunction, so we know something is damaging their guts. High fructose corn syrup, ubiquitous in processed food, is often manufactured in a way that actually allows mercury residues to remain in the final product.[5]

Although 95 percent of our genes are identical, critical variations take place in that remaining 5 percent that differentiates one person from another. Glutathione is a protein that is produced by the body for the purpose of detoxification of foreign compounds. Levels are low in many autistic children, either because they are less able to produce the protein, or because they have used up their stores in the process of getting rid of toxins to which they have been exposed. Both may well be a factor – we know that autistic children are generally unable to excrete toxins as well as other non-autistic children.

Unfortunately many vaccines contain an aluminum adjuvant which is neurotoxic, although less so than mercury. Neil Z. Miller of the Thinktwice Global Vaccine Institute points out that the number of vaccines with aluminum has increased:

> The hepatitis B vaccine given at birth contains 250 mcg of aluminum – 20 times higher than safety levels ... Babies who have followed the CDC immunization schedule are injected with nearly 5000 mcg (5 mg) of aluminum by 18 months of age.[6]

You will also find that MSG, another neurotoxin, is a component of some vaccines. The flu vaccine continues to be preserved with mercury, and is recommended by official governmental policy most strongly for the very young and the very old, precisely those least able to deal with the extra toxic load.

Some biological dentists will say that no child should be vaccinated until all the "adult" teeth have erupted. Before then, the theory goes, the immature immune system cannot handle vaccines well.

Dr. Natasha Campbell-McBride, an outspoken British pediatrician, believes that the link between learning disabilities and the condition of our digestive system is the key to understanding autism.

> We really started prescribing antibiotics for everything and anything in the '70s and '80s," she says. "That's when we started to get generations of people with compromised gut flora. Antibiotics wipe out the beneficial bacteria as well as the pathogenic bacteria... Between 95-100% of mothers of children with autism, hyperactivity, asthma, eczema and other problems, also have conditions that are related to abnormal gut flora. I hardly ever see healthy mothers.[7]

These kinds of factors give rise to the "toxic assault" theory. Today's children are burdened with toxins from day one. The Environmental Working Group and the CDC studied umbilical cord blood and found babies are loaded with chemicals – fire retardants, pesticides, and more.[8] Many parents will say their child turned autistic immediately after a vaccination, but it may be too simple to blame just the vaccines. Many different elements combined to weaken today's children such that the vaccinations in one "well baby visit" can be the final straw.

What do we know about the expression of autism?

Autistic children are easy to recognize. They are the children who do not play with other children. They have poor eye contact and little or no ability to speak. They sometimes have verbal understanding, but it is very difficult to get through to them. They have repetitive movements like hand flapping, staring at ceiling fans, and hitting themselves. They are sometimes thought to be deaf because they often do not respond when their names are called. They may communicate through grunts, or screams, or pulling at parents' arm or clothes.

The DSM-IV (the American Psychiatric Association's Diagnostic and Statistical Manual of Mental Disorders) recognizes the following as criteria for diagnosis of autism:

- The disease is defined by symptoms that appear before the age of three which reflect delayed or abnormal development in language, social skills and behavioral repertoire
- Impaired social interaction (at least 2 manifestations)
- Impaired communication
- Repetitive behaviors, activities, and interests

Children with autism have a heightened sensitivity to all sensory input. The parietal lobes, where sensory input is integrated, are out of balance; they are not properly connected to other parts of the brain like the temporal lobes, where language is processed. The autistic child's "stimming", or repetitive activities like rocking, humming, hitting themselves, may well be simply their way of creating "white noise" to shut out the excessive sensory input.

A few children are autistic from birth. These are the babies who do not cuddle, who do not look at the mother, who do not like to be touched. Most autistic children manifest their disability around the age of 15-18 months.

Autism seems to be a disease on the severe end of a spectrum of chronic diseases which includes Asperger's disease, developmental disorders, Attention deficit (hyperactivity) disorder, childhood asthma, juvenile rheumatoid arthritis, and other autoimmune diseases. The incidence of these illnesses has also increased dramatically since the 1960s, most likely due to a combination of genetic susceptibility with ever-increasing pollution of our atmosphere, food, water and soil.[9]

What about Asperger's?

𝒜sperger's syndrome (AS) got its name from Viennese physician, Hans Asperger, who published a paper in 1944 that described a pattern of behaviors in several young boys who had normal intelligence and language development, but who also exhibited autistic-like behaviors and marked deficiencies in social and communication skills. In 1994 Asperger's

Syndrome was added to the DSM-IV and only in the past few years has AS been recognized by professionals and parents. Until then, those with AS were seen usually as brilliant, eccentric, absent minded, socially inept, and a little awkward physically.

AS is a lifelong disability that affects how a person makes sense of the world, processes information, and relates to other people.

Children with AS may show no delays in language development; they usually have good grammatical skills and an advanced vocabulary at an early age. However, they may be very literal, and they may have trouble using language in a social context. Often there are no obvious delays in cognitive development or in age-appropriate self-help skills such as feeding and dressing themselves.

You cannot tell that someone has Asperger's syndrome just by looking at them. When we meet a person, we make judgments. From their facial expression, tone of voice and body language, we can usually tell whether they are happy, angry, or sad and respond accordingly.

People with AS can find it harder, if not impossible, to read the signals that most of us take for granted. This can lead to high levels of anxiety and confusion. They desire interaction with others but have trouble knowing how to make it work. They do not understand why people misinterpret what they say. They tend to interpret everything in a very literal way.

AS is not caused by emotional deprivation or the way a person has been brought up. Because some of the behaviors exhibited by a person with AS may be seen by others as intentionally rude, many people wrongly assume that AS is the result of bad parenting – it isn't.

There is a general impression that Asperger's syndrome carries with it superior intelligence and a tendency to become very interested in and preoccupied with a particular subject. Often this preoccupation leads to a specific career at which the adult is very successful. At younger ages, one might see the child being a bit more rigid and apprehensive about changes or about adhering to routines. This can lead to a consideration of OCD (obsessive compulsive disorder) but it is not the same phenomenon.

How do we approach those on the autistic spectrum?

$\mathscr{A}$re these children best served, as the conventional medical community tells parents, by controlling their behavior with pharmaceuticals and just "giving them a lot of love"?

Of course, all children need love, autistic or not. But drugs add to the chemical burden and all drugs come with side effects.

If the neural processing is defective, is there no way to help it develop correctly? If children are unable to detoxify heavy metals by themselves, is there no way to help them rid their bodies of these neurotoxic metals? If they have chronic diarrhea, or chronic constipation, is there no way, outside of pharmacology, to help them improve their quality of life?

If the answers were easy, there would not be such a proliferation of self-help parent groups, and there would be agreement among physicians treating this disorder. There does not appear to be a single "one size fits all" answer.

But there are answers – they just have to be discovered and individualized to the child. Some of the answers lie in the area of virology and gastroenterology. It has been shown conclusively that some children who get the measles virus through a vaccine are unable to eliminate the virus from their systems. Instead, the virus lives on in the intestinal tract, giving rise to lymphoid hyperplasia (swelling of the lymphatic glands in the GI tract) and chronic GI symptoms with which parents of autistic children are so familiar.[10, 11, 12,13]

Some of the answers lie in the area of biochemistry. Autistic children typically have significant difficulty with detoxification of viruses, organic pollutants, heavy metals, and often pharmaceutical medications. Many of these children have somewhat abnormal genes controlling the initial detoxification pathways, through methylation and sulfation and synthesis of glutathione. Glutathione[14] is produced by all mammals, and is found all over the body. It is a powerful antioxidant, and plays a key role in liver detoxification of all kinds of chemicals and viruses.

124

Some of the answers lie in the area of clinical metal toxicology. Mercury is one of the most toxic substances known to humankind. Lead comes right on its heels. Arsenic, cadmium, and aluminum are not far behind. Toxicity is the major cause of chronic illness in our 21st century world. One out of every six women in the United States today is mercury toxic, according to data from the NHANES study in 2002.[15] Infants are born with an average of more than 200 toxic chemicals in their blood.[16] In order to remove toxicity, it is necessary to clean up both the intestinal tract and the liver, so that they can function as the toxic filters and excretors they are meant to be. Sometimes it is not possible to restore the intestinal tract to health unless we deal with the heavy metals first.

Treatment for heavy metal toxicity is accomplished through several means, including oral EDTA, various creams rubbed on the skin – both DMPS and EDTA – oral DMSA, oral penicillamine, and other agents. Many of these medications can also be given intravenously. Measurement of the heavy metal body burden is sometimes difficult, as autistic children have difficulty excreting these heavy metals.[17] They may require treatment for up to a year before the heavy metals start to be excreted in measurable quantities.

Once neural development is defective, is there any way to restore the normal pathways and normal function? Primitive reflexes appear to be retained in children with both autism and Asperger's syndrome.[18] In fact, movement disturbances in children later diagnosed as autistic seem to appear early in life, as early as 4-6 months, and are at least potentially diagnostic.[19] Neurofeedback has been helpful in the treatment of some autistic children.[20, 21, 22]

From the point of view of neurodevelopment, the brain appears to be in a hyperexcitable state, reacting to many stimuli in an accelerated fashion, all the while being unable to process these stimuli in any coherent way. Often the parietal lobes, where sensory input function is coordinated, perceive the information in a distorted fashion, resulting therefore in a distortion of perceived reality. This distortion no doubt prompts some of the behaviors associated with autism – the stimming, for example.

Many children diagnosed with autism suffer from environmental overload. How we see the world is determined by how our brain interprets information through our five senses. Each sensory channel can be affected in different ways, hyperactive, hypoactive, or disrupted by "white noise" interference from within the system.

Neurotherapy like BrainAdvantage™ can assist in stimulating those areas of decreased function, calming those areas of increased function, and modifying some of the distorted information pathways in the brain, allowing the brain to receive distortion-free sensory input. The brain then has the potential to re-set itself, re-establishing more normal neural connections.

Missed stages of neurodevelopment need to be corrected, through a series of training exercises which are done at home.

Personalizing the Treatment

Determining the metabolic pathways that are dysfunctional is best done through genetic testing, but it can be accomplished also simply by adding supplements on the "trial and error" principle – if they get better we keep the supplement; if they get worse we eliminate it.

We modify the diets, to ensure that children are not sensitive to any of the foods they are eating. We prefer to do allergy testing first, because it is much easier to eliminate a favorite food if it becomes clear that the food is causing behavioral or physical reactions. Since so many children (more than 50%) are sensitive to the break-down products of gluten (wheat, rye, barley, kamut, spelt, and most baked goods) and casein (cow's milk, cheese, yogurt and most baked goods), even if testing is negative, this is the first step of many in therapeutic dietary modification. This is NOT child abuse, as has been the accusation thrown at some moms of autistic children. It is a therapeutic trial.

We may treat children for heavy metal toxicity. For those whose initial provocation tests are negative, we may use other means to determine whether mercury toxicity may be a significant part of their disease.

There are no easy fixes. But caring physicians do not give up. We walk the journey with you, investigate new things that you bring to us, and together with you, we determine the best course of action for your child.

RESOURCES

Valley of the Sun Autism Network (www.vsan.org) – serves parents of children with autism who live in Phoenix, Arizona and surrounding areas. They provide information on topics of interest including doctors, co-op, meetings, forums, providers, therapists, and ideas for living a healthy and toxic-free life.

Autism Research Institute – **(www.autism.com)** – involved with research and teaching for the past 40 years. They have conferences annually for parents and clinicians, and a wonderful summary to biomedical treatments for autism, available on the web at

http://www.autism.com/pdf/providers/adams_biomed_summary.pdf

---

[1]Overloaded? New science, new insights about mercury and autism in susceptible children. Environmental Working Group. December, 2004.

[2]Mutter J, Naumann J. Mercury and autism: accelerating evidence. *Neuro Endocrinol Lett.* 2005 Oct 30;26(5)

[3]Mark R. Geier and David A. Geier. The potential importance of steroids in the treatment of autistic spectrum disorders and other disorders involving mercury toxicity. *Medical Hypotheses*, Vol. 64, No. 5, 2005, 946-54.

[4]Ziff MF. Documented clinical side-effects to dental amalgam. *Adv Dental Res* 6;1:131-34.

[5] Dufault R, LeBlanc B et al. Mercury from chlor-alkali plants: measured concentrations in food product sugar. *Environ Health.* 2009 Jan 26; 8:2.

[6]Neil Z Miller. Aluminum in Vaccines – A Neurological Gamble. Thinktwice Global Vaccine Institute. 2009

[7]Dr. Natasha Campbell-McBride. *Gut and Psychology Syndrome.* Medinform Publishing, 2008

[8]Environmental Working Group. Body Burden – the Pollution in Newborns. July 14, 2005. Downloaded from http://www.ewg.org/reports_content/bodyburden2/pdf/bodyburden2_final-r2.pdf

[9]Sengler C, Lau S, et al. Interactions between genes and environmental factors in asthma and atopy: new developments. *Respir Res* 2002, 3:7

[10]Ashwood P, Anthony A et al. Intestinal lymphocyte populations in children with regressive autism: evidence for extensive mucosal immunopathology. *J Clin Immunol.* 2003 Nov;23(6):504-17.

[11]Horvath K, Papadimitriou JC et al. Gastrointestinal abnormalities in children with autistic disorder . *J Pediatr.* 1999 Nov;135(5):559-63.

[12]Wakefield AJ, Murch SH et al. Ileal-lymphoid-nodular hyperplasia, non-specific colitis, and pervasive developmental disorder in children. *The Lancet* 351 (Feb 28, 1998):637-641).

[13]Horvath K, Perman JA. Autism and gastrointestinal symptoms. *Curr Gastroenterol Rep.* 2002 Jun;4(3):251-8.

[14]Glutathione (GSH): Technical Monograph. Alternative Medicine Review – 6;6 (December 2001).

[15]N H A N E S - National Health and Examination Survey – N H A N E S 2001-2002.

[16]Body Burden – the Pollution in Newborns. Environmental Working Group.

[17]Holmes AS, Blaxill MF et al. Reduced Levels of Mercury in First Baby Haircuts of Autistic Children. *Int J Toxicol.* 22;4:277-85 (Jul-Aug 2003).

[18]Teitelbaum O, Benton T et al. Eshkol–Wachman movement notation in diagnosis: The early detection of Asperger's syndrome . *PNAS* 101;32: 11909-11914. (Aug 10, 2004).

[19]Teitelbaum P, Teitelbaum O et al. Movement analysis in infancy may be useful for early diagnosis of autism. *PNAS* Vol. 95, Issue 23, 13982-13987, November 10, 1998.

[20]Scolnick, Barbara. Effects of electroencephalogram biofeedback with Asperger's syndrome. *Int J Rehab Res* 28(2):159-163, June 2005.

[21]Jarusiewicz B. Efficacy of Neurofeedback for Children in the autistic spectrum. *Journal of Neurotherapy,* 2002. 6(4), 39-49.

[22]Sichel AG, Fehmi LG et al. Positive Outcome With Neurofeedback Treatment In a Case of Mild Autism. *J Neurother* 1;1:60-64.

Autoimmune Diseases

$\mathcal{A}$utoimmune diseases are the third most common category of disease in the United States after cancer and heart disease.[1] Conservative estimates indicate that three-quarters of the persons with autoimmune diseases are women.[2]

The statistics keepers tell us one in 12 Americans will develop an autoimmune disorder. Compare that to the estimate that one in 20 adult Americans will have heart disease.[3] Yes, autoimmune diseases are more common than heart disease, the number one killer. Clearly, many people are finding that their immune system is failing them.

Autoimmune disease refers to a group of more than 80 serious chronic illnesses that can manifest in many different places in the body, with many different diagnoses. Their common thread is that the body makes antibodies to its own tissues. The body's immune system becomes misdirected, attacking the very organs it was designed to protect.

Most common autoimmune diseases

Rheumatoid arthritis, juvenile rheumatoid arthritis, lupus, scleroderma, multiple sclerosis, Hashimoto's thyroiditis, Graves' disease, type 1 diabetes, Sjögren's syndrome, Crohn's disease, celiac disease, ulcerative colitis, Addison's disease, Guillain-Barré syndrome, temporal arteritis, Ménière's disease

---

Autoimmune diseases tend to cluster in families and in individuals – a person with one autoimmune disease is more likely to acquire another one. This indicates that common mechanisms are at work. Studies of the prevalence of autoimmune disease in monozygotic (identical) twins show that genetic as well as environmental factors are necessary for the disease to develop.[4] Also, infections play a big role in the development of autoimmune disease.

Why would the body become "allergic" to itself?

$\mathcal{I}$mmunity begins at birth. Soon after giving birth, female mammals produce colostrum, which is a milk-like substance that jump-starts a newborn's immune system. Human breast milk contains large quantities of secretory IgA, lysozyme-secreting macrophages, and lymphocytes (T cells and B cells). The lymphocytes release compounds that strengthen the immune response of the infant. There is evidence that the protection given by breast milk lasts for years.[5]

Our lymphocytes react to *all* our tissues. Why, then, does the process sometimes become pathologic? Why don't we react to our own tissues all the time? Because these self-reactive cells are normally destroyed before they get into the circulation – when they are not destroyed, we get autoimmune disease.

Our immune system is designed to protect us against that which is foreign, while recognizing that which is native. If, for some reason, our own tissues become contaminated with something foreign which attaches itself to the proteins of the tissues and changes the configuration of the proteins, the body could very well become confused and think protection is needed. An inflammatory process begins, and we are on the road to developing autoimmune disease.

So... is the treatment answer to suppress the immune system, with steroids or immune-suppressant drugs, so that we no longer react to our own tissues? Or attempt to kill every bacterium, virus or cancer cell that happens to come down the pike?

Mounting a war against our own bodies is probably not the best answer.

A better treatment answer is to discover what caused the abnormal response in the first place, and remove that trigger, allowing the body to restore itself to health.

The first place to look is in the gut because 75 percent of the body's immune system activity comes from the gut.[6]

We can identify foods and other substances (chemicals, pollens, molds) which cause gut inflammation and work to eliminate the responsible foods from your environment. We look at your body burden of heavy metals like mercury, arsenic and lead, and make every effort to eliminate these as well, since they can be a significant cause of inflammatory response. We can provide supplements and remedies to correct the dysfunctional information systems in the body, and to heal the GI tract and improve its overall health. We can give you natural substances which modulate (or change toward the "normal") the immune system. We show you how colonics and probiotics work to replace the damaging bacteria in the gut with ones which are actively helpful. And finally, we look at brain function, to help modify the effect of the autonomic nervous system (the stress system) on the gut. Once the GI tract is restored to health, many symptoms are cleared, and health may return to the entire body.

Most Americans today have weakened and impaired immune systems that are unable to function as Nature designed them. Experts estimate that many allergies and immune-system diseases have doubled, tripled or even quadrupled in the last few decades. Some studies indicate that more than half of the U.S. population has at least one allergy.[7]

Some researchers suspect the rise in immune system dysfunctions may have a common explanation rooted in aspects of modern living.

First, we have undergone a revolutionary change in how we fuel our body. For tens of thousands of years, mankind ate unprocessed, truly natural food. In the last 150 years or so, our diets have changed dramatically. Our genes simply cannot adapt that quickly. The human body is not designed to run on 150 pounds per year of processed sugar, nor is it designed to run on baby formula, aspartame, pesticides, hydrogenated oils or meat from animals fed unnatural diets and hormones. Sugar for example, impairs the intestinal microflora and undermines a strong immune system.

Second, there is the "hygiene hypothesis," which suggests germ-free homes and childhood vaccinations have eliminated challenges to our immune systems so they don't learn how to defend us properly when we are young. The immune system is sort of like a muscle – use it or lose it. We eat food inoculated with antibiotics. Our children stay indoors more, play outside less. Studies suggest that children who are raised with pets, have older siblings or play with livestock on the farm, are less likely to develop allergies, probably because they are exposed to more microbes than those living in overly sterile homes. "The data are very strong," said Erika von Mutius of the Ludwig-Maximilians University in Munich. "If kids have all sorts of exposures on the farm by being in the stables a lot, close to the animals and the grasses, and drinking cow's milk from their own farm, that seems to confer protection." Researchers believe the lack of exposure to potential threats early in life leaves the immune system with fewer command-and-control cells known as regulatory T cells, making the system more likely to overreact or run wild.[8]

Third, environmental pollution and sedentary lifestyles may play more of a role than we understand. One reason that many researchers suspect something about modern living is to blame is that the increases in allergies and auto-immune diseases show up largely in highly developed countries in Europe and North America. The illnesses have only started to rise in other countries as they have become more developed. Donna Jackson Nakawaza, author of *The Autoimmune Epidemic*, implicates the bioaccumulation of toxins that pervade our home, food, and environment, as a primary cause of autoimmune diseases. What effect are plastics and other persistent organic pollutants having on human health? "Rising levels of autoimmune disease may well prove to be the next environmental disaster – only in this case, the changes taking place degree by degree are in the interior landscapes of our bodies," Nakawaza writes. "Our immune systems may be less prepared because we're confronting fewer natural pathogens, but we're also encountering an endless barrage of artificial pathogens that are taxing our systems to the maximum."

Autoimmune diseases have common patterns

$\mathcal{A}$utoimmune diseases occur because the metabolism goes awry. The dysfunction manifests as some 80+ different diseases that we know of, but the contributions to the breakdown seem to have common patterns:

- Autoimmune diseases seem to develop in people who have experienced an ongoing lack of nutrients in their diet.
- Autoimmune diseases seem to be associated with environmental toxicity.
- The susceptible individual has very likely experienced significant and prolonged chronic stress.
- The immune system in the susceptible individual may have been fighting on more than one front – for example dealing with a root canal infection as well as multiple amalgam (mercury) fillings – and does not have enough activity left to overcome a serious infection or inflammatory state.
- The body starts to experience inflammation and eventually breaks down; genetics will determine where the weakness occurs, and thus the timing and location of the breakdown.
- Steroids and other drugs may suppress the inflammatory symptoms for a time, but do not have the capacity to heal. In fact, they certainly contribute to overall suppression of the immune system.

The various forms of arthritis, for example, bring many of the common patterns into play.

Osteoarthritis, characterized by destruction of cartilage within the joint, is a case of the cells which produce cartilage failing to maintain the balance between production and destruction of normal cartilage tissue. Compounds called proteoglycans form the cartilage itself, and these proteins are found to be deficient in cartilage from patients with osteoarthritis. Other compounds called metalloproteinases are also found in high concentration in osteoarthritic cartilage. These compounds digest proteoglycans. So for unknown reasons, the body has turned, you might say, on its own cartilage. It is possible that the imbalance is due to vitamin and/or nutrient deficiency. One study demonstrated that niacinamide, vitamin B3, improved the global impact of osteoarthritis, improved joint flexibility, reduced inflammation, and allowed for reduction in standard anti-inflammatory medications when compared to placebo.[9]

Rheumatoid arthritis is associated with several genes, the most familiar of which is the HLA gene.[10] Other factors come into play, including bacterial infection,[11] diet,[12,13] inflammation, and heavy metals. With an RA patient, determination of food sensitivities and heavy metal toxicities is crucial. For many, remission has not been possible without dietary changes, particularly elimination of sugar and grains. The Mediterranean diet has been shown to have significant impact of the symptoms of rheumatoid arthritis,[14] as does treatment with y-linoleic acid (GLA).[15]

Additionally, chronic mycoplasma infections must be investigated; some patients treated with antibiotics for months have improved their arthritis symptoms.[16] And some patients diagnosed with rheumatoid arthritis actually have symptoms from infection with a different organism – Borrelia burgdorferi, or Lyme disease. The use of long term steroids and other anti-inflammatories have led to suppressed immune system, candida overgrowth, peptic ulcers and other problems.

Spondyloarthropathies occur with peripheral joint inflammation, mainly of the knees or hips, rather than the hands as typically seen in osteoarthritis. This form of arthritis is frequently associated with inflammatory bowel disease, inflammation of the eye (uveitis), and skin diseases like psoriasis. Genetics are thought to play a significant role in this form of arthritis. HLA B27 is found in 90% of patients with ankylosing spondylitis.[17]

Nutrient deficiencies, infections, pathologic gene expression, environmental pollution, stress… all scourges of our modern day world.

Leaky gut's ugly cascade invites autoimmune diseases

*F*ood is fuel for the body, and most of us don't eat well. We may eat a lot of calories, but we are still malnourished. We eat genetically modified corn, soy, canola, and cottonseed oil which impacts our guts in ways science is just beginning to understand. We use antibiotics which drastically alter gut flora. We eat sugar to calm our stress levels, sugar which then plays havoc with our immune system. We become sensitive to some foods, often ones we crave. Since this picture describes so many people's lifestyle, you can imagine (correctly) that gut problems are widespread.

It is well documented that patients with increased intestinal permeability – leaky gut – have a higher incidence of arthritis.[18] In ten years, it may be very common that we hear about leaky gut syndrome or LGS. Today, mainstream medicine doesn't talk about it much, the pharmaceutical industry has no drugs for it, and it is rarely looked for. But it is likely a very common problem.

In simple terms, the lining of the intestines becomes inflamed and permeable, like a piece of Swiss cheese. Large spaces develop between the cells of the gut wall, and then things that were never meant to get out of the gut, such as partially digested foods and bacteria, pass though the small intestine into the blood stream. The body senses something foreign now in the blood, so the immune system is called in to attack it. Antibodies are formed against once harmless, innocuous foods.

When the gut is leaky, a cascade of problems ensues. The body fails to properly absorb vitamins and minerals, so the person becomes depleted. The leakage of toxins overburdens the liver so that the body is less able to handle everyday chemicals. Additionally, the body loses its ability to ward off protozoa, bacteria, viruses and fungi. Bacteria and yeasts are able to pass through the gut into the bloodstream and set up infection elsewhere in the body.

With LGS, the protective coating of the IgA family of antibodies normally present in a healthy gut is disabled. IgA antibodies help defend against the invasion of microorganisms through body surfaces lined with a mucous membrane. When they are not on the job, viruses, bacteria, parasites and yeast are then able to invade the bloodstream and colonize almost any body tissue or organ. When this occurs in the gums, periodontal disease results. When it occurs in the synovial lining of the joints, arthritis results. And so on.

One particularly ugly part of that cascade is the overgrowth of yeast. Candida, a yeast normally present in the gut in low levels, typically overgrows in this unhealthy environment and is thought to grow pseudopods, kind of like roots, which penetrate the gut lining, creating even more permeability.[19]

LGS is almost always associated with autoimmune disease. Conversely, reversing autoimmune disease depends on healing the lining of the gastrointestinal tract.

A number of patients with LGS also find dramatic improvement with colonics because by removing toxins, they help heal the gut, allowing the immune system to reset itself.

What else besides leaky gut?

*S*ome patients and doctors have discerned that there is nearly always a stressful event that triggers the outbreak of rheumatoid arthritis, lupus or scleroderma. Researchers evaluated several hundred studies on stress and concluded that the kind of stress that most negatively compromises the immune system is chronic stress.[20]

A study published in the April 1, 2007 edition of *Nature Immunology* concluded that allergic and inflammatory diseases may actually trigger autoimmune diseases by relaxing the controls that normally eliminate newly produced, self-reactive B cells.[21] This is important because many autoimmune diseases are caused by self-reactive antibodies produced by such B cells.

Vitamin D deficiency has been strongly linked to autoimmune disease.[22] Nearly every auto-immune patient tested will be found to be very deficient in this nutrient. Vitamin D status affects chemicals that modulate the immune system called cytokines. Vitamin D keeps cells in check. When the body has too little D, cell regulation can go haywire, causing cells to become overly active or multiply too quickly. It is well-known that in higher latitudes where there is less sun exposure, there is a higher risk for multiple sclerosis (MS). Higher sun exposure during childhood and early adolescence is associated with a decreased risk of MS.[23]

Vaccines by their very design stimulate the immune system. They also may contain mercury and aluminum which are immunosuppressive and neurotoxic. Mercury actually causes changes in the lymphocyte activity and decreases lymphocyte viability.[24] Vaccines deplete our body of vital immune-enhancing nutrients, like vitamin C, vitamin A and zinc.[25] Nutrients like these boost the immune system, and feed white blood cells and macrophages which become the immune system "soldiers."

Soy products, including soy-based baby formulas, contain a plant estrogen called genistein which is a hormone-like compound that appears to impair immune function. The Proceedings of the National Academy of Sciences reported in 2002 that when the plant estrogen genistein found in soy was injected in mice, levels of several immune cells dropped and the thymus, a gland where immune cells mature, shrank.[26]

Root canal fillings can become a lifetime bacteria "factory" which sows the seeds of disease throughout the body.[27] A strong immune system will control the germs that escape from teeth into other areas of the body. But this defensive action may tie up so many of the immune system's "soldiers" that when it comes time to fight off a Candida overgrowth, for example, there may not be enough immune system lymphocytes (white blood cells) remaining to do it. Dr. Weston A. Price documented how entrenched dental bacterial can contribute to heart and circulatory diseases, as well as autoimmune diseases of the joints, the brain and nervous system.[28]

After World War II, we traded animal and tropical fats for vegetable oils. Only now is the conventional medical community coming to realize that those veggie oils are inflammatory and deficient in omega-3 fatty acids, high in omga-6 fatty acids. The omega-3s and their derivative, DHA (docosahexaenoic acid), are critical to correct development of a child's nervous system and immune system. We have a generation of children born during a time of omega-3 deficiency.

Gluten is thought to be one trigger for autoimmune disease.[29] Indeed gluten sensitivity may be a major trigger for autoimmune disease.[30] Researchers have found an association between gluten enteropathy and/or celiac disease and thyroiditis,[31,32] Alzheimer's brain tissue,[33] diabetes,[34] and auto-immune disease in general.[35]

We have now learned that children who frequently use antibacterial soaps are not exposed to common bacteria that may protect them from allergies and asthma. Indeed, exposure to bacteria and viruses acts as a natural vaccine to boost the ability of the immune system to fend off invaders. Farmers used to eat carrots and other vegetables right out of the field during the day as a snack. They might wipe off the dirt on their pants, but wash and scrub the vegetables? No. They got a small dose of dirt with its population of good microorganisms. Today's kids spend most of their time indoors, and are warned away from germs.

Patterns of dysfunctions that begin in childhood affect autoimmune diseases. The recent identification of major immune-based disease patterns beginning in childhood suggests that the immune system may play an even more important role in determining health status and health care needs across a lifetime than was previously understood.[36] Heavy metals, in particular mercury, are thought to be another trigger for autoimmune disease.[37,38,39] Other metals are similarly implicated.[40,41,42]

Most of the risk of autoimmunity comes from environmental exposures rather than from genetic susceptibilities. Global chemical production is expected to double in the next 24 years.[43] Donna Jackson Nakazawa writes:

> It has taken several decades for the many researchers in the autoimmune disease field to come to the conclusion that our contaminated environment is causing the human immune system to run amok.
>
> We are our environment. What we put into it, we also put into ourselves. The way in which our bodies are turning against themselves when autoimmune disease strikes serves, sadly, as a disturbing modern analogy for what we are doing to ourselves as a society as we continue to dump thousands of chemicals ... whose properties we do not yet fully understand.[44]

Healing Answers

*R*eversing autoimmune disease is a process of education and medical assistance regarding:

- Identification of foods which cause an allergic reaction.
- Identification of molds, pollen and other airborne allergens.
- Identification and elimination of heavy metals.
- Identification of malfunctioning information systems within the body and use of supplements and energetic medicine to re-establish healthy function.
- Learning how to eat a nutrient dense diet.
- Learning how to heal the GI tract and promote good intestinal flora.
- Learning about household and personal care chemicals.
- Reduction of stress.

Patients typically go on an anti-inflammatory diet. Alternative anti-inflammatory herbs can be used. Acupuncture can treat specific arthritic joints, as well as decrease the inflammatory potential of the entire body. Immune system modulating substances are prescribed.

The most common themes running through treatment of an autoimmune disease are education, and cleaning up our individual corners of the world.

RESOURCES

Our Toxic World by Dr. Doris Rapp
From electromagnetic pollution and chemicals, to mold and food, Dr. Rapp will increase your awareness of the largely unseen hazards in our world.

The Autoimmune Epidemic by Donna Jackson Nakazawa

"Nearly 24 million Americans are suffering from an autoimmune illness, yet nine out of ten Americans cannot name a single one of thee diseases. It boggles the mind."

---

[1]National Institutes of Health Autoimmune Disease Coordinating Committee Report, 2002. Bethesda (MD): The Institutes; 2002.

[2]Jacobson DL, Gange SJ, Rose NR, Graham NMH. Epidemiology and estimated population burden of selected autoimmune disease in the United States. *Clin Immunol Immunopathol.* 1997;84:223–43.

[3]Donna Jackson Nakazawa. *The Autoimmune Epidemic.* Simon & Schuster, 2008

[4]Rose NR. Mechanisms of autoimmunity. *Semin Liver Dis.* 2002;22:387–94.

[5]Hanson, LA. Ann. *All.Asth Imm.*1998 Dec; 81(6):523-33

[6]Downloaded on September 12, 2020 from http:/www.accessmedicine.com/popup.aspx?aID=2858456&print=yes_chapter

[7]Rob Stein. Immune Systems Increasingly On Attack. *The Washington Post*, March 4, 2008

[8]Ibid

[9]Jonas WB, Rapoza CP et al. The effect of niacinamide on osteoarthritis: a pilot study. *Inflamm Res.* 1996 Jul;45(7):330-4.

[10]Weyand CM, Hicok KC, et al. The influence of HLA-DRB1 genes on disease severity in rheumatoid arthritis. *Ann Intern Med.* 1992 Nov 15;117(10):801-6.

[11]Ebringer A, Khalafpour S. Rheumatoid arthritis and Proteus: a possible aetiological association. *Rheumatol Int.* 1989;9(3-5):223-8.

[12]Remans PH, Sont JK. Nutrient supplementation with polyunsaturated fatty acids and micronutrients in rheumatoid arthritis: clinical and biochemical effects. *Eur J Clin Nutr.* 2004 Jun;58(6):839-45.

[13]Kjeldsen-Kragh J. Mediterranean diet intervention in rheumatoid arthritis. *Ann. Rheum. Dis* 2003;62;193-195

[14]Kjeldsen-Kragh J. Mediterranean diet intervention in rheumatoid arthritis. *Ann Rheum Dis* 2003;62;193-195.

[15]Leventhal LJ, Boyce EG. Treatment of Rheumatoid Arthritis with Gammalinolenic Acid. *Ann Int Med* 119;9:867-873 (1 November 1993).

[16]Kloppenburg M, Breedveld FC, et al. Minocycline in active rheumatoid arthritis. A double-blind, placebo-controlled trial. *Arthritis Rheum.* 1994 May;37(5):629-36.

[17]Mielants H, De Keyser F. Gut inflammation in the spondyloarthropathies. *Curr Rheumatol Rep.* 2005 Jun;7(3):188-94.

[18]Mielants H, De Vos M, et al. Intestinal mucosal permeability in inflammatory rheumatic diseases. II. Role of disease. *J Rheumatol.* 1991 Mar;18(3):394-400.

[19]John Trowbridge and Morton Walker. *The Yeast Syndrome.* Bantam Books, 1986, p39-40. Bharati C. Purohit et al, The formation of germtubes by Candida albicans, when grown with staphylococcus pyogenes, Escherichia coli, klebsiella pneumoniae, lactobacillus acidophilus, and proteus vulgaris, *Myopathologia*, 1977, 62, 3:187-189

[20]Segerstrom, Suzanne C., Miller, Gregory E. Psychological Stress and the Human Immune System: A Meta-Analytic Study of 30 Years of Inquiry. *Psychological Bulletin.* 130(4), Jul 2004, 601-630.

[21]Astrakhan A, Omori M et al. Local increase in thymic stromal lymphopoietin induces system alterations in B cell development. *Nat Immunol* 8, 522-531 (2007)

[22]Cantorna MT, Mahon BD. Mounting Evidence for Vitamin D as an Environmental Factor Affecting Autoimmune Disease Prevalence. *Experimental Biology and Medicine* 229:1136-1142 (2004).

[23]I A F van der Mei, et al. Past exposure to sun, skin phenotype, and risk of multiple sclerosis: case-control study, *British Medical Journal.* August 9, 2003;327:316

[24]Windham, Bernard. Annotated Bibliography: Adverse health effects related to mercury and amalgam fillings and clinically documented recoveries after amalgam replacement, berniew1@earthlink.net
Shenker, BK; Berthold, P; Immunotoxic effects of mercuric compounds on human lymphocytes and monocytes. II. Alterations in cell viability, *Immunopharmacol Immunotoxicol.*, 1992;14(3):555-77

[25]Megson MN. Is autism a G-alpha protein defect reversible with natural vitamin A? *Medical Hypotheses,* Volume 54, Issue 6, June 2000, Pages 979-983

[26]Proceedings of the National Academy of Sciences, May 21, 2002;99:7616-7621

[27]George E. Meinig. *Root Canal Cover-up.* Published by Price Pottenger Nutrition Foundation

[28]Dr. Weston Price, *Dental Infections Oral & Systemic and Dental Infections and the Degenerative Diseases, Volumes I and II,* Price Pottenger Nutrition Foundation library

[29]Tlaskanova-Hagenova H, Tuckova L et al. Involvement of innate immunity in the development of inflammatory and autoimmune disease. *Ann NY Acad Sci* 1051:787-98 (2005).

[30]Kumar V, Rajadhyaksha M et al. Celiac Disease-Associated Autoimmune Endocrinopathies. *Clin Diag Lab Immunol* 8;4:678-85 (July 2001).

[31]Volta U. Coeliac Disease in Patients with Autoimmune Thyroiditis. *Digestion* 2001;64:61-65.

[32]Valentino R, Savastano S. Markers of potential coeliac disease in patients with Hashimoto's thyroiditis. *Eur J Endocrinol* 146:4(479-83).

[33]D'Andrea MR. Evidence linking neuronal cell death to autoimmunity in Alzheimer's disease. *Brain Research* 982 (2003) 19-30.

[34]Not T, Tommasini A, et al. Undiagnosed coeliac disease and risk of autoimmune disorders in subjects with Type I diabetes mellitus. *Diabetologia* 44;2:151-55 (Feb 2001)

[35]Ciacci C, Iovino P, et al. Grown-up coeliac children: the effects of only a few years on a gluten-free diet in childhood. *Aliment Pharmacol Ther.* 2005 Feb 15;21(4)421-9.

[36]Dietert RR, DeWitt JC, Germolec DR, Zelikoff JT. Breaking Patterns of Environmentally Influenced Disease for Health Risk Reduction: Immune Perspectives. *Environ Health Perspect.* August, 2010. 118:1091-1099. doi:10.1289/ehp.1001971

[37]Silbergelt FK, Silva IA et al. Mercury and autoimmunity: implications for occupational and environmental health. *Toxicol Appl Pharmacol.* 2005 Sep 1;207(2 Suppl):282-92.

[38]Holtman P, Johansson U et al. Adverse immunological effects and autoimmunity induced by dental amalgam and alloy in mice. *FASEB* 8:1184-90 (Nov 1994).

[39]Prochazkova J, Sterzl I, et al. The beneficial effects of amalgam replacement on health in patients with autoimmunity. *Neuroendocrinol Let* 3;25:211-18 (June 2004).

[40]Stejskal J, Stejskal VDM. The role of metals in autoimmunity and the link to neuroendocrinology. *Neuroendocrinol Let* 20;6:351-64 (1999).

[41]Bigazzi PE. Autoimmunity and heavy metals. *Lupus.* 1994 Dec;3(6):449-53.

[42]Subat-Dezulovic M, Slavic I, et al. Drug-induced acute tubulointerstitial nephritis: a case with elevated urinary cadmium. *Pediatr Nephrol.* 2002 May;17(5):382-5.

[43]Chemicals Policy Gap: Toward Stronger Regulation in the United States. *Environ Health Perspect.* August, 2009. 117:A358-A358. doi:10.1289/ehp.117-a358b

[44]Donna Jackson Nakazawa. *The Autoimmune Epidemic.* Simon & Schuster, 2008

Cancer

Every one of us has cancer. Every single one of us. Our bodies, as part of the normal metabolic process, produce anywhere from a few hundred to perhaps 10,000 cancerous cells each day. The immune system has the ability to recognize every one of those aberrant cells and remove them – if it is functioning properly. There is universal agreement that cancer is a failure of the immune system.

Cancer has shifted from being rare to being commonplace. Its growth parallels the growth of industrialized economies which introduced heavy metals and unnatural chemicals into the environment, and began to industrialize and process food. Our immune systems were not designed to handle the bombardment of modern toxins combined with lack of nutrient-dense food.

In 1971, President Richard Nixon announced a "war on cancer" with the goal that cancer would be cured by 1976. Since then, the National Cancer Institute, the federal government's main cancer research entity, has spent more than $105 billion. And other government agencies, universities, drug companies and philanthropies have spent billions more. Yet the death rate for cancer, adjusted for the size and age of the population, dropped only five percent from 1950 to 2005.[1]

Today, according to the National Cancer Institute, cancer will affect 1 in 2 men and 1 in 3 women in the United States. Cancer is now the number one cause of death in children between the ages of 1 and 14.

For well over half a century mainstream medicine has promised that a cure or major breakthrough for cancer was just around the corner. This has not happened. Perhaps we are attempting to fight the wrong battle.

Cancer is an Environmental Disease

𝒪n 2007, information that cancer is largely an environmentally-caused disease, and thus can be prevented, almost made it to the mainstream news. Almost.

The Susan G. Komen (SGK) organization and the Silent Spring Institute published "Environmental Factors in Breast Cancer," described as the most comprehensive review to date of scientific research on environmental factors and breast cancer risk. As the *Los Angeles Times* reported, researchers concluded that environmental pollutants contribute by "damaging DNA, promoting tumor growth, or increasing susceptibility by altering mammary gland development." Because breast cancer is so common and the chemicals so widespread, they said, "if even a small percentage is due to preventable environmental factors, modifying these factors would spare thousands of women. Regulators have not paid much attention to potential mammary carcinogens." The study concluded that cancer is an environmental disease.[2]

This conclusion, however, conflicts with many of SGK's sponsors. The organization virtually buried the report. A public education campaign to prevent cancer was never launched.

In 2007, one of SGK's million dollar sponsors was M&M candies. Otto Warburg won the Nobel Prize in the 1930s by demonstrating that cancer cells use much more sugar than normal cells. Hence the phrase: sugar feeds cancer.

According to a 2009 report in the *International Journal of Occupational and Environmental Health*:

> A substantial body of scientific evidence indicates that exposures to common chemicals and radiation, alone and in combination, are contributing to the increase in breast cancer incidence observed over the past several decades... A review of the scientific literature shows several classes of environmental factors have been implicated in an increased risk for breast cancer, including hormones and endocrine-disrupting compounds, organic chemicals and

144

by-products of industrial and vehicular combustion, and both ionizing and non-ionizing radiation.[3]

Suzanne Somers' 2009 book about cancer entitled *KNOCKOUT* quickly became a best seller. She was attacked by many in the mainstream media, but the public welcomed her like a breath of fresh air. Many people agree with her message about curing cancer:

> The present template of medicine is not working... the public needs to know there are real alternatives to chemo, radiation and surgery, and that a world without cancer is possible today. You have options.

In 2010, the panel that advises the president on cancer released a watershed report. It said that Americans are facing "grievous harm" from chemicals in the air, food, and water that have largely gone unregulated and ignored. The report said:

> U.S. regulation of environmental contaminants is rendered ineffective by five major problems: (1) inadequate funding and insufficient staffing, (2) fragmented and overlapping authorities coupled with uneven and decentralized enforcement, (3) excessive regulatory complexity, (4) weak laws and regulations, and (5) undue industry influence. Too often, these factors, either singly or in combination, result in agency dysfunction and a lack of will to identify and remove hazards.

Records from the 19th and 20th centuries show people in traditional societies, such as the Hunza and Eskimo, living to great ages and in good health, free of cancer. Researcher Dr. Weston Price found in the 1930s that cancer was unknown to the Eskimos until traders came and set up stores with jams and jellies, and sacks of sugar and refined flour.

The average person now has hundreds of groups of novel compounds in their bodies that weren't there 70 years ago. We have even changed the chemical environment of the womb. According to tests of umbilical cord blood done by Environment Working Group, babies marinate in a toxic strew and are born with more than 200 synthetic chemicals in their blood including BPA, pesticides, mercury, and fire retardants.[4] Through medical tests and electronic networks, we are exposed to cancer-causing radiation more than ever before. And as the epidemic of obesity will attest, processed food sends all the wrong signals to our body and fails to deliver the basic nutrients needed for healthy metabolism.

Environment or Genetics?

Cancer is what doctors call a multi-factorial disease – something resulting from the interaction of genetic factors with environmental factors. There are more than 200 different cancers. What they have in common is that they all start in the same way – with a change in the normal make-up of a cell.

According to the National Cancer Institute, "most cancers come from random mutations that develop in body cells during one's lifetime – either as a mistake when cells are going through cell division or in response to injuries from environmental agents such as radiation or chemicals."[5]

When a gene is damaged by radiation or chemicals, or receives misinformation from a chemical messenger, and the mistaken signal is not corrected, the result is inappropriate or uncontrolled growth. Normal cells have a finite lifespan – they divide many times, do what they are supposed to, and then die by committing cell suicide (apoptosis). Cancerous cells have mutated and do not follow the rulebook. They don't die; they divide endlessly and wander where they are not supposed to go. They are uniquely adapted to thrive in today's high-sugar diet and acidic internal environment.

When cells divide, their DNA is often copied with mistakes. Nature handles this by supplying proteins to fix those mistakes. The mutations that cause cancer disable the fail-safe mechanism of those mistake-fixing proteins.

By decoding nearly 40,000 genes in the human body, the Human Genome Project opened up an entirely new spectrum of knowledge. In two decades, for example, the BRCA1 and BRCA2 mutations were identified.

Recent studies suggest that BRCA1 mutations account for about 5% of inherited breast cancers, and that BRCA2 mutations account for half this fraction of families. Environment is, by far, the bigger factor.

So why does one woman with the BRCA1 gene get breast cancer and another does not? Because we influence how our genes *express* themselves. This is the science of epigenetics. We cannot change the fact we have the BRCA1 gene (or any of the other genes we have). Although only about five percent of us carry the BRCA1 gene, those who carry it tend to express it in today's world. In other words, if you have the gene, you are much more likely than the rest of us to develop breast cancer. Nevertheless, how we eat, the environmental pollution to which we are exposed, our stress level, and our mindset, can determine whether we get the best or the worst case scenario from various genes.

For example, we know that your odds of coming down with lung cancer greatly increase if you smoke. Farmers who apply certain pesticides to farm fields are twice as likely to contract melanoma, a deadly form of skin cancer.[6] If you took synthetic HRT – hormone replacement therapy – you have an increased chance of heart disease, breast cancer, and ovarian cancer.[7]

Genetics loads the gun; environment pulls the trigger.

We can undergo genetic testing to find out which genes we have, and how we might modify how we live to reduce the chance that we will become a cancer statistic.

Genetic Testing

*G*enetic testing gives you the ability to understand your body's vulnerabilities, your unique genetic predispositions. Genetics are playing an increasingly important role in the diagnosis, monitoring, and treatment of diseases.

Genetic testing plays a big role in the efficient diagnosis and treatment of cancer. To diagnose cancer, tissue is the gold standard – look at it under the microscope. But tissue isn't always available and it doesn't always tell the whole story; blood is always available and it can tell us a lot. Tumors shed what are called circulating tumor cells (CTCs) into the blood stream. These are potential metastatic cancer cells because tumors spread by shedding cells. The BioFocus Analysis can see if CTCs are present in the blood.

Like all cells, tumor cells have a genetic makeup. The BioFocus Analysis also shows us the genetic fingerprint of your specific CTCs. Looking at circulating tumor cells is critically important, since it is the spread of cancer to other parts of the body – and not the primary cancer – that is often responsible for the death of a person with cancer. When we know the genetics of your specific CTCs, then we can find out which treatments are going to work and which aren't. The BioFocus Analysis can predict, for example, which men with prostate cancer are more or less likely to benefit from chemotherapy.[8] Also, metastatic cancer cells can vary genetically from the primary tumor. At least two studies with breast cancer patients have demonstrated that CTCs can be HER2 positive while the primary breast tumor can be HER2 negative.[9, 10]

The BioFocus Analysis lets us be "smart" about how we design the regimen to defeat cancer. Think back to a time when you had a bladder infection. The lab tested your urine sample against different antibiotics to find out which ones were most effective at killing the bacteria. We can use the same concept when custom designing cancer treatments.

Treating Cancer

The conventional treatment for cancer is the familiar trio of chemotherapy, radiation, and surgery. Chemotherapy drugs are administered in doses high enough to kill a large number of cancer cells without (in theory) killing the body's immune system and intestinal tract. Patients are given as much chemotherapy as their body can tolerate. It is like killing flies with a cannonball instead of fly swatter. You get rid of some flies, yes, but you have a lot of collateral damage. Good cells die along with the bad. Over time (and sometimes a fairly short period of time, days rather than weeks), this massive bombardment can lead to low blood counts, organ failure, and death. Because an already poorly functioning immune system is subjected to radiation and toxic drugs, it is difficult to deliver a "cure."[11]

It is also a one-size-fits-all approach.

A study published in the *Journal of the National Cancer Institute* in 2008 measured the effectiveness of an anthracycline-based chemotherapy regimen in 5,354 women with early-stage breast cancer. Anthracyclines are a class of chemotherapy drugs of which Adriamycin® is a key member. Scientists determined that women with early-stage breast cancer who were HER2 negative derived absolutely no benefit from taking Adriamycin® or other anthracycline drugs.[12] Given that approximately 80% of breast cancers are HER2 negative, then only 1 out of 5 women with breast cancer can benefit from these drugs that have considerable toxicity associated with their use. In another study, 7% of patients treated with Adriamycin® developed congestive heart failure.[13]

There is a more enlightened, less toxic paradigm that tailors treatment towards the individual uniqueness of your cancer. And it works by exploiting cancer's fundamental weakness: sugar.

A key difference between cancer cells and healthy cells is that cancer cells run exclusively on sugar. Cancer cells have a ravenous need to consume the glucose (sugar) found in the blood stream. Glucose is their unique source of energy, and because of the relatively inefficient way cancer

149

cells burn this fuel, they use up a great deal of it. This is why cancer patients lose so much weight. Because cancer cells require so much glucose, they virtually steal it away from the body's normal cells, thus starving them.

To help sugar get inside the cancer cells, they are equipped with 10-16 times as many insulin receptors as healthy cells.[14] Insulin manages the delivery of glucose across cell membranes into the cells. Put another way, insulin escorts glucose through the cell membrane, into the interior where the glucose provides energy to keep the cell alive.

If you have had a PET/CT scan, you have seen this connection between sugar and cancer cells at work. A PET scan is performed by injecting a radioactive agent attached to a glucose molecule into a vein. The cancer cells, always ravenous for sugar, take up the glucose much faster than healthy cells. The radioactive agent gets into the cell along with the glucose. Bingo – the scan produces a three-dimensional picture of a cancerous mass.

Targeted Therapy

*N*ow, what would happen if, in addition to glucose, you add a little bit of chemotherapy to the mixture? Bingo – the chemotherapy drugs are taken up into the cancer cells. The healthy cells are not bombarded.

This paradigm is called IPT, Insulin Potentiation Therapy. Some people call it IPTLD, or Insulin Potentiation Targeted Low Dose therapy.

IPT uses about one-tenth the dosage of a conventional chemotherapy regime, and employs other complementary therapies to defeat your cancer while rebuilding your immune system. IPT provides a safer, much gentler alternative to conventional chemotherapy. Patients do not experience the severe side effects of conventional therapy – they generally do not go bald, nor do they experience severe nausea or organ damage. When combined with complementary therapies to nurture the body, it is also more effective. It is a smart way to approach cancer based on what makes cancer cells vulnerable.

IPT uses only 10% - 15% of the standard dose of chemotherapy agents.

The word "potentiate" means to make stronger or more effective. In this case, it means that insulin makes the chemotherapy more effective. A 1981 study conducted at George Washington University showed that when the chemotherapy drug, methotrexate, is combined with insulin, the drug's cell-killing effect increased by a factor of 10,000.[15] Because insulin enhances the effectiveness of the drugs, IPT uses only 10% – 15% of standard dose drugs. There is no need to overwhelm a patient with large quantities of drugs in the hope that the drugs will kill the cancer before they kill the patient's immune system.

There is a second way that insulin helps us defeat cancer. Insulin stimulates cells to grow, which they do by dividing.[16] Cancer cells are most vulnerable to many chemotherapeutic agents when they are dividing. With IPT, we use insulin's stimulating properties to catch more cancer cells in the process of dividing, so the drugs can be more effective than if division had not been encouraged.

A third way insulin helps is with detoxification. Insulin increases "cellular permeability." Glucose goes in easier, and the low dose chemo goes in easier. The door swings both ways – toxins and debris from dying tumor cells also pass out much easier. Insulin facilitates the detoxification so necessary with cancer.

IPT has been in use for more than 70 years, and is a standard form of cancer therapy all over Europe. In the United States, IPT has been largely ignored by conventional oncology.

Strengthen the Immune System

With IPT, we don't rely just on chemotherapy drugs to do the job. Therapeutic doses of vitamin C, administered intravenously, have been proven to defeat cancer cells, for example. The National Institutes of Health confirmed in 2005 that vitamin C is selectively toxic to cancer cells and that tumor-toxic levels of vitamin C can be attained using intravenous administration.[17]

Poly-MVA, or lipoic acid palladium complex, defeats cancer on an energetic level while helping the liver filter out spent chemo agents from the body.[18,19]

We make use of nutritional IVs, anti-oxidants like glutathione, various herbs and botanical preparations, coffee enemas, and chelation. Special attention is paid to nourishing the liver, the key organ for that all-important job of detoxification.

The culprit behind perhaps half the cancer deaths is a wasting syndrome called cachexia (pronounced "ka-**kek**-see-ah"). Patients lose weight and literally starve to death. Because cancer cells need even more energy than regular cells, the cancer cells gobble up the incoming nutrition first. Your healthy cells get what is left over which can mean the rest of your cells starve when conventional treatment leaves you too nauseated to eat. The tumor stays strong, but the patient wastes away. The hypoglycemic pulse that occurs with the administration of insulin actually helps the body assimilate the nutrition in food – vitamins, minerals, and enzymes.

Those of us who use IPT strongly believe it is more effective than conventional chemotherapy because IPT does not inflict the severe damage to the immune system that conventional chemo and radiation do; cancer is first and foremost a failure of the immune system. When combined with the chemosensitivity test, your physician is treating you with drugs to which the circulating tumor cells are sensitive. If your physician is also working simultaneously to rebuild the immune system, you've got the best of all worlds.

CASE STUDY

Although "Carole" had experienced GI issues for years, she had been doing a gluten-free diet and feeling fine. But one morning she passed out at the breakfast table. Surgery subsequently removed half her colon. I sent off a piece of the tumor to Germany for the BioFocus test so we would know what drugs and complementary therapies would be most effective.

As I write this, Carole has finished her twelfth IPT treatment, and we just did a blood test. She has a white blood cell count (WBC) of 4.2 and an absolute neutrophil count (the white cells that knock out infection) of 2.8. Both values are well within normal limits. Her initial WBC was 7.6 with 5.7 absolute neutrophils count, so she really did not lose much ground with the treatments.

This tells me the IPT has spared her immune system. After conventional chemo, within about 2 weeks you typically see a WBC of 1.0 or less. The white blood cells tend to get killed en masse by the bombardment of so much chemo; conventional chemo sessions are scheduled about 3-6 weeks apart because it kills so many neutrophils and they must regenerate before the chemo can be administered again; infection is a large and growing problem in conventional chemotherapy.

Carole has experienced no nausea, vomiting, hair loss, heart arrhythmias, ulcerations of the mucus membranes – all standard side effects of the chemotherapy drug Fluorouracil. She called me the day after her first treatment and said, "Martha, I feel wonderful." She often takes a nap after her treatments, but she is always up and about the next day – and she is in her 90s!

Prevention or Detection?

When you look at the array of organizations that concern themselves with cancer, you see a lot of emphasis on raising money for the cure and "awareness." For example, the National Breast Cancer Foundation (NBCF) says its mission "is to save lives by increasing awareness of breast cancer through education and by providing mammograms for those in need. The best way to fight breast cancer is to have a plan that helps you detect the disease in its early stages."[20]

So, in the world of conventional medicine, it's about detection and fighting it (chemotherapy) once you have cancer.

"Awareness of breast cancer": We are awash in pink ribbons every fall. Is anyone in the world not aware that breast cancer is a problem?

"Through education": That means an explanation of the signs, symptoms, and stages of breast cancer, according to the NBCF website. This is merely cancer 101, textbook information about the mechanics of cancer. There is nothing about how to prevent breast cancer, almost nothing about the environmental connection.

"Providing mammograms": They recommend an annual blast of radiation. Meanwhile, the only cause of cancer officially recognized by the American Cancer Society is radiation.

We didn't "fight" lung cancer. We insisted that the vested interests selling cigarettes finally tell the truth after 20-plus years of denial. We exposed the memos that covered up the dangers. We educated people about the harm of smoking so they would stop. We put warning labels on the cigarette packages. We stopped letting cigarettes be advertised on TV. We limited where cigarettes could be smoked in public. Because of all that, the incidence of lung cancer fell.

Taking on "Big Tobacco" was a huge undertaking. On behalf of cancer, one would need to take on "Big Food," "Big Pharma," the powerful chemical industry, and maybe the telecommunications industry. That's a tall order. No wonder so many people wanted to hear what Suzanne Somers had to say about standing up to the cancer establishment.

The Inconvenient Truth About Cancer Screenings

We do not have regular echocardiograms for heart disease, the number one killer in the United States. Yet breast cancer screening with mammography and prostate cancer screening with prostrate specific antigen (PSA) blood test has captured more customers than all other efforts combined. More than $20 billion is spent annually on screening for these two diseases. Campaigns have been so effective that about 75 percent of men have had a routine PSA test and about 70 percent of women older than 40 report they have had a recent mammogram.[21]

The U.S. Preventive Services Task Force revised the mammography guidelines in 2009, backing off on regular mammography exams. The

American Cancer Society tightened up their guidelines on PSA tests. Those were both good calls.

But the mammography recommendations triggered an uproar in large part because breast and prostate cancer screening runs counter to everything people have been told about cancer: The screenings are finding cancers that may well not need to be found because they would never spread and kill or even be noticed if left alone. That has led to a huge increase in cancer diagnoses and treatment because, without screening, those innocuous cancers would go undetected. Most cases of prostate cancer advance so slowly that a man will die of other causes before he would die of cancer.

The Task Force said the modest benefit of mammograms must be weighed against the harms — false positives, overtreatment, and radiation exposure. Research shows that although some lives are saved by early detection, many more may be damaged by biopsies and medical intervention applied to tumors that otherwise would disappear 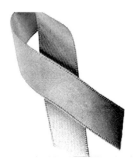 spontaneously. About three-quarters of the biopsies turn out to be benign, so three out of four women endure the needless fear that they have breast cancer — which is no small fear.[22]

Dr. John W. Gofman, an authority on the health effects of ionizing radiation, estimates that 75 percent of breast cancer could be prevented by avoiding or minimizing exposure to the ionizing radiation. This includes mammography, X-rays and other medical and dental sources.[23]

Let's see... Everyone admits radiation causes cancer... compression (squeezing) that takes place during a mammogram can spread cancerous cells... a cancerous mass is pretty far along by the time mammography can see it... So what if you could see the cancer forming years earlier without using radiation and compression?

This is the benefit of thermography.

As a tumor forms, it develops its own blood supply to feed its accelerated growth and this increased blood flow can increase the surface temperatures of the breast. Pre-cancerous tissues can start this process well in advance of the cells becoming malignant. Thermography measures the skin's autonomic response to that inflammation – its "heat signature." Modern thermography can detect suspicions of cancer's formation sometimes 10 years earlier than mammography.

Mammograms look at structure; they detect a cancerous mass. Thermograms look at systems; they can detect early suspicions of cancer formation. Thus thermography is clearly the better early warning system.

Thermography	Mammography
A functional test which detects the body's cutaneous sympathetic response to underlying inflammation.	An anatomic test which detects calcification and/or fairly large masses
Inflammation is detectable by thermography almost immediately	Does not detect early inflammatory change which eventually results in cancer
Early detection is best prevention	Tumor is detectable generally after it has been in the body for 10 years
No ionizing radiation – no radiation at all	Ionizing radiation
No compression (squeezing)	Compression (squeezing)
No problem with fibrous and dense breasts, or implants	Problem with fibrous and dense breasts, and with implants

In general, breast cancers come in three types: aggressive cancers that spread before they can be detected, cancers that spread slowly enough to be detected and treated early, and cancers that spread so slowly they pose no threat. Unfortunately, mammograms are best at detecting cancers in that last category and not in the first two, and there is no way to distinguish the cancers from each other without watching them progress. Thermography can detect the progression of early inflammation many years before mammography can detect a lesion.

Thermography has a lot going for it. Unfortunately, it is on the wrong side of the political divide.

Many people invested early on in mammography; thermography was viewed as a competitor. Lobbying efforts some years ago at the American Medical Association's House of Delegates and at Medicare brought 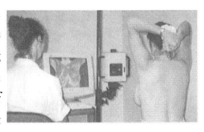 about the removal of thermography coverage by insurance companies. To this day, the American Cancer Society still promotes only mammography, despite its dangers.

Recent advances in technology have brought thermography to the point where it is now used as one of the diagnostic tools in two cancer research centers in North America.[24,25] Today, there are very strict protocols both for testing and interpreting. Perhaps due to these guidelines, thermography (unlike digital mammography) has exploded in its technique and capabilities. Thermography is increasingly the first choice for many women for early detection of breast disease.

Education is Prevention

An enlightened medical practitioner will spend a lot of time with patients educating them about environmental factors that can precipitate cancer, and how they can make lifestyle changes to reduce the risk of cancer in the future. You should hear about sugar, vitamin D, minerals, fats and oils, chemicals, dental toxicity, depleted thyroid and iodine, low levels of B vitamins, a deficiency of vitamin K, hormone-mimicking chemicals, oral contraceptives, obesity, pesticides, radon, heavy metals, mold, airport screening and medical X-rays, how EMFs from wireless technology interfere with the body's normal chemical signaling… Knowledge is power, and prevention is the best medicine.

Illness develops because the body is sending us a message. The message may be as simple as chemical toxins too numerous to handle (lung cancer in a smoker) or as complex as emotional toxins too hard to handle (childhood sexual abuse or rejection by the mother). Some stress has caused some of the cells in our body to stop responding to the normal traffic control. We express the illness in whatever organ is the most vulnerable either because of genetics or because of the message which needs to be delivered. Understanding and resolving that message can be key to keeping cancer from coming back for a second or third round.

RESOURCES

Breast Cancer Fund (www.breastcancerfund.org) – Not all organizations follow the money. The Breast Cancer Fund's stated mission: "To expose and eliminate the environmental causes of cancer. We can stop this disease before it starts." Yes we can. Kudos for staying on message and on task. The Breast Cancer Fund has a very well-designed website for education. And we absolutely love their "State of the Evidence," an easy to read, thoroughly-researched booklet on environmental causes of cancer and how to avoid them. We give it to our patients. It is a downloadable PDF file at their website.

Thermography Arizona (www.thermograpyArizona.com) is a source of all kinds of information about the use of this technology to identify cancer. Thermography can also look for changes in the abdomen which could indicate inflammatory bowel disease like colitis, ileitis or Crohn's disease. In sports medicine and pain management, it can map inflammation from neurologic or musculoskeletal dysfunction. It can also be of assistance in the evaluation of deep vein thrombosis or insufficiency of the blood supply.

---

[1]Gina Kolata. Forty Years War-Advances Elusive in the Drive to Cure Cancer, *New York Times*, April 23, 2009

[2]http://articles.latimes.com/2007/may/14/nation/na-cancer14

[3]Janet Gray, Nancy Evans, Brynn Taylor, Jeanne Rizzo, Marisa Walker. State of the Evidence-the Connection between Breast Cancer and the Environment. *International Journal of Occupational and Environmental Health*, Vol 15, No 1, 2009

[4]Environmental Working Group. Body Burden – the Pollution in Newborns. July 14, 2005. Downloaded from http://www.ewg.org/reports_content/bodyburden2/pdf/bodyburden2_final-r2.pdf

[5]http://www.cancer.gov/cancertopics/understandingcancer/genetesting/Slide27

[6]Leslie K. Dennis, Charles F. Lynch. Pesticide use and cutaneous melanoma in pesticide applicators in the Agricultural Heath Study. *Environ Health Perspect* :-. doi:10.1289/ehp.0901518

[7]http://mensnewsdaily.com/2009/07/19/hormone-replacement-therapy-hrt-ovarian-cancer

[8]CA Olsson, GM De Vries, et al. The use of RT-PCR for prostate-specific antigen assay to predict potential surgical failures before radical prostatectomy: molecular staging of prostate cancer. *Br J Urol.* March 7, 1996;7(3):411-7.

[9]S Meng, D Tripathy, et al. HER-2 gene amplification can be acquired as breast cancer progresses. *Proc Natl Acad Sci U S A.* June 22, 2004;101(25):9393-8.

[10]P. Wülfing, J Borchard, et al. HER2-positive circulating tumor cells indicate poor clinical outcome in stage I to III breast cancer patients. *Clin Cancer Res.* March 15, 2006;12(6):1715-20.

[11]Morgan G, Ward R et al. The contribution of cytotoxic chemotherapy to 5-year survival in adult malignancies. *Clin Oncol (R Coll Radiol).* 2004 Dec;16(8):549-60.

[12]A Gennari, MP Sormani, et al. HER2 status and efficacy of adjuvant anthracyclines in early breast cancer: a pooled analysis of randomized trials. *J Natl Cancer Inst.* January 2, 2008; 100(1):14-20.

[13]SM Swain, FS Whaley, MS Ewer. Congestive heart failure in patients treated with doxorubicin: a retrospective analysis of three trials. *Cancer.* June 1, 2003; 97(11):2869-79.

[14]Papa V, Pezzino V et al. Elevated insulin receptor content in human breast cancer. *J Clin Invest.* 1990 November; 86(5): 1503–1510.

[15] Lasalvia-Prisco E, Cucchi S et al. Insulin-induced enhancement of antitumoral response to methotrexate in breast cancer patients. *Cancer Chemother Pharmacol.* 2004 Mar;53(3):220-4.

[16]Scavo LM, Karas et al. Insulin-Like Growth Factor-I Stimulates Both Cell Growth and Lipogenesis during Differentiation of Human Mesenchymal Stem Cells into Adipocytes. *J Clin Endocrin Metab* 89;7:3542-3552.

[17] Casciari JJ, Riordan NH et al. Cytotoxicity of ascorbate, lipoic acid, and other antioxidants in hollow fibre in vitro tumours. *Br J Cancer.* 2001 Jun 1;84(11):1544-50.

[18] Lieberman S, Forsythe JW. Poly-MVA for Treating Prostate Cancer. *Alternative and Complementary Therapies.* August 2005, 11(4): 203-207. doi:10.1089/act.2005.11.203.

[19]Lieberman S, Forsythe JW. Poly-MVA for Treating Non–Small-Cell Lung Cancer: A Case Study of an Integrative Approach. Alternative and Complementary Therapies. April 2006, 12(2): 77-80. doi:10.1089/act.2006.12.77.

[20] http://www.nationalbreastcancer.org

[21]L Esserman, Y Shieh, I Thompson. Rethinking screening for breast cancer and prostate cancer, *JAMA.* 2009 Oct 21;302(15):1685-92.

[22]Saving Women's Lives: Strategies for Improving Breast Cancer Detection and Diagnosis. National Academy of Sciences 2005 publication.

[23]John W. Gofman, M.D., Ph.D. Radiation from Medical Procedures in the Pathogenesis of Cancer and Ischemic Heart Disease, C.N.R. Book Division, Committee for Nuclear Responsibility, Inc., San Francisco, 1999

[24]Arora N, Martins D et al. Effectiveness of a noninvasive digital infrared thermal imaging system in the detection of breast cancer. *Am J Surg.* 2008 Oct;196(4):523-6.

[25]Agnese DM. Advances in breast imaging. *Surg Technol Int.* 2005;14:51-6.

Cholesterol

$\mathcal{I}$t may be that 2008 will be remembered as the year the high cholesterol tune began to change and the old mantras began to give way to a more accurate understanding of heart disease.

The January 17th, 2008 cover story of *Business Week* openly questioned whether high cholesterol causes heart disease:[1]

> People like to have a metric, such as cholesterol levels, that can be monitored and altered. "Once you tell people a number, they will be fixated on the number and try to get it better," says University of Texas' Dr. Howard Brody. Moreover, "the American cultural norm is that doing something makes us feel better than just watching and waiting," says Brody. That applies to doctors as well. They are being pushed by the national guidelines, by patients' own requests, and by pay-for-performance rules that reward physicians for checking and reducing cholesterol. "I bought into it," Brody says. Not to do so is almost impossible, he adds. "If a physician suggested not checking a cholesterol level, many patients would stomp out of the office claiming the guy was a quack."
>
> Yet Brody changed his mind. "I now see it as myth that everyone should have their cholesterol checked," he says. "In hindsight it was obvious. Duh! Why didn't I see it before?"

It Started with Rabbits

$\mathcal{T}$he idea that cholesterol causes coronary heart disease started in the early 1900's when extremely high amounts of dietary cholesterol were fed to rabbits. Their blood cholesterol rose twenty-fold and a soft plaque-like substance formed on the coronary arteries. Cholesterol levels returned to normal and the plaque disappeared when the feeding was stopped.

In the early 1950s autopsies were done on heart attack victims and their arteries were found clogged with plaques containing high concentrations of cholesterol. And among servicemen who died in battle in Korea and Vietnam, more than 75 percent were found to have hardening and narrowing of the arteries. More evidence that cholesterol causes atherosclerosis.

> Arteries are normally smooth and unobstructed on the inside, but as you age, a sticky substance called plaque forms in the walls of your arteries. Plaque is made of lipids (cholesterol) and fibrin circulating in your blood. As more plaque builds up, your arteries can narrow and stiffen. Eventually, the soft plaque becomes calcified, and enough of it may build up to reduce blood flow through your arteries. Atherosclerosis increases your risk of heart disease, stroke, and other vascular diseases.

In the late 1950s, Ancel Keys proposed that the more saturated fat you ate, the higher your cholesterol. This gave birth to the "lipid theory" that dietary cholesterol is downright dangerous because it directly causes atherosclerosis. Based on this idea, people were told to eat a low fat diet and to embrace "heart-healthy" vegetables oils, despite the fact most were hydrogenated. A time-honored breakfast of steak and eggs, biscuits and gravy was now described as "a heart attack on a plate."

Yet despite increased sales of margarine and corn oil, rates of heart disease continued to climb.

Look again at those rabbits. They were given a synthetic form of cholesterol that easily oxidized when exposed to air. Oxidation makes cholesterol toxic to the body. Another key point – rabbits also do not metabolize cholesterol the way humans do. That's why mice are usually used in lab studies.

What might have accounted for atherosclerosis in American servicemen? The water given to servicemen was so heavily chlorinated it was virtually undrinkable. Chlorine is a powerful oxidizing agent that is capable of causing severe damage to blood vessels. There are few, if any, communities around the world with chlorinated drinking water that have a low incidence of atherosclerosis. In animal studies, chlorine has been found to promote the development of atherosclerosis.[2]

What of Ancel Keyes' findings? His data was seriously flawed. Probably the most painstaking analyses of the Keyes data was published in 2001 in a book entitled *The Cholesterol Myths* by Dr. Uffe Ravnskov:

> People with high cholesterol live the longest. This statement seems so incredible that it takes a long time to clear one's brainwashed mind to fully understand its importance. Yet the fact that people with high cholesterol live the longest emerges clearly from many scientific papers.[3]

For many years, researchers uncovered – and published – evidence that ran contrary to the "saturated fat and high cholesterol will kill you" mantra. For example, in 1994, Dr. Harlan Krumholz of the Department of Cardiovascular Medicine at Yale University reported that old people with low cholesterol died twice as often from a heart attack as did old people with high cholesterol.[4]

The Herd Mentality

But that kind of finding didn't make the evening news. Instead, the high cholesterol myth kept going and going and going like the Energizer Bunny. Why?

Here's an inside look at how things sounded in the 1980s from Mary Enig, a world renowned expert on fats (lipids) and oils:[5]

> The 1984 Cholesterol Consensus Conference final report [contained] no mention of the large body of evidence that conflicted with the lipid hypothesis. One of the blanks was filled with the number 200. The document defined all those with cholesterol levels above 200 mg/dL as "at risk" and called for mass cholesterol screening, even though the most ardent supporters of the lipid hypothesis had surmised in print that 240 should be the magic cutoff point. Such screening would, in fact, need to be carried out on a massive scale [because] the federal medical bureaucracy, by picking the number 200, had defined the vast majority of the American adult population as "at risk."

The Consensus Conference also provided a launching pad for the nationwide National Cholesterol Education Program, which had the stated goal of "changing physicians' attitudes." NHLBI-funded studies had determined that while the general population had bought into the lipid hypotheses, and was dutifully using margarine and buying low-cholesterol foods, the medical profession remained skeptical. A large "Physicians Kit" was sent to all doctors in America, compiled in part by the American Pharmaceutical Association, whose representatives served on the NCEP coordinating committee. Doctors were taught the importance of cholesterol screening, the advantages of cholesterol-lowering drugs and the unique benefits of the Prudent Diet. NCEP materials told every doctor in America to recommend the use of margarine rather than butter.

In 1988, the American Medical Association's Executive Vice-President, Dr. James Sammons, promised physicians their financial rewards, stating:

The AMA's campaign against cholesterol will bring both old and new patients to you for necessary testing, counseling and care.[6]

And many doctors took it to heart. As David S. Goodman of the Institute of Human Nutrition wrote in 1989:

... the current cholesterol campaign represents a rare concordance of interests on the part of many constituencies. ... Physicians will benefit because they will be providing better medical care to their patients and incidentally will have a new and expanded market of patients for preventive medical care. The pharmaceutical industry will benefit from the greatly expanded market for cholesterol lowering drugs that will result from even the most careful application of the guidelines on a national scale. The public will benefit from reductions in coronary risk...[7]

Ah, the silver bullet theory of medicine. A simple, convenient pill will fix everything.

Dr. Uffe Ravnskov put that in perspective:[8]

This is a dream come true for doctors. All that's necessary to prevent heart disease is a prescription pad and a gadget for measuring cholesterol – and no time-consuming fuss with diet counseling. And what a bonanza for the drug producers! A lifetime lowering of cholesterol with expensive drugs in a substantial proportion of the population.

In 2004, the National Cholesterol Education Program recommended that those "at risk" of cardiovascular events decrease their LDL levels to between 70 and 100 mg/dl.

The following year, sales of statin drugs ballooned 46% to over $22 billion.

"But besides real diseases, we are subject to many that are only imaginary, for which the physicians have invented imaginary cures; these have several names, and so have the drugs that are proper for them."   —Jonathan Swift (1667-1745)

Caught at the Scene of the Crime

Imagine your home security alarm system goes off, police respond. You arrive, determine you have been robbed – and blame the police officers still at the scene.

That is basically what happened to cholesterol.

Cholesterol is used by the body like a bandage for the healing process. When lesions are formed in arterial walls, LDL is dispatched to the site carrying cholesterol to mend the lesion and restore the waterproof feature to prevent clotting within the blood vessel. Serious damage to arteries can cause high amounts of cholesterol in a blockage due to the amount of cholesterol necessary to heal the lesions. This is why cholesterol has been associated with blockage of arteries. Cholesterol buildup may be part of the mechanism of blockages, but it is not the cause of the coronary disease resulting in blockages.

Half the people who have heart attacks have "normal" cholesterol levels. "If you follow the guidelines, you may be treating people who will never get coronary disease and you may not be treating people with coronary disease," said Carlos Ayers, director of the University of Virginia's vascular medicine and preventive cardiology program as long ago as 2001. [9]

Cholesterol is a response to something attacking the arteries.

Free Radicals Committed the Crime

Free radicals are unpaired electrons looking for a mate. They roam your body like a burglar looking to steal electrons from tissues. They are part of the body's immune mechanism that kills viruses and bacteria, and destroys toxins. An excess of them can cause tears and irritation in the artery walls. Excess free radicals are generated by the detoxification of environmental toxins like cigarette smoke, vehicle exhaust, and insecticides. Free radicals are also generated by what we eat like sugar, preservatives, aspartame, trans-fats, and vegetable oils.

We ingest free radicals when we eat foods prepared with processed vegetable oils – French fries, fried food, non-fat dried milk and homogenized milk,[10] powdered or liquid coffee creamer, most salad dressings, crackers, cookies, chips, and a plethora of other processed and convenience foods. Margarine, heavily promoted since the 1940s, was a tub of lethal trans fats until just recently. As some put it, we've been poisoning ourselves with vegetable oils, which mankind never ate in great quantity before. The dietary use of vegetable oils became widespread in America in the 1930s, about the same time atherosclerotic heart disease began to climb. Not only do corn and soy oils provide the oxidized fats that cause heart disease, they raise cholesterol levels in the process.[11] Processed vegetable oils have an unstable chemical structure. They are a free radical waiting to happen. When free radicals come in contact with the blood vessel, they cause lesions which trigger inflammation. LDL cholesterol molecules are dispatched to the scene to repair the lesion and stop the inflammation.

Free radicals from vegetable oils, however, are not the only reason for arterial plaque and lesions. There likely were lots of other "accomplices to the crime." Here are a few:

(1) Chlorine

During the 1960s Dr. Joseph Price wanted to know why cardiovascular heart disease, such as heart attacks, strokes, and atherosclerosis, had become so prevalent during that decade, when prior to 1900 it was virtually non-existent. His search led him to chlorine.[12]

Dr. Price reported that the Japanese people, who have a heart attack rate one-sixth that of the United States, develop atherosclerosis when they move to Hawaii and drink chlorinated water. When the Japanese were rebuilding their cities after WWI, they installed water purification systems using chlorine recommended by American engineers. Prior to this time they had never used it. Shortly thereafter, the Japanese medical community began to notice that the Japanese people were starting to have a lot of heart attacks. Their investigation led them to chlorine as the source of the causative factor. They discontinued the use of chlorine.

Chlorination of water supplies first began in 1908 in the United States, but it wasn't until 10 to 20 years later that heart attacks first began to increase. That's because unlike the soldiers in the Korean and Vietnam Wars who drank very high concentrations of chlorinated water, causing a faster rate of developing plaques on the blood vessel walls within a year or less, the public water supplies had much lower amounts which produced a slower rate of developing plaques over a 10 to 20 year period. It is also interesting to note that women with breast cancer have been found to have 50% to 60% more organochlorines in their breast tissue than women without breast cancer.[13] Does this reflect absorption of pesticides? Creation of organochlorine compounds within the breast tissue itself because of high chlorine levels in the water? We can only speculate.

(2) Low thyroid

Since the 1930s, it has been clearly established that suppression of the thyroid raises serum cholesterol while increasing mortality from infections, cancer, and heart disease. Restoring thyroid function often brings cholesterol down to normal.[14,15] By some estimates, more than half the population is running low on thyroid, and on the iodine required for production of thyroid hormone.[16,17] When thyroid function is poor, the body floods the blood with cholesterol as an adaptive and protective mechanism, providing a superabundance of materials needed to heal tissues and produce protective steroids. Why are we so low on iodine? One reason is because so much non-organic commercially produced bread since the 1980s contains bromide as a dough conditioner; bromide is a chemical cousin to chlorine. The body uses bromide as a substitute for the (unavailable) iodine, but it makes thyroid hormone that the body cannot use. Corn oil and soybean oil also suppress thyroid function.[18]

(3) Lack of Sunshine

Sunlight lowers cholesterol levels. Since the 1980s, we've been subject to an erroneous public relations campaign to stay out of the sun for fear of skin cancer. Sunlight converts the cholesterol on your skin to hormone precursors which are used to make steroid hormones like vitamin D. The cholesterol in your bloodstream then migrates to the surface of the skin, to replace the cholesterol that was converted. Staying out of the sun and routine use of sunscreens is an invitation to increased cholesterol levels.[19]

(4) Lack of Vitamin C

Dr. Linus Pauling met Dr. Matthias Rath, a German cardiologist, in July of 1983 at a Nobel Laureates meeting in Germany. Dr.

Rath shared with Dr. Pauling his hunch that if you were low in vitamin C you produced more LDL cholesterol. The reverse is also true; if you have more vitamin C, you produce less LDL cholesterol. Atherosclerosis appears to be a defensive mechanism so we don't bleed to death from scurvy – scurvy weakens blood vessels. Instead, we die later from heart disease. The formation of cholesterol plaques is the body's way of "patching" the vessel walls, weakened by a deficiency of vitamin C, zinc, copper and magnesium.[20]

Vitamin C is also the recycler of vitamin E which shields cells, fats, cholesterol and LDL from oxidation. Vitamin E is also a potent stimulant for production of prostanoids which dilate the arteries. Long-term or periodically low vitamin C weakens the connective tissue (made of collagen, elastin and 'cartilage proteoglycans') which then allows blood to enter the artery walls, thickening and hardening them with repair and clotting materials, with calcium and with cholesterol crystals. Muscle cells then multiply inside the connective tissue to strengthen the wall. Such thickened artery walls increase the risk for stroke and heart disease.[21]

(5) Stress

Some of those hormones made by cholesterol are the ones that help you handle stress. The more stress you have, the more corticosteroid hormones you need. When you lower cholesterol with drugs, you get more stress-related problems. High cholesterol in young and middle-aged men could, for instance, reflect the body's need for more cholesterol because cholesterol is the building material of many stress hormones. Any possible protective effect of high cholesterol may therefore be counteracted by the negative influence of the artificially lowered levels of cholesterol on the vascular system.

(6) Infection

For many years scientists have suspected that viruses and bacteria, in particular Cytomegalovirus and Chlamydia pneumoniae, participate in the development of atherosclerosis.

The role of infections in chronic heart failure has been studied by Dr. Mathias Rauchhaus of Martin Luther University in Halle, Germany. His research team found that the strongest predictor of death for patients with chronic heart failure was the concentration of cytokines in the blood, in particular in patients with heart failure due to coronary heart disease.[22] To explain their finding they suggested that bacteria from the gut may more easily penetrate into the tissues when the pressure in the abdominal veins is increased because of heart failure. In keeping with this theory, they found more endotoxin in the blood of patients with congestive heart failure and edema than in patients with chronic heart failure without edema, and endotoxin concentrations decreased significantly when the heart's function was improved by medical treatment.[23]

"Saturated fat and cholesterol in the diet are not the cause of coronary heart disease. That myth is the greatest scientific deception of this century, perhaps of any century."

—George V. Mann, M.D.
professor of Medicine and Biochemistry at Vanderbilt University

---

Statin Drugs — Bring 'em On

Statin drugs, which promise to lower cholesterol, are the best selling drugs on the market.

It appears their anti-inflammatory effects are the main source of their cardiac benefits, rather than their ability to lower cholesterol. Atheroscleosis is fundamentally an inflammatory disease.

"What the shrewd marketing people at Pfizer and the other companies did was spin it to make everyone with high cholesterol think they really need to reduce it," says Dr. Bryan A. Liang, director of the Institute of Health Law Studies at the California Western School of Law and co-director of the San Diego Center for Patient Safety.[24]

An estimated 25 million Americans take statin drugs at the constant urging and heavy pressure of the mainstream medical establishment.

Muscle pain and weakness are common side effects of statin drugs. To a lesser extent, so is diabetes. The JUPITER clinical trials first linked an increase in diabetes to Crestor®; a 2010 analysis of statin clinical trials suggests that some increased diabetes risk is linked to *all* statins.[25]

We have conclusive evidence of statins' profoundly destructive impact on the brain. A University of California-San Diego study found statins can provoke symptoms similar to Alzheimer's.[26] No wonder. Cholesterol is crucial to brain function. It protects nerve cells and literally speeds up your brain's operation in all areas, including your thought processes, recall, and speech. It's also the building block for synapses, the areas between nerve cells that transmit messages.

Some of the UCSD study subjects reported memory loss to the point where they couldn't recognize people they'd known for decades. Others found that statins had stripped them of their ability to concentrate, work, think clearly or even talk.

A February, 2008 column in the *Wall Street Journal* underscores the concern:

Cognitive side effects like memory loss and fuzzy thinking aren't listed on the patient information sheet for Lipitor ... [but] some doctors theorize that lowering cholesterol would slow the connections that facilitate thought and memory. ... "This drug makes women stupid," Oril Etingin, vice-chairman of medicine at New York Presbyterian Hospital, declared ... Anecdotes linking statins to memory problems have been rampant for years.[27]

Statin use may lead to cancer. Cholesterol-lowering drugs cause cancer in rodents at the equivalent doses used by man.[28] The extrapolation of evidence of cancer from rodent to human is very uncertain. This is the argument of those in favor of using cholesterol-lowering drugs. However, evidence from the cholesterol-lowering drug trial known as CARE (Cholesterol And Recurrent Events) showed that Pravachol (a cholesterol-lowering drug made by Bristol-Myers Squibb) was associated with a 1500% increase in breast cancer among women taking it. An increase in cancer rates among Pravachol users was also shown in the drug trial known as PROSPER. Many feel this side effect continues to fly below the radar because cancer typically takes a long time to develop and most of the statin trials do not go on longer than two or three years.

A 2008 paper published in the *American Journal of Cardiovascular Drugs* cites nearly 900 studies on the adverse effects of statins.[29]

In 2010, a research paper in the *British Medical Journal* warned doctors to think more carefully about prescribing cholesterol-lowering drugs because of their wide range of "unintended" side effects that include liver problems, kidney failure, muscle failure, and cataracts.[30]

Also in 2010, researchers re-examined the extremely influential JUPITER trial and found it was both flawed and biased – nine of 14 authors of the JUPITER trial had financial relationships with AstraZeneca, which sponsored the trial. The JUPITER trial basically said that if you give people who have not yet had heart trouble 20 mg of a statin drug, you will see a 44% reduction in nonfatal heart attacks and strokes, and confirmed death from cardiovascular causes. But when researchers re-examined the JUPITER data, they found no evidence of the "striking decrease in coronary heart disease complications" reported in the trial. "The results of the trial do not support the use of statin treatment for primary prevention of cardiovascular diseases and raise troubling questions concerning the role of commercial sponsors," the authors wrote.[31]

But most of all, why lower cholesterol by force when it is not the cause of heart disease?

Can't Live Without It

𝒞holesterol is something humans simply need – a lot.

Mother's milk contains a high ratio of cholesterol and saturated fat. It is critical for proper brain development of fetuses and growing children. Women in China have a tradition of eating perhaps 30 eggs a day when they are pregnant so they will have healthy, smart babies.

During puberty, the brain sprouts all sorts of new nerve cells. These cells have to make connections with each other, and the body needs the right kind of fats and cholesterol to do this.

Cholesterol is "the mother of all hormones." It is the precursor to all steroid hormones, including mineralocorticoids, glucocorticoids, and sex hormones. Thus cholesterol is a major player in athletic performance, regulating blood sugar, controlling blood pressure, regulating mineral balance, maintaining libido, building muscle mass, and more.[32]

It is also the raw material from which vitamin D and CoQ-10 are made. Vitamin D boosts the immune system and protects us from cancer; CoQ-10 acts like the catalytic converter in the mitochondria, removing excessive free electrons from the energy factory line.

All living creatures use cholesterol to make cells waterproof, a mechanism vital for proper function. The fact that cells are waterproof is especially critical for normal functioning of nerves and nerve cells. Thus, the highest concentration of cholesterol in the body is found in the brain and other parts of the nervous system.

Cholesterol forms 50 percent of the nervous system. A deficiency of cholesterol results in fatigue, obesity, nervous and emotional disturbances, digestive difficulties, impotence or inability to conceive and/or complete a pregnancy, menstrual syndromes and masculine traits in women, effeminate traits in men, blood pressure irregularities, fluid imbalances, nutritional deficits and imbalances, and more.

In addition to acting like the body's ever-ready bandage for arterial lesions, cholesterol is a potent antioxidant. It scavenges free radicals. It is flooded into the bloodstream when we take in too many harmful free radicals – usually from damaged and rancid fats in margarine and highly processed vegetable oils. This is the likely explanation for the fact that cholesterol levels go up with age. As an antioxidant, cholesterol protects us against free radical damage that leads to heart disease and cancer.[33] Those who have very low levels of cholesterol have a greater incidence of cancer.[34, 35, 36, 37, 38, 39]

Researchers at Texas A&M University found that lower cholesterol levels result in reduced muscle mass among older adults engaging in resistance exercise. Cholesterol serves as an essential building block for repair of the "micro-tears" that occur in muscle membranes stressed by exercise.[40]

You'll find about five ounces of cholesterol in the average person. Approximately seven percent of that, or one tablespoon, circulates in the blood. The less cholesterol comes from food, the more the body produces. Adults probably absorb only about 25 percent of the dietary cholesterol they consume.

Cholesterol is not water-soluble so it needs to travel through the bloodstream in little round orbs made of protein and fats called lipoproteins. These lipoproteins are categorized according to their density.

HDL means a High Density Lipoprotein and LDL means a Low Density Lipoprotein. HDL carries cholesterol to the liver from body tissues. LDL carries cholesterol away from the liver, where it is produced, to tissues including blood vessel walls.

Cholesterol is a poor risk factor for heart disease. Dr. Ronald M. Krauss, director of atherosclerosis research at the Oakland Research Institute, explained that higher LDL levels do help set the stage for heart disease by contributing to the buildup of plaque in arteries. But something else has to happen before people get heart disease. "When you look at patients with heart disease, their cholesterol levels are not that [much] higher than those without heart disease," he says. Compare countries, for example. Spaniards have LDL levels similar to Americans', but less than half the rate of heart disease. The Swiss have even higher cholesterol levels, but their rates of heart disease are also lower. Australian aborigines have low cholesterol but high rates of heart disease.[41]

Saturated Fat

Along with cholesterol, saturated fat has also been wrongly blamed for heart disease. The "lipid hypothesis" said saturated fat and cholesterol from animal sources raise cholesterol levels in the blood, leading to deposition of cholesterol and fatty material as pathogenic plaques in the arteries.

Saturated fat was a mainstay of mankind's diet for tens of thousands of years; atherosclerosis was not a problem until just recently. This part of the story has been well documented with research over the years, but still has not broken through the mainstream news barrier.

Heart disease is unknown today among the Eskimos who eat their traditional diet, primarily blubber. Heart disease is unknown today among the Masai of Africa who eat their traditional diet, primarily milk and meat, a diet rich in cholesterol and saturated fat.[42] George Mann's independent studies of the Masai in Africa, had convinced him that the lipid hypothesis was "the public health diversion of this century ... hundreds of millions of tax dollars are wasted by the bureaucracy and the self-interested Heart Association."[43]

In the early 1900s, half of all Americans lived on farms and ate lots of meats, raw whole milk, cream, butter, and eggs. Heart attacks were rare. But the nature of saturated fat has been changed by modern farming methods into a form which is unhealthy for the structure of the cell wall. Saturated fat has no strong links with disease, while industrially produced trans fats do.

Cattle, like all other ruminants, grow up eating green leafy plants, mostly grass. But industrialized farming puts them in feedlots toward the end of their lives where they eat grain, much of it genetically modified. Jo Robinson, an investigative journalist and best-selling writer, explains that red meat is not bad, it's the grain-fed, commercial cattle with 20:1 ratios of omega-6s to omega-3s that are the problem. Grass-fed beef ratios are about 1:1. Cultures who ate meat from grass-fed cattle didn't know what heart disease was.

Asking the Wrong Question?

$\mathcal{M}$illions of people have had their cholesterol levels tested, but only a tiny fraction ask about their triglycerides or understand why high triglycerides levels warrant more attention than high cholesterol levels. Why are most people – and many doctors – in the dark about triglycerides? Perhaps because there is no quick prescription pad answer for lowering triglycerides, the amount of fat circulating in the bloodstream.

When you eat, your body uses the calories it needs for quick energy. Excess calories are stored as fat regardless of what kind of food you eat – fat, carbohydrate, or protein. If you regularly eat more calories than you burn, you may have high triglycerides.

Also, kidney disease, obesity, and an underactive thyroid (hypothyroidism) may cause high triglycerides. Alcohol and sugar have a particularly strong effect on triglycerides.

In normal amounts, triglycerides are important to good health. When triglyceride levels are high, it is not clear whether these high levels directly increase your risk for heart disease. But high triglycerides are often part of a group of conditions called metabolic syndrome.

An elevated triglyceride blood level in and of itself is a strong and independent risk factor for heart attack among middle-aged and elderly men. In fact, studies have shown that blood triglyceride level was a stronger risk factor than total cholesterol alone. It is not known why women appear to be immune to this other than postulations that the high level of estrogen acts as a protective factor.

Triglycerides 101:[44]

- There are two main lipids found in the blood, cholesterol and triglycerides.

- A normal triglyceride level is less than 150 milligrams per deciliter (mg/dL), according to the National Cholesterol Education Program guidelines.
- When triglyceride levels reach 200 mg/dL, coronary artery disease risk doubles.
- Heart disease risk is considerably higher among women than men when triglyceride levels top 200 mg/dL.
- Extremely high levels of triglycerides may result in kidney disease and pancreatitis – a severe inflammation of the pancreas that may be life-threatening.
- Sepsis, a life-threatening condition caused by bacterial growth in the blood, is associated with a high level of triglycerides. The high level of triglycerides seen in sepsis is a normal immune response to infection.

Triglyceride levels are strongly influenced by diet. While cholesterol levels remain pretty constant over a month or so and aren't terribly affected by meals, triglycerides respond quickly to a meal, particularly one with a lot of fat, sugar, or alcohol.

There are two ways to control triglycerides: 1) Exercise regularly, and 2) eat a balanced diet that's low in sugar, simple carbohydrates, and processed foods.

Prevention is the Best Medicine

Drugs induce a false sense of security. You might force the body to stop making cholesterol, but do you really want to?

When you stop the manufacture of cholesterol, you also stop the manufacture of Coenzyme Q-10 (CoQ-10) which is crucial for function of the cell's energy factories known as mitochondria. This is one explanation for the muscle fatigue, muscle pain and congestive heart failure which can develop as a "side effect" of lipid-lowering drugs. Let us not forget that the heart is a muscle.

How to prevent arterial lesions and the resulting inflammation? Here is our Top Ten List:

1. Pick low glycemic foods like veggies, fruits, fish, and meat. Say no to chips of all kinds, ice cream, and potatoes and grains.

2. Think in terms of what causes free radicals. The short list of what to avoid includes trans fats, refined and synthetic sugars, food additives and preservatives, cigarette smoke, chlorine, and pesticides.

3. Increase your intake of vitamins B12, B6, and folic acid which can reduce levels of homocysteine, which damages the arteries and set the stage for disease. Fish oil helps curb inflammation, a most significant risk factor for heart attack. Increase your intake of vitamins C and E which neutralize free radicals that oxidize LDL cholesterol.

4. Stick with unrefined olive oil, unrefined coconut oil, butter, fish oils, and flax oil. Avoid margarine and vegetable oils like the plague.

5. Consider bringing your own butter and salad dressing to the office lunchroom and when you eat out.

6. Feed your thyroid. Virgin coconut oil has wonderful antimicrobial properties, and it stimulates your metabolism and increases thyroid function. Buy organic breads that do not use bromide. Use honest-to-goodness sea salt for its mineral content, including absorbable iodine; minerals influence thyroid activity.

7. Increase your exposure to sunlight. Your body needs about 15 minutes a day (without sunscreen and in a bikini bathing suit) to make enough vitamin D.

8. Come to terms with the sugar habit. Sugar increases triglyceride storage and cellular oxidative damage. This assaults the vascular wall, leading to micro-leakages in the endothelial wall of blood vessels, leading to the self-repair mechanism of

cholesterol. In medical lingo, sugar is a significant contributory factor to oxidative stress. Cuba, for example, has one of the highest levels of sugar use, and has a higher death rate from heart attacks in men between ages 55 and 64 than the U.S.[45]

9. Reduce systemic inflammation by searching out the triggers – allergies, leaky gut, and toxicities like chemicals and heavy metals.

10. Laugh more, stress less.

Treating abnormalities of blood chemistry requires effort and takes time.

A nutrition program can help people kick the sugar habit and migrate toward a diet that lessens inflammation overall in the body and heals the gut.

IV nutritional therapies can get a jumpstart on nutritional deficiencies. Intravenous vitamin C is excellent for reducing free radicals. We can treat heavy metal toxicity with chelation. We can determine allergies (food, pollen, chemical, etc) and treat those, to lessen the overall burden of inflammation and toxicity in the body.

Yes, the end result is worth it – a healthy lifestyle, a longer and healthier life... healthy old age... what could be better?

RESOURCES

The Weston A. Price Foundation's website is a source of many great articles on food and nutrition, including:

- Cholesterol and Heart Disease – A Phony Issue
- The Benefits of High Cholesterol
- Dangers of Statin Drugs: What You Haven't Been Told About Popular Cholesterol-Lowering Medicines
- What Causes Heart Disease?
- The Skinny on Fats

- The Oiling of America
- Dietary Recommendations for Children
- Milk Homogenization and Heart Disease
- Ancient Dietary Wisdom for Tomorrow's Children

BOOKS

Cholesterol Facts & Fantasies
by Judith A. DeCava, CNC, LNC, 2005

Coconut Oil Miracle
by Bruce Fife, 2004

The Cholesterol Myths
by Uffe Ravnskov, 2002

Eat Fat, Look Thin
by Bruce Fife, N.D., 2002

Know Your Fats: The Complete Primer for Understanding the Nutrition of Fats, Oils and Cholesterol
by Mary G. Enig, 2000

Cholesterol Conspiracy
by Russell L. Smith, Edward R. Pinckney, 1991

---

[1] John Carey. Do Cholesterol Drugs Do any Good? Research suggests that, except among high-risk heart patients, the benefits of statins such as Lipitor are overstated. *Business Week*, January 17, 2008

[2] Joseph G. Hattersley. The negative health effects of chlorine. *Townsend Letter for Doctors and Patients*, May 2003

[3] Uffe Ravnskov. The Benefits of High Cholesterol. *The Quarterly Journal of the Weston Price Association*

[4] H.M. Krumholz HM, et al. Lack of association between cholesterol and coronary heart disease mortality and morbidity and all-cause mortality in persons older than 70 years. *Journal of the American Medical Association* 272, 1335-1340, 1990.

[5] Mary Enig, PhD, and Sally Fallon. Oiling of America, 1999. Accessed at

http://www.westonaprice.org/knowyourfats/oiling.html

[6]Ray Gebauer. The Cholesterol Myth, accessed February 2008 at http://freehealthcontent.com/article_1722.shtml

[7]D.S. Goodman. Cholesterol Revisited: Molecule, Medicine and Media. *Arteriosclerosis*, 9, 430-438, 1989"

[8]Uffe Ravnskov. *The Cholesterol Myth*, p. 166

[9]Tara Parker-Pope. Tests Can Effectively Screen For Early Signs of Heart Disease. *Wall Street Journal*, June 22, 2001

[10]Weston A. Price Foundation

[11]Bruce Fife. *The Coconut Oil Miracle*. 2004

[12]Dr. Joseph M. Price. *Coronaries/Cholesterol/Chlorine*. Pyramid, NY. 1969.

[13]Charlie Skeen. Chlorine – A Crippler and Killer, Live Well Naturally Newsletter, September 24 , 2006

[14]Raymond Peat, Ph.D. Coconut Oil, newsletter of 1996, accessed February 2008 at www.efn.org/~raypeat/coconut.rtf

[15]Dr. Mark Starr. *Hypothyroidism Type 2-The Epidemic*. Mark Starr Trust, 2005

[16]Ibid

[17]Barnes, Broda, and L Galton. *Hypothyroidism, The Unsuspected Illness*, 1976, T Y Crowell, New York, NY

[18]Bruce Fife. *Eat Fat, Look Thin*. Picadilly Books, 2002

[19]Z.R. Kime, MD, MS. *Sunlight Could Save Your Life*, World Health Pubns, 1980

[20]Daniel P. Reardon, DDS, with Information from Harry S. Wilbur, DDS. Dentistry, Antioxidants and Atherosclerosis Have Strong Links. Price Pottenger Nutritional Foundation. Accessed February 2008 at http://www.ppnf.org/catalog/ppnf/Articles/Dent_Antiox_Arter.htm

[21]Daniel H. O'Leary, MD. et al; Carotid-Artery Intima and Media Thickness as a Risk Factor for Myocardial Infarction and Stroke in Older Adults, *New England Journal of Medicine*, Volume 340:14-22, January 7, 1999

[22]Rauchhaus M and others. Plasma cytokine parameters and mortality in patients with chronic heart failure. *Circulation* 102, 3060-3067, 2000.

[23]Niebauer J and others. Endotoxin and immune activation in chronic heart failure. *The Lancet* 353, 1838-1842, 1999.

[24] Carey, John. Do Cholesterol Drugs Do Any Good? *Business Week*, January 17, 2008

[25]Cannon CP. Balancing the benefits of statins versus a new risk-diabetes. *The Lancet* 2010; DOI:10.1016/S0140-6736(09)60234-6.

[26]B.A. Golomb. Impact of statin adverse events in the elderly. *Expert Opinion on Drug Safety*. 2005;4(3):389-397.

[27]Melinda Beck. Can a Drug That Helps Hearts Be Harmful to the Brain? *Wall Street Journal*, Health Journal. February 12, 2008

[28]Thomas B. Newman, et al. Carcinogenicity of Lipid-Lowering Drugs. *JAMA*, January 3, 1996-Vol 275, No. 1.

[29]Golomb BA, Evans MA. Statin adverse effects : a review of the literature and evidence for a mitochondrial mechanism. *Am J Cardiovasc Drugs*. 2008;8(6):373-418. doi: 10.2165/0129784-200808060-00004.

[30]Hippisley-Cox J, Coupland C. Unintended effects of statins in men and women in England and Wales: population based cohort study using the QResearch database. *British Medical Journal*, 2010 May 20;340:c2197. doi: 10.1136/bmj.c2197.

[31]Michel de Lorgeril, Patricia Salen et al. Cholesterol Lowering, Cardiovascular Diseases, and the Rosuvastatin-JUPITER Controversy. *Arch Intern Med*. 2010;170(12):1032-1036.

[32]Judith A. DeCava. *Cholesterol Facts and Fantasies*. Selene River Press, 2005

[33]Mary Enig, PhD, and Sally Fallon. *The Truth About Saturated Fat*. Weston A. Price Foundation

181

[34]G.N. Stemmermann et al. Sereum cholesterol and colon cancer incidence in Hawaiian-Japanese men. *Journal of the National Cancer Institute*, 67, 1179-1182, 1982

[35]D.L. Morris et al. Serum cholesterol and cancer in the hypertension detection and follow-up program. *Cancer*, 52, 1754-1759, 1983

[36]R. W. Sherwin et al. Serum cholesterol level and cancer mortality in 361,662 men screened for the multiple risk factor intervention trial. *Journal of the American Medical Association*, 257, 943-948, 1987

[37]C.G. Isles et al. Plasma cholesterol, coronary heart disease, and cancer in the Renfew and Paisley survey, *British Medical Journal.* 298, 920-924, 1989

[38]S.J. Winawer et al. Declining serum cholesterol levels prior to diagnosis of colon cancer. A time-trend, case control study. *Journal of the American Medical Association*, 263, 2083-2085, 1990

[39]L.D. Cowen et al. Cancer mortality and lipid and lipoprotein levels. The Lipid research Clinics' program mortality follow up study. *American Journal of Epidemiology*, 131, 468-482, 1990

[40]Riechman SE, Andrews RD, MacLean DA, Sheather S. Statins and dietary and serum cholesterol are associated with increased lean mass following resistance training. *J Gerontol A Biol Sci Med Sci.* 2007 62: 1164-1171.

[41]John Carey. Do Cholesterol Drugs Do any Good? Research suggests that, except among high-risk heart patients, the benefits of statins such as Lipitor are overstated. *Business Week*, January 17, 2008

[42]Mann, G V, et al. "Atherosclerosis in the Maasai." *Am J Epidemiol,* 1972, 95:26-37

[43]Coronary Heart Disease. The Dietary Sense and Nonsense, George V Mann, ed. 1993. Veritas Society, London

[44]Harris HW, Gosnell JE, Kumwenda ZL. The lipemia of sepsis: triglyceride-rich lipoproteins as agents of innate immunity. *Journal of Endotoxin Research* 6, 421-430, 2001.

[45]Judith DeCava. *Cholesterol, Facts and Fantasies*, Selene River Press, 2005

Chronic Disease and Inflammation

*C*hronic inflammation feeds a smorgasbord of chronic diseases. If you don't have a chronic disease yourself, you know someone who does. An estimated 80 percent of visits to doctor's offices are for issues relating to chronic disease. The CDC tells us 7 of every 10 Americans die of a chronic disease.

Chronic inflammation gradually destroys an otherwise beautiful machine.

If you hit your thumb with a hammer, the resulting swelling and inflammation is obvious, painful, and short lived. Your immune system sends white blood cells and other hormone-like substances to help start the healing process. Inflammation serves a healthy purpose.

Inflammation is the life-saving component of your immune system that helps fend off bacteria, viruses, fungi, and other microbial invaders. Without inflammation we would be sitting ducks in a very hostile world, with no way to repair the damage that we sustain.

But inflammation has a dark side if it isn't turned off.

CHRONIC DISEASE

- Persistent or recurring disease, usually affecting a person for three months or longer
- Generally triggered by diet and environmental contaminants
- Standard allopathic medicine believes such diseases can be managed but rarely cured
- Includes allergies, Alzheimer's, arthritis, asthma, cancer, COPD, Crohn's, chronic fatigue, cystic fibrosis, diabetes, emphysema, fibromyalgia, Gulf War Syndrome, heart disease and stroke, high blood pressure, Lyme, lupus, multiple sclerosis, obesity, osteoporosis, depression, anxiety, PTSD, ulcerative colitis and more.

The Persistent Stimulus

*I*nflammation goes chronic when there is a persistent stimulus. The stimulus might come from an army of free radicals launched every day when we eat foods made with inflammatory processed vegetable oils. The stimulus might be an allergy to wheat (gluten) which inflames the gut. Or a growing body burden of heavy metals, pesticides, and chemicals. Or a low-grade, lingering infection from an old injury, insect bite or root canal. There is a lot of opportunity in today's contaminated, junk food-filled world for a combination of factors to constantly impede the body's normal functions.

Chronic inflammation falls below the threshold of perceived pain. You don't feel sick – in fact, you don't even think about it – but a fire is quietly smoldering within you, upsetting the delicate balance among the major systems: endocrine, central nervous, digestive, and cardiovascular/ respiratory. In a healthy body, these systems communicate with each another. With chronic inflammation, that communication becomes distorted.

Medical schools don't teach much about the inflammatory effects of food, toxic chemicals, and electrosmog (EMF) so the medical profession has been slow to appreciate the extent of the problem. "Researchers are linking inflammation to an ever-wider array of chronic illnesses," reported *Newsweek*'s Anne Underwood in 2005. "Suddenly medical puzzles seem to be fitting together, such as why hypertension puts patients at increased risk of Alzheimer's, or why rheumatoid-arthritis sufferers have higher rates of sudden cardiac death. They're all connected on some fundamental level."[1]

Dr. Barry Marshall and Dr. Robin Warren turned medical dogma on its head by proving that bacteria — not stress — caused ulcers. Some 20 years after their discovery, having endured a storm of criticism from the medical establishment, the pair was awarded the Nobel Prize for Medicine. Their work stimulated research into inflammatory role microbes may have with other chronic inflammatory conditions, such as rheumatoid arthritis and atherosclerosis.

Heart Attacks, Cancer, Alzheimers, Arthritis…

*C*hronic inflammation has a damaging effect on arteries, which can lead to heart attacks and strokes. Microorganisms and viscous (thick, sticky) blood cause inflammation and tiny wounds within the lining of the blood vessels. Immune cells are dispatched to heal the wounds, and then cholesterol is laid down over the wound like a bandage, to allow the wound to heal. However, the inflammation is still active under that bandage. In time, the bandage bulges. In time, maybe a small part of the blood vessel gives way. Whoops! Now the body has to put a finger in the dyke. It uses a blood clot to do that. But if the clot breaks loose and goes to the brain, you have a stroke. If it goes to the heart, you have a heart attack. If it goes to the leg, you have emergency bypass surgery to salvage the leg – or else you just have a dead leg, without blood supply.

Statin drugs were developed to limit cholesterol. But suppressing cholesterol production is not a good way to address the problem. Recently, we are hearing that statins' best asset may be their anti-inflammatory properties. Although drugs can suppress the inflammation, they do not put out the fire. They don't bring a cure.

Chronic inflammation depresses the immune system and helps promote the formation of cancerous tumors. A substantial body of evidence supports the conclusion that chronic inflammation can predispose an individual to cancer as demonstrated by the association between chronic inflammatory bowel diseases and the increased risk of colon carcinoma. The longer the inflammation persists, the higher the risk of associated carcinogenesis.[2]

Chronic inflammation can play out in numerous ways. In some people, it destroys nerve cells in the brains – Alzheimer's patients. The inflammation in a joint can eat away at cartilage and you've got a serious case of arthritis. In rheumatoid arthritis, the inflammation is systemic, eating away at the entire body, an autoimmune disorder. Inflammation of kidneys is known as nephritis and may cause kidney failure or high blood pressure. Unchecked inflammation in the pancreas can cause both pancreatitis, a potentially fatal disease, and type 1 diabetes, in which the pancreatic islet cells that produce insulin are destroyed. Inflammation of the small airways that transport air to the lungs may cause an asthma attack or chronic bronchitis.

What determines how inflammation will affect you? Your genes play a part. If arthritis runs in your family, then you very possibly have a genetic weak link in that regard and you are likely prone to arthritis. For someone else, the genetic weak link may make them prone to cancer or Crohn's Disease.

The Obesity Connection

Not all body fat is the same. The fat we use as energy in between meals, and the fat that pads our organs, is different from the kind of fat that collects around our middle and makes us overweight. In the overweight fat, the cells become more biochemically active, churning out inflammatory compounds. As obesity ratchets up inflammation, inflammation in turn promotes insulin resistance, a central feature of diabetes and the metabolic syndrome that precedes it.

Some of the excess weight comes from excess calories, and some comes from toxins stored in our fat cells. Our bodies have become virtual dumping grounds for the tens of thousands of toxic compounds that invade our everyday world, setting the stage for a slow decline in health.

Getting rid of that hormonally active belly fat is often crucial for people with a chronic disease because it fuels the slow burning fires of chronic inflammation. Detoxification is something best done under skilled medical supervision. Toxins not only need to be released, but they have to be "escorted" out of the body or they merely resettle in other locations. Additionally, the various organs of the body need to be well supported throughout the process.

C-Reactive Protein

$\mathcal{A}$ critical inflammatory marker is C-reactive protein. This marker measures inflammation in the arteries that can cause heart attacks. A study reported in the *New England Journal of Medicine* showed that people with high levels of C-reactive protein were almost three times as likely to die from a heart attack.[3] C-reactive protein is regulated by proinflammatory cytokines, such as interleukins IL1 and TNF-α.

In a study published in the July 18, 2001 issue of the *Journal of the American Medical Association*, a group from the famous Women's Health Study was evaluated to ascertain what risk factors could predict future development of type 2 diabetes.[4] The findings showed that baseline levels of C-reactive protein and interleukin-6 were significantly higher among those who subsequently developed diabetes compared to those who did not.

In January, 2003, the American Heart Association and CDC jointly endorsed the C-reactive protein test to screen for coronary-artery inflammation to identify those at risk for heart attack.

However, those who partake of medicine as dictated by insurance companies usually do not get tested. Insurance companies have been reluctant to reimburse for the test.

Food is Information

$\mathcal{F}$ood is a big key to chronic inflammation.

Consider what our great-grandmother had to eat; she lived in a time when chronic inflammation and chronic diseases were almost unheard of. Everything came from a farmer's field, nothing from a food chemist's laboratory. Nothing was homogenized, refined, or processed. There was no need for "nutrition labels" because food was not so altered and compromised that it required labels to be recognizable as food.

Your great-grandmother's food had *information*. Eat the wrong information and you give your genes instructions to make you fat. Eat the

187

right information and you give your genes instructions to lose weight. Our great-grandmother ate lots of butter, eggs, raw milk, and grass-fed meats. Fat and cholesterol? If she lived on a farm, she ate a lot of it. Her pantry bore almost no resemblance to the modern pantry full of food "products" in bags with a long shelf life. And she got lots of sunshine – vitamin D is anti-inflammatory and anti-cancer.

An anti-inflammatory diet is rich in vegetables, antioxidants like fruits, and anti-inflammatory spices like curcumin, ginger, and turmeric.[5] Gluten grains – wheat, rye, barley – are inflammatory for many people so they are not included in an anti-inflammatory diet. Nor are refined carbohydrates (pasta, chips, crackers, cookies) and homogenized milk. The acidity of coffee and soda is thought to contribute to chronic inflammation in many people. Processed meats like hot dogs and sausages contain chemicals associated with increased inflammation and chronic disease.

AGEs – advanced glycation end products (also called glycotoxins) – are naturally present in our bodies, but we drastically add to them by eating foods cooked at high temperatures. AGEs are excreted by the kidneys, whose capacity may be easily exceeded. As the level of AGEs builds up, cells start to signal the production of inflammatory cytokines. In general, frying, roasting, broiling, and "blackened" (not the spices, but the heat used for cooking) BBQ result in increased formation of AGEs.

It goes without saying that health requires you to cut out the junk foods. But it is difficult to get the straight story on good versus bad fats.

Good Fats are Anti-Inflammatory

Good fats cleanse and lubricate the body. They provide the building blocks for cell membranes and a variety of hormones and hormone-like substances which we need. Fats act as carriers for vitamins A, K, D & E. Good fats enhance immune function. They also defend against depression because so much of our brain is fat. They also are a concentrated source of energy and give us that feeling that we are "full" and should stop eating.

Here is an easy chart to go by:

188

Good Fats	Bad Fats
Butter, tallow (from beef), and coconut oil are the best anti-inflammatory fats.	Shortening, margarine, and "spreads."
Lard (from pork). This is what grandma cooked with before the vegetable oil industry kicked into gear. She did not use fats preserved with BHT.	Anything hydrogenated or partially hydrogenated. Higher levels of trans fatty acids are strongly associated with systemic inflammation in patients with heart disease.[6] Have also been implicated in cancer.
Traditional vegetable oils – coconut oil and palm oil are both rich sources of lauric acid, which has strong antifungal and antimicrobial properties. Extremely stable with high smoking points, so they can be used in baking, frying, sautéing. Also sesame oil, another traditional vegetable oil.	Vegetable oils (corn, soy, canola, safflower, cottonseed). Produced with toxic chemicals and high temperatures. High in inflammatory omega-6s. Canola oil and soy oils – lots of negative research. Most of these products are extracted from genetically modified plants.
The monounsaturated oils (olive, avocado) in small amounts - can be inflammatory if there is too much. Olive oil – a good base for salad dressings, smoking point is too low.	Commercial salad dressings are typically made from processed vegetable oils. (Make your own with olive oil and balsamic vinegar and a dollop of honey mustard.)
Cod liver oil - High in vitamins A and D. Omega-3 fatty acids are the building blocks of anti-inflammatory hormones. Flax oil – good source of omega-3 fatty acids, but take in small amounts. Not good for cooking.	Fish oil – usually an industrial product.
Whole cheeses, eggs, grass-fed meat.	Skim milk cheeses, low fat yogurt, soybean imitation products.
Nuts – walnuts, almonds, pecans, macadamia nuts have a mix of good fats.	Peanuts – often carry a mold that causes allergies, generally roasted in a vegetable oil.

Getting a Bum Steer on Diet

For years, Americans have been given inaccurate information on diet – remember the carbs-are-good-for-you and resulting pasta craze of the 1980s? Today, we are still being given inaccurate nutrition advice on fats. Studies done after World War II comparing coconut oil to the new vegetables oils made coconut oil look awful. However, those studies used hydrogenated coconut oil.[7] Until recently saturated fats were usually lumped together with trans fats in the various U.S. databases that researchers use to correlate dietary trends with disease conditions.[8]

Butter is bad for you, eat margarine, says the American Heart Association (AHA). We know soda pop is not good for us – the phosphoric acid weakens bones, and the sweeteners are much to blame for the obesity epidemic. Yet the American Dietetic Association proudly states, "PepsiCo: License to Snack. PepsiCo and ADA are working together to develop education programs that help consumers make improved choices and promote healthful, active lifestyles." For several years, the ADA had a nutrition fact sheet on "Balancing Calories and Optimizing Fats" sponsored by two makers of mayonnaise. Their fact sheet on canola oil, "Good for Every Body," was sponsored by the Canola Council. Their fact sheet on dietary fats was sponsored by the company that makes Promise margarine. These drew criticism. In 2009, this kind of over-the-top corporate influence disappeared from their fact sheets.

But the take-home message is the following: know that there are lots of corporate sponsorships that heavily influence the messages in TV ads and on websites. Don't confuse objective information with marketing efforts. Organizations dependent upon sponsorship from food and drug manufacturers are often marketing vehicles for those manufacturers. In the public relations business, this is called a third party endorsement. If you want objective nutritional advice based upon solid expertise, you often need to go elsewhere.

Holistic versus Component Approaches to Medicine

Conventional medicine tends to specialize. A cardiologist looks at your heart, a pulmonologist looks at your lungs, and so on. Treatment is symptom-specific and targets one component of your body. Conventional treatment makes use of pharmaceutical drugs to suppress the inflammatory mechanism. Although pain medications can be very effective at providing temporary relief, they are powerless to stop what's causing the inflammation in the first place.

It takes an integrative approach to put out the fire:

- Test for allergies to food and chemicals.
- With chelation, you can reduce the heavy metal and viral burden in your body.
- With nutritional guidance, you can create an anti-inflammatory diet for a lifetime.
- With acupuncture, many find a drug-free alternative to alleviate pain.
- With colonics, you can reduce the overall toxic burden by emptying and washing out the colon which then frees it to accept more of what needs to be eliminated.

Sometimes the triggers for chronic disease are on the energetic level. It is often said, for example, that rheumatoid arthritis befalls people who are self critical and heart attacks befall the type A personalities who are always pushing themselves. Depression can occur as the result of *in utero* exposure to a mother's depression – the child comes to think that the level of hormones associated with depression are normal and attempts to mirror the same level via its own neurotransmitters.

The Chinese describe fire as one of the five elements in the body that foster life. Just as summer gives way to fall, fire represents the height of activity before a decline and rest. It is a necessary part of a balanced system.

But if the balance is upset and fire takes over, then the system burns itself out. The result is early disease and decline into chronic illness.

The benefits of reducing inflammation are immediate as well as long term. You will notice that your skin looks younger, your joints feel better, and your allergy symptoms improve. At the same time, when you reduce inflammation, you also reduce your risk of chronic disease and complications of aging.

RESOURCES

The Price Pottenger-Nutrition Foundation and the Weston A. Price Foundation is a favorite source of dietary wisdom.

You can watch a YouTube video describing a traditional diet by searching YouTube for "Weston A Price Foundation – Educational Television"

---

[1]Anne Underwood. Quieting a Body's Defenses-Researchers are linking inflammation to an ever-wider array of chronic illnesses but treatments that block the inflammatory response can backfire. *Newsweek*, June 10, 2005

[2]Emily Shacter. Chronic Inflammation and Cancer, *Oncology*, 16:217-232, 2002

[3]Ridker PM, Rifai N et al. Comparison of C-Reactive Protein and Low-Density Lipoprotein Cholesterol Levels in the Prediction of First Cardiovascular Events. *N Engl J Med* 2002; 347:1557-1565

[4]Pradhan AD, Manson JE et al. C-Reactive Protein, Interleukin 6, and Risk of Developing Type 2 Diabetes Mellitus. *JAMA.* 2001;286:327-334.

[5]Anne Underwood. Quieting a Body's Defenses-Researchers are linking inflammation to an ever-wider array of chronic illnesses but treatments that block the inflammatory response can backfire. *Newsweek*, June 10, 2005

[6]Dariush Mozaffarian, Eric B Rimm, Irena B King, Richard L Lawler, George B McDonald, and Wayne C Levy. *trans* Fatty acids and systemic inflammation in heart failure. *Am J Clin Nutr* 2004 80: 1521-1525.

[7]Enig, Mary G, PhD. *Nutr Quarterly*, 1993, 17:(4):79-95

[8]Enig, Mary G, PhD. *Trans Fatty Acids in the Food Supply: A Comprehensive Report Covering 60 Years of Research*, 2nd Edition, Enig Associates, Inc, Silver Spring, MD, 1995, 148-154; Enig, Mary G, PhD, et al, *J Am Coll Nutr*, 1990, 9:471-86

Chronic Fatigue and Fibromyalgia

Chronic fatigue syndrome (CFS) and fibromyalgia have intertwined symptoms and can be virtually indistinguishable. The British call these two conditions encephalomyalgia (head and muscle achiness) and the Chinese call them energy trapped between the skin and the muscle – the energy is stuck there. You are tired and you hurt.

The simplest way to put it is that both of these conditions are products of living in a polluted world. Both are characterized by fatigue – the body cannot generate enough energy to keep us going. And both are characterized by pain – the body's call for help because something is wrong. Both CFS and fibromyalgia can devastate people's lives.

Both can be overcome by removing the blockages to healing – whatever is holding the body back from righting itself. It may mean getting rid of inflammatory foods – some common food allergies like gluten (wheat) and casein (milk) attack the nervous system and make you tired. Many people feel hopelessly "brain fogged" because they have leaky gut from poor diet and the neurotransmitters in the gut are not functioning well. Other people have had so many courses of antibiotics, their gut flora can't support a reasonable immune system. Some people turn around dramatically when they reduce their heavy metals load with chelation. Others need to remove solvents (VOCs) from their tissues. And evidence is growing that the electromagnetic frequencies which bombard us every day weaken the ability of our cells to do their job.

Healing comes when we reverse the downward spiral of various dysfunctions that show up as fatigue and pain.

Chronic Fatigue Syndrome

Chronic fatigue (immune deficiency) syndrome, CFIDS, is not a condition which fits neatly into the allopathic model of illness. Diagnosis is made by ruling out all other "treatable" causes of fatigue. The symptoms make the diagnosis. Patients describe debilitating fatigue, persistent for more than six months. Patients also describe problems with focus and memory – they are often diagnosed with depression or other neuro-psychiatric labels.

The syndrome is estimated to affect almost 1% of the population, and is not limited to white Caucasian middle aged females, as previously thought, but is found in all age groups, races, and economic strata.[1] About twice as many women as men are affected.

Diagnostic criteria, as defined by the International Chronic Fatigue Syndrome Work Group:[2]

clinically evaluated, unexplained, persistent or relapsing chronic fatigue that has not been lifelong; that is not the result of ongoing exertion; is not substantially alleviated by rest; and results in substantial reduction in previous levels of occupational, educational, social, or personal activities;

and

four or more of the following symptoms, all of which must have persisted or recurred during six or more consecutive months of illness and must not have predated the fatigue:

- self-reported impairment in short-term memory or concentration severe enough to cause substantial reduction in previous levels of occupational, educational, social, or personal activities
- sore throat
- tender cervical or auxilliary lymph nodes
- muscle pain
- multi-joint pain without joint swelling or redness
- headaches of a new type, pattern, or severity
- unrefreshing sleep
- postexertional malaise lasting more than 24 hours

CFS is often a mixed bag of infections, allergies, food and chemical sensitivities, hormonal imbalance, nutritional imbalances, and abnormal immune system activity with the production of too many inflammatory cytokines.

One school of thought is that CFS is a free radical disease involving damaged mitochondria. We have some 60 trillion cells in our body and each one has a large number of "generators" inside called the mitochondria. To make energy, these mitochondria send electrons in the form of ATP to the muscles. If the muscles don't have enough fuel, we feel very tired, achy, and depressed. The mitochondria can be damaged by toxins in our modern world – damaged by chemical sensitivities, allergic reactions, exposure to electrosmog, viruses, bacteria, yeast toxins, chronic hypothyroidism, and more.

Mitochondrial dysfunction results in oxidative stress and excess generation of free radicals which are damaging to the cell and to its DNA.[3,4,5] We can relieve oxidative stress by taking antioxidants like CoQ-10, glutathione, vitamin C, vitamin E and other similar substances. This simple approach can go a long way toward improving mitochondrial function and relieving the symptoms of chronic fatigue.[6,7]

CFS patients typically have an excessive body burden of heavy metals. Heavy metals can reduce the ability of enzymes to do their job. When enzymes cannot fulfill the needs of the cells' biochemical reactions, the body experiences fatigue. Mitochondrial function is significantly disturbed by heavy metals.[8] Chelation can reduce the level of heavy metals.

Food intolerance has been shown to increase inflammatory mediators in the body[9] and to activate the immune system.[10] Food intolerance has also been shown to be related to several other dysfunctions commonly associated with chronic fatigue syndrome: asthma or respiratory distress,[11] inflammatory bowel disease,[12] irritable bowel syndrome (IBS).[13] Intolerance to gluten (wheat, barley, rye and a few other grains) can result in neurologic symptoms like extreme fatigue without any intestinal symptoms at all. An investigation of gluten intolerance and other food sensitivities should be part of an initial work-up.

Decreased production of neurotransmitters in the central nervous system is often a factor.[14] People with CFS seem to have abnormal levels of some chemicals regulated in the brain system known as the hypothalamic-pituitary-adrenal axis. Some patients with CFS have abnormally high levels of serotonin and low levels of cortisol.

Chronic viral infection plays a big role in CFS.[15] When health declines, pathogens move in and set up housekeeping. Some commonly performed tests look for Epstein-Barr virus and other viruses, Candida albicans (yeast), and immunologic functions.

Many people, including author Dr. William Crook, feel yeast is the missing link to both CFS and fibromalgia. "People with these disorders seem to develop them because their immune systems are weakened (by yeast overgrowth), viruses are activated, yeasts multiply, food and chemical allergies become activated, and nutritional deficiencies develop."[16] Prior use of birth control pills and antibiotics, and a diet high in sugar play a big role in the overgrowth of Candida albicans.

"CFS will disappear when we are smart enough to diagnose all the different infections and all the different toxicities that can cause chronic fatigue," says Dr. Murray Susser who wrote one of the first groundbreaking books on CFS. "Lyme is a perfect example. Lots of these people we've labeled with CFS have Lyme disease."[17]

Other factors that appear to play a role in CFS

- Anesthesia and surgery – many people see that their CFS started after an operation; anesthesia is a selective and reversible toxin that puts enormous demands on the immune system
- Degenerative diseases such as cancer and heart disease
- Drug reactions (including addiction) – drugs are poisons which use up nutrients required by the immune system
- Fibromyalgia

- Low thyroid and thyroiditis – thyroid controls our metabolism, the rate at which our cells burn oxygen and fuel
- Chronic exposure to low level electromagnetic radiation – microwave ovens, call phones, electric alarm clocks, and medical X-rays all appear to suppress the immune system in vulnerable people

Fibromyalgia

Fibromyalgia (FMS) was first recognized by the American Medical Association as an illness and a cause of disability in 1987. A physician named Don Goldenberg named the syndrome "fibromyalgia" in an article in the *Journal of the American Medical Association* that same year.

The universal symptom of fibromyalgia is pain. FMS is characterized by widespread, debilitating pain involving the muscles, the joints – almost any area of the body.

Usually when the body has pain, inflammation is present. But this is not necessarily the case with fibromyalgia. People with FMS can experience pain throughout their entire body without any damage or apparent inflammation of the peripheral tissues.

According to the National Fibromyalgia Association, 10 million Americans suffer from it. Most of them are women.

There is no blood or X-ray test that can diagnose fibromyalgia. The diagnosis is based upon the patient's history and physical examination. Widely accepted criteria created by the American College of Rheumatology define fibromyalgia by two things:

- A history of widespread pain lasting more than 3 months and affecting all 4 quadrants of the body (left side, right side, below the waist, above the waist).
- Upon examination, a finding of pain at 11 or more of 18 defined "tender points."

While these criteria for classification of patients were originally established for research purposes, they have become the de facto diagnostic criteria.

Fibromyalgia is characterized by diffuse pain, but is often accompanied by other "functional" conditions like irritable bowel syndrome, migraine headaches, chemical sensitivity, Raynaud's phenomenon[18] and chronic fatigue, making it often difficult to reach a definitive diagnosis.

Because of the difficulty of diagnosis, and because so many patients also reported cognitive difficulties, for years the conventional medical community was quick to tell patients that "it's in your head." But patients instinctively knew better. So they shuffled from one doctor to another as they continued to search for what was wrong. Many physicians believed that FMS was mainly a disguised form of psychological distress or depression.

The Pain is Real

New research since 2003 demonstrates that FMS is indeed real, not imagined.

Daniel Clauw, M.D., of the University of Michigan, has done much to legitimize the pain of FMS. He used magnetic resonance imaging (MRI) to look into the area of the brain that registers pain. Dr. Clauw observed that the area of the brain that registers pain showed an increase of blood flow when FMS patients were given a low-pressure stimulus. The identical stimulus produced no change in the brains of control group subjects. But when a more intense stimulus was administered to the control group, the blood flow increased in the same way as it had when the FMS group received the low-pressure stimulus. Dr. Clauw says his research finally offers visual proof that FMS patients experience hypersensitivity in the pain processing areas of their brains.

Dr. Clauw's work provided visual evidence that FMS patients really do experience pain differently than people who don't have the disorder. Clauw states:

Pain is always a subjective matter, but everything that we can measure about the pain in fibromyalgia shows that it is real. We think that one of the primary abnormalities in fibromyalgia is an imbalance between the levels of neurotransmitters in the brain that affect pain sensitivity. Although right now there are no drugs approved to treat fibromyalgia, within three years it its likely that there will be three, if not four, drugs specifically approved to treat the condition. This is not an inflammatory disorder and this is not a primary psychological condition. ... A person is about eight times more likely to develop fibromyalgia if one of their relatives has it. But there are also certain environmental triggers. For example, people develop fibromyalgia after motor vehicle accidents, or after certain types of infections or biological stress.[19]

In a 2003 paper in the journal *Science*, a University of Michigan team reported that a small variation in the gene that encodes the enzyme called catechol-O-methyl transferase, or COMT, made a significant difference in the pain tolerance, and pain-related emotions and feelings, of healthy volunteers. Researchers also have found that individual mutations in the COMT gene are related to the future development of temporo-mandibular joint disorder, also known as TMJ, a condition related to fibromyalgia.

In 2006, the University of Michigan team concluded:

It is increasingly clear that fibromyalgia is a central nervous system disorder and that patients experience hypersensitivity to pain. There also appears to be a fairly strong genetic component to fibromyalgia and related conditions. These studies indicate that fibromyalgia patients have abnormalities within their central brain structures. ... It is time for us to move past the rhetoric about whether these conditions are real, and take these patients seriously as we endeavor to learn more about the causes and most effective treatments for these disorders.[20]

National Fibromyalgia Association president and founder Lynne Matallana said that doctors who treat fibromyalgia patients face a unique challenge. "This is a new paradigm for medical professionals to understand," she says. "It isn't a tumor or something else that you can see.

It is a problem within the pain-processing center of the central nervous system."[21]

And It's More Than Just Pain

People with FMS can be sensitive to changes in barometric pressure and temperature. Rain beating on the windowpane may feel as if it were beating on the walls of their cells. Noise emitted by fluorescent lights can be very irritating, and they may have to avoid overcrowded areas such as malls. FMS sensitizes nerve endings as well as the rest of the autonomic nervous system. The actual ends of the nerve receptors may have changed shape, turning touch and other receptors into pain receptors. Pain signals then bombard the brain. The brain knows that pain is a danger signal — an indication that something is wrong and needs attention — so it mobilizes its defenses. Then, when those defenses are not used, because there has been no apparent threat, the brain thinks it must have missed something, and becomes anxious.

If you have FMS, you may have insomnia or a host of other sleep-related problems. You may have sleep apnea, or your heightened sensitivity does not allow you to sleep deeply. Our body heals and many neurotransmitters are balanced during deep sleep. If our sleep is of poor quality, or frequently interrupted, we soon suffer from the effects of sleep deprivation.

You may experience skin mottling. Your finger and toe nails may have vertical ridges — a typical sign of endocrine imbalance. Fingernails may break off, often in crescent-shaped pieces. If nails do grow, some may start to curve under the fingertip.[22]

You may experience "brain fog" and thus you may develop a cognitive overload, memory dysfunction, and an inability to do more than one thing at once. The brain "feel good" chemical, dopamine, and the overall master controlling neurotransmitter, serotonin, are typically low in patients with fibromyalgia. Since a firm diagnosis of fibromyalgia is difficult, and no confirmatory laboratory tests are available, FMS patients are often misdiagnosed with depression.

People with a diagnosis of rheumatoid arthritis and other autoimmune diseases are particularly likely to develop fibromyalgia. To the good, patients with fibromyalgia do not develop deformity as happens with rheumatoid arthritis. Fibromyalgia also does not cause damage to internal body organs. Therefore, fibromyalgia is different from many other rheumatic conditions.

Many medical conditions can cause pain in different areas of the body, mimicking fibromyalgia. These conditions include:

- low thyroid hormone level (hypothyroidism)
- parathyroid disease (causing elevated blood calcium level)
- muscle diseases causing muscle pain (polymyositis)
- bone diseases causing bone pain (Paget's Disease)
- infectious diseases

Even though there is no blood test for fibromyalgia, blood tests are important to exclude other medical conditions.

Is Fibromyalgia Sometimes Lyme Disease?

*M*any people with Lyme disease suffer the same widespread pain and tender points as fibromyalgia sufferers do. There is no great test for Lyme disease, so things get confusing. According to some in the Lyme community, as many as half the people diagnosed with fibromyalgia actually have Lyme disease.

Lyme disease and fibromyalgia have very similar symptoms. Lyme disease is an infection caused by the spirochete Borrelia burgdorferi, an organism originally transmitted to animals and then humans by ticks. Lyme disease can cause a host of different symptoms because it affects a number of different systems within the body, including the heart, brain, and musculoskeletal systems.

One school of thought says that many fibromyalgia patients have unrecognized infections caused by atypical bacteria or viruses, including mycoplasma, chlamydia, Lyme disease and HHV-6. They claim beneficial results from long-term antibiotics. Several studies support these claims, but none was large or well-designed enough to put skepticism to rest. Breakthrough research on HHV-6 virus as a cause of chronic fatigue syndrome was reported recently. Transfer Factor, a cow's milk colostrum made from cows especially immunized to produce antibodies against HHV-6, was reported to help about two-thirds of patients. This same approach, in theory, could also help fibromyalgia.[23]

Fibromyalgia can affect every aspect of a person's life. The chronic pain associated with fibromyalgia is pervasive and persistent and can severely curtail social activity and recreation. As many as 30% of those diagnosed with fibromyalgia are unable to maintain full-time employment. Like others with disabilities, individuals with FMS often need accommodations to fully participate in their education or remain active in their careers.

How to Treat

Traditionally, the most effective prescription drugs have been the tricyclic antidepressants. In treating fibromyalgia, tricyclic antidepressants are taken at bedtime in doses that are a fraction of those used for treating depression. Tricyclic antidepressants appear to reduce fatigue, relieve muscle pain and spasm, and promote deep restorative sleep in patients with fibromyalgia. Scientists believe that tricyclics work by inhibiting the reuptake of all three catecholamine neurotransmitters, serotonin, norepinephrine and dopamine, making the body think that it has plenty of the neurotransmitters available.

The degree of benefit differs very much for each individual.

Several drug companies are testing new drugs for the treatment of fibromyalgia that target the central nervous system. These drugs fall into two general classes. One class raises the levels of neurotransmitters that normally stop the spread of pain, while another class lowers the levels of neurotransmitters that normally increase the spread of pain.

In 2007, pregabalin (Lyrica) became the first drug approved specifically for treating fibromyalgia.

Local injections of analgesics and/or cortisone medication into the trigger point areas can also be helpful in relieving painful soft tissues, while breaking cycles of pain and muscle spasm.

Non-Pharmaceutical Treatments

Limit the dietary stimulants. Just say no to caffeine and sugar. Avoid excitotoxins, especially MSG (monosodium glutamate) and artificial sweeteners like aspartame. Both glutamate (in MSG) and the amino acid aspartic acid (in aspartame) stimulate pain augmenting receptors within the spinal cord. These are called NMDA receptors. Some individuals with fibromyalgia improve very much on a fibromyalgia diet that avoids MSG and aspartame. Occasionally, people with fibromyalgia improve with the elimination of foods to which they personally are sensitive. Wheat/gluten, milk, yeast, and sugar can be culprits.

One patient had been diagnosed with fibromyalgia since 1996. In 2007 he came to us. One week after we took him off gluten, his pain was completely gone. Gluten, the protein in wheat, is notorious for creating chronic inflammation in many people.

Acupuncture is effective in treating some patients with fibromyalgia. Dr. Clauw's University of Michigan team is attempting to quantify just how helpful it is.

Exercise helps many patients. While exercise improves the symptoms of FMS, pain and fatigue often prevent individuals from beginning an exercise regimen in the first place. Because of the known benefits of exercise on FMS, it is important to find new ways for individuals with FMS to increase their physical activity. Lifestyle physical activity, which involves any type of moderate-intensity activity such as walking, housecleaning, shopping, and gardening, may be more doable than structured exercise like what you find at a gym.

Irritable Bowel Syndrome often goes hand in hand with fibromyalgia. Detoxification of the body is especially beneficial at the beginning of treatment. Colon hydrotherapy cleans out the colon, initiating the detoxification process. The first step in any detoxification process is to make sure the toxin has someplace to go that is outside the body.

As is true with so many autoimmune diseases, stress plays a big role and learning how to handle stress can make living with the disease easier. Hypnosis can be extremely helpful to learn how to defuse stress.

Everything hurts, you feel you have been beaten up, and that there is no way out. This can relate emotionally to current or past experiences. Energetically, the fibromyalgia may be serving as a signpost to get us to look at those experiences and deal with them in a way that does not make us ill, and that allows for escape in a way that we might not have seen before – the famous "door in the ceiling" phenomenon. Energetic medicine is an excellent choice in these situations.

One thing which may distinguish fibromyalgia is its brain activity. It does appear that people with fibromyalgia have a hyperactive pain sensitivity, with significant elevations of substance P, a pain neurotransmitter, in the cerebro-spinal fluid.[24] Differences in blood flow to specific areas of the brain have been noted in patients with fibromyalgia.[25]

You can retrain your autonomic nervous system to respond differently, and more appropriately, to signals coming from your body and from the environment, using the techniques of BrainAdvantage™ to enable you to make new and more efficient connections in the brain, lessening the hypersensitivity to external stimuli.

FMS dysfunctions may be simply points on a spectrum of chemical sensitivity or autonomic nervous system imbalance,[26] through a mechanism called "neurogenic switching."[27] This is a process whereby a signal from the brain, in response to an inflammation from a given site in the body, causes inflammation at a second site elsewhere in the body, apparently not related to the first site. Fibromyalgia is an excellent example of the "switching" phenomenon – we may ingest a food which causes inflammation in the intestinal tract, sending signals to the brain, which are then expressed as diffuse pain in the muscles. This phenomenon happens because the body uses many of the same neurotransmitters and hormones to activate pathways in many different organ systems. It is not surprising that, with an overwhelming stimulus, the system itself may become overwhelmed.[28]

RESOURCES

BrainAdvantage™ (www.BrainAdvantage.com) – bringing more oxygen to the brain and developing new neural connections, to decrease the hypersensitivity to various stimuli. This non-drug approach can improve fibromyalgia and other disorders.

---

[1]Jason LA, Richman JA et al. A Community-Based Study of Chronic Fatigue Syndrome. *Arch Intern Med.* 1999;159:2129-2137.

[2]Fukuda K, Straus SE et al. The Chronic Fatigue Syndrome: A Comprehensive Approach to Its Definition and Study. *Ann Int Med* 121;12:953-59 (15 Dec 1994).

[3]Ojo-Amaize EA, Conley EJ, et al. Decreased natural killer cell activity is associated with severity of chronic fatigue immune dysfunction syndrome. *Clin Infect Dis.* 1994 Jan;18 Suppl 1:S157-9.

[4]Paul ML, Satterlee JD. Elevated Nitric Oxide/Peroxynitrite Mechanism for the Common Etiology of Multiple Chemical Sensitivity, Chronic Fatigue Syndrome, and Posttraumatic Stress Disorder. *Annals of the New York Academy of Sciences* 933:323-329 (2001)

[5]Liu JK, Atamna HT et al. Delaying Brain Mitochondrial Decay and Aging with Mitochondrial Antioxidants and Metabolites. *Annals of the New York Academy of Sciences* 959:133-166 (2002).

[6]Fulle S, Mecocci P, et al. Specific oxidative alterations in vastus lateralis muscle of patients with the diagnosis of chronic fatigue syndrome. *Free Radic Biol Med.* 2000 Dec 15;29(12):1252-9.

[7]Pall ML. Elevated, sustained peroxynitrite levels as the cause of chronic fatigue syndrome. *Med Hypotheses.* 2000 Jan;54(1):115-25.

[8]Quig DW. Cysteine metabolism and Metal Toxicity. *Alt Med Review* 3;4:262-70.

[9]Jacobsen MB, Aukrust P et al. Relation between food provocation and systemic immune activation in patients with food intolerance. *The Lancet* 356;9227:400-401 (29 July 2000).

[10]Kitts D, Yuan Y, et al. Adverse reactions to food constituents: allergy, intolerance, and autoimmunity. *Can J Physiol Pharmacol.* 1997 Apr;75(4):241-54.

[11]Baker JC, Ayres JG. Diet and asthma. *Resp Med* 94;10:925-34 (October 2000).

[12]Magee EA, Edmond LM et al. Associations between diet and disease activity in ulcerative colitis patients using a novel method of data analysis. *Nutr J.* 2005 Feb 10;4:7.

[13]Nanda R, James R et al. Food intolerance and the irritable bowel syndrome. *Gut,* Vol 30, 1099-1104.

[14]Georgiades E, Behan WM, et al. Chronic fatigue syndrome: new evidence for a central fatigue disorder. *Clinical Science* (2003) 105, (213–218).

[15]Preedy VR, Smith DG et al. Biochemical and muscle studies in patients with acute onset post-viral fatigue syndrome. *J Clin Pathol.* 1993 August; 46(8): 722–726.

[16]William Crook, MD. *The Yeast Connection*, Vintage Books, 1986

[17]Michael Rosenbaum, Murray Susser. *Solving the Puzzle of Chronic Fatigue.* Life Science Press. 1992

[18]Vaerøy H, Helle R. Elevated CSF levels of substance P and high incidence of Raynaud phenomenon in patients with fibromyalgia: new features for diagnosis. *Pain.* 1988 Jan; 32(1):21-6.

[19] Press release: *Fibromyalgia: the Misunderstood Disease*, University of Michigan Health System, June 4, 2007, accessed at http://www.newswise.com/articles/view/530528/

[20]Harris, R. and Clauw, D. *Current Pain and Headache Reports*, December 2006

[21]Salynn Boyles. Fibromyalgia Pain: It's for Real. *WebMD Health*, Nov. 30, 2006

[22]Devin J. Starlanyl and Mary Ellen Copeland. *Fibromyalgia and Chronic Myofascial Pain Syndrome: A Survival Manual.* © by the authors, revised 2/4/04

[23]Dr. Richard N. Podell. How We Approach Fibromyalgia Treatments, accessed September 2007 at http://www.drpodell.org/fibromyalgia_treatments.shtml

[24]Russell IJ, Orr MD. Elevated cerebrospinal fluid levels of substance P in patients with the fibromyalgia syndrome. *Arthritis Rheum.* 1994 Nov;37(11):1593-601.

[25]Mountz JM, Bradley LA. Fibromyalgia in women. Abnormalities of regional cerebral blood flow in the thalamus and the caudate nucleus are associated with low pain threshold levels. *Arthritis Rheum.* 1995 Jul;38(7):926-38.

[26]Buchwald D, Garrity D. Comparison of patients with chronic fatigue syndrome, fibromyalgia, and multiple chemical sensitivities. *Archives of Internal Medicine* 154;18 (September 26, 1994).

[27]Meggs W. Neurogenic Switching: A Hypothesis for a Mechanism for Shifting the Site of Inflammation in Allergy and Chemical Sensitivity. *EHP* 103;1 (1995).

[28]Rowat SC. Integrated Defense System Overlaps as a Disease Model: With Examples for Multiple Chemical Sensitivity. *EHP Supplements* 106;S1 (Feb 1998).

Depression and Anxiety

Depression can range anywhere from "the world is grey today" to "the world is intolerable today and I want out." The only emotion is greyness and sadness, hopelessness and helplessness – it feels as though there is no hope of anything changing in the foreseeable future.

When depression is combined with anxiety – a constant feeling of agitation, where nothing ever settles down, the nerves are always on edge – it is even more difficult to deal with, because there is never a time of quiet. For those who have anxiety, having to perform at work, going shopping, cooking breakfast, reading the newspaper – almost anything can stop them in their tracks.

Depression affects approximately 10-15% of our population in any given year, and up to 20% of the population as a whole, at some time in their lifetime. Three times more women than men are diagnosed with depression. Average duration of illness is 10 years.[1] It is estimated that 15-20% of older adults suffer from depression.[2]

Many symptoms of depression are associated with things which we are "supposed to" be able to control – mood swings, focus on self, concentration, ability to experience pleasure. "Just pull yourself together!" "Get over it!" Once a person has been treated successfully, and has experienced remission of symptoms (one hardly dares say cure), it becomes quite clear that they were in fact incapable of "pulling themselves together" prior to the treatment.

Conventional Western treatment for depression used to involve cognitive/behavioral therapy – let's sit on the couch and talk. Increasingly in these days of HMOs, standard treatment comes from the prescription pad – antidepressants, anticonvulsants, anxiolytics (anti-anxiety agents), stimulants, and other psychotropic (mind-changing) pharmaceuticals.

Drugs sometimes calm the anxiety, sometimes they merely make people feel brain fogged. Antidepressants do not work for everyone. A 50%

relief of symptoms is called "treatment success." Many patients have experienced that over time their anti-depressant doesn't seem to work anymore and they have to switch to an ever stronger cocktail of pharmaceuticals. If you are way low on serotonin – the hormone that is a master neurotransmitter – the drugs may not work much at all. Up to 20% of patients fail to respond to any form of conventional therapy for depression.

Dr. David Rubinow, in an excellent editorial in the *New England Journal of Medicine* in 2006,[3] talks about the National Institutes of Health funded trials which were also reported in the same issue, and laments that at least half the patients treated for depression with standard antidepressant medication continue to have symptoms of depression despite treatment. Seventy-five percent of the patients in those studies had suffered from depression for 15 years or more, and over half of them waited for over a year before receiving their first treatment.

Findings from the Women's Health Initiative Study revealed that post-menopausal women taking antidepressants were 45 per cent more likely to suffer a stroke than those of the same age not on the medicines. The research also found that overall death rates were 32 per cent higher in women on the drugs.[4]

Because therapy is so ineffective and the condition so prevalent, it just makes sense to look for more effective alternative therapies.

Depression can be caused by many things. If it has a spiritual basis, then acupuncture and hypnosis can be helpful. A sudden spiritual awakening is enough to lift the veil – but those awakenings are hard to orchestrate. More often, depression and anxiety have an organic cause. You may have very poor neural function, meaning your brain doesn't work very well because some wires are crossed or don't even exist.[5] Your neurotransmitters could be misfiring because of low levels of serotonin and dopamine[6] – your brain functions like a truck running on two cylinders instead of eight. For some people, food allergies trigger the blues. For others, a body burden of heavy metals inhibits neural functions to the point nothing works and you feel depressed.

Other physiologic factors implicated in depression include low levels of vitamin D,[7] hormonal imbalance,[8] head injury,[9] vitamin deficiency,[10] and fatty acid deficiency.[11, 12]

A five-year study involving 3,500 people showed that people who eat a diet high in processed food increase their chances of depression. Conversely, those who avoided processed food and instead ate a healthy amount of vegetables, fruit and fish, or what is known as the Mediterranean diet, actually lowered their risk of depression.[13]

We can start by looking at hormone levels because they affect all the neurotransmitters. Then we look to see if there is merit in desensitizing environmental allergies with smart testing and homeopathy, removing heavy metals with chelation, and identifying food allergies.

Is there any exercise in the picture? The January 2005 issue of the *American Journal of Preventive Medicine* reported a study on the effects of exercise and found results comparable to studies in which patients with mild to moderate depression were treated with antidepressants. "The effect you find using aerobic exercise alone in treating clinical depression is similar to what you find with antidepressant medications," said Dr. Madhukar Trivedi, a study author and professor of psychiatry and director of University of Texas Southwestern Medical Center's mood disorders research program. "The key is the intensity of the exercise and continuing it for 30 to 35 minutes per day. It's not for the faint of heart."

How are the vitamin D levels? How is the omega 3/omega 6 balance in the diet? Vitamin D, the "sunshine vitamin" and fish oils with omega-3 oils have been found to provide some benefit. Vitamin D deficiency is associated with low mood and worse cognitive performance in older adults.[14] Consumption of omega-3 fats is especially low in the United States, and we have one of the highest depression rates in the world. Dr. Joseph Hibbeln of the National Institutes of Health has shown that higher national consumption of fish for a nation equates with lower rates of depression.[15]

What are the sleep patterns? The body does most of its healing as we sleep, so adequate sleep is important too.

In sum, you want to create a good terrain from the neck down.

Then it is time to go to work on the brain. The frontal lobe is key to depression because it usually isn't working right. Your right frontal lobe looks at the big picture and puts the past and the future in perspective. When the frontal lobes are not working well, it is harder for people to cope. You get slow or garbled transmission of impulses to the limbic system in the brain. This is often the source of the fight or flight response in the brain. The anxiety makes you want to run away, and depression makes you want to freeze. You are quivering between the proverbial rock and the hard place.

We all have different reactions to dysfunctional transmission of nerve impulses. If we look at the temperaments as described in Chinese Medicine:

- Wood – angry and anxious and depressed
- Water – fearful and depressed (frozen)
- Metal – rigid and obsessed
- Earth – soggy and weepy and depressed
- Fire – anxious and depressed

The Traditional Chinese Medicine Theory of Five Elements

The theory says wood, fire, earth, metal, and water are the basic elements of the material world.

Each element possesses distinct characteristics. These elements are in constant movement and change. We all have each of these elements in us.

On the basis of the elements' different characteristics, functions, and forms, the complex links between physiology and pathology as well as the correlation between the human body and the natural environment were explained.

We can give a patient more serotonin for example, but odds are the brain wouldn't know what to do with it. We can increase the brain's processing speed by increasing neural connections with the BrainAdvantage™ program that uses HEG (hemoencephalography) to increase oxygen flow, and then exercising the brain to teach it to make new connections.

The brain operates on a use it or lose it principal. Blood brings oxygen and the basic nutrient, glucose, to all parts of the brain. The more blood flow you have, the more oxygen and glucose you will have on board and the more neural connections you can make. The less blood flow you have, the less processing power you have.

CASE STUDY

One 42-year old professional woman was incapacitated with depression and anxiety. She had been unable to work for two years and spent most of her days crying. Within 3 ½ weeks of starting BrainAdvantage™ Combined therapy, she was off her meds, had stopped crying, and was able to see the "light of day." Within six weeks she was done with therapy, done with meds, and looking at going back to work. She had previously tried biofeedback, which does not stimulate blood flow, but her depression and anxiety were not relieved. She said she began to see changes within three days of starting therapy.

Incapacitating anxiety is one of the most difficult things to deal with on any level. The anxiety becomes a global state of being. It can relate to misinterpretation of physical signals like falling blood sugar. Depending upon the personality, that can advance to a state where everything triggers anxiety.

Looking at things energetically can help. Sometimes things are hidden in the cellular biology of our body. There may be a latent reason for the anxiety that has become an integral component of the person and the ego. A skilled energetic healer can sometimes see what is going on behind the scenes and help bring it to the surface so the conscious mind can deal with it and get rid of it. Hypnosis is another option for getting at the root cause. Psychotherapy used to be a (somewhat cumbersome and lengthy) way of unroofing latent issues – before psychiatrists were reduced to treatment by prescription pad.

"Just pull yourself together!" is not a realistic demand of someone with depression and anxiety. Solving depression is not as easy as tackling any one thing. And sometimes the prescription pad leads to tragedy. I am in mind of a woman who had been on an antidepressant for years – initially prescribed to help her deal with the unexpected and traumatic death of her first husband, some 25 years before I first saw her. She decided to come off the medication because things were falling apart physically. Unfortunately she stopped abruptly rather than gradually, because she did not know any better. Within three weeks she was frantic with withdrawal symptoms. And when she went back on the medication, she had worse symptoms. Despite all efforts to help her system stabilize, and although she appeared to improve somewhat, she soon died in a single-car accident. We never knew whether it was suicide or an accident brought on by poor judgment caused by neurotransmitter imbalance.

Would things have turned out differently had she been encouraged to work through the initial tragedy of her first husband's death? Perhaps... Perhaps not... She was completely dysfunctional, incapable of taking care of either herself or her small children. So the medication did serve a purpose – back when. Would it have been easier to come off the medication earlier in the course of her illness? Again, perhaps... we will never know. It is possible that coming off the medication would have hastened her death. Had she never been on medication, she might have simply died... or she might have learned to cope with her situation.

There are no easy answers. I am pretty sure that the relatively easier ones are found in the prescription pad. We can attempt to modify our body's efforts at controlling our environment by manipulating the chemistry. Or we can tackle the harder issue of figuring out what causes the biochemistry to become distorted in the first place. It may be a physical issue (chemical or heavy metal toxicity, food intolerance). It may be an electrical issue (abnormal neural pathways in the brain, abnormal connections). It may be an emotional issue (reaction to overwhelming stress, or abuse). It may be an issue which (if you play on that game board) has manifested itself over many lifetimes.

It is all experience – and we do have the ability to choose what we experience. We may have come into this lifetime with the purpose of exposing ourselves to situations where we learn to deal with specific experiences. We do not know for certain. But this is a philosophy espoused by millions of people in the world. Perhaps we do not have all the answers. But at the very least, we can be open to possibilities… Quantum physics tells us that possibilities are infinite – photons are always popping in and out of existence. Photons are particles of light, shining on our darkness.

Who knows what they may illuminate?

[1]Murphy JM, Olivier DC et al. Incidence of depression and anxiety: the Stirling County Study. *Am J Publ Hlth* 78; 5 534-540.

[2]Gallo JJ, Lebowitz BD. The Epidemiology of Common Late-life mental disorders in the Community: Themes for the New Century. *Psychiatric Services* 50:1158–1166, 1999.

[3]Rubinow DR. Treatment Strategies after SSRI Failure — Good News and Bad News. *NEJM* 354.12:1305-07 (March 23, 2006).

[4]J Smoller, MD et al. Antidepressant Use and Risk of Incident Cardiovascular Morbidity and Mortality Among Postmenopausal Women in the Women's Health Initiative Study, *Arch Intern Medicine*, 2009;169(22):2128-2139. See also: http://www.psychologytoday.com/blog/charting-the-depths/201001/the-womens-health-initiative-study-firebell-in-the-night-0

[5]Mayberg HS. Modulating limbic-cortical circuits in depression: targets of antidepressant treatments. *Semin Clin Neuropsychiatry*, 2002;7:255-268.

[6]Papakostas G. Dopaminergic-based pharmacotherapies for depression. *European Neuropsycho-pharmacology*, Volume 16 , Issue 6, Pages 391 - 402.

[7]Gloth FM 3rd, Alam W, et al. Vitamin D vs broad spectrum phototherapy in the treatment of seasonal affective disorder. *J Nutr Health Aging*. 1999;3(1):5-7.

[8]Walf AA, Frye CA. A Review and Update of Mechanisms of Estrogen in the Hippocampus and Amygdala for Anxiety and Depression Behavior. *Neuropsychopharmacology* (2006) 31, 1097 - 1111.

[9]Jorge RE, Robinson RG et al. Major Depression Following Traumatic Brain Injury. *Arch Gen Psychiatry*. 2004;61:42-50.

[10]Morris MS, Fava M. Depression and folate status in the US Population. *Psychother Psychosom*. 2003 Mar-Apr;72(2):80-7.

[11]Hibbeln JR, Salem N. Dietary polyunsaturated fatty acids and depression: when cholesterol does not satisfy. *AJCN*, Vol 62, 1-9.

[12]Puri BK, Counsell SJ et al. Eicosapentaenoic acid in treatment-resistant depression associated with symptom remission, structural brain changes and reduced neuronal phospholipid turnover. *Int J Clin Pract.* 2001 Oct;55(8):560-3.

[13]T Akbaraly, E Brunner, et al. Depression link to processed food, *British Journal of Psychiatry.* February 2009, 195: 408-413

[14]C.H Wilkins. Vitamin D Deficiency Is Associated With Low Mood and Worse Cognitive Performance in Older Adults. *Am J Geriatr Psychiatry,* 14:1032-1040, December 2006.

[15]Hibbeln JR. Fish consumption and major depression. *The Lancet,* 1998; 351: 1213.

Diabetes and Metabolic Syndrome

$\mathcal{D}$iabetics have a problem with insulin, the hormone that keeps blood sugar within healthy levels.

An estimated 85-90 percent of those who have diabetes have type 2 diabetes. It used to be called the "adult" version of the disease because it came after decades of eating an unhealthy diet. However, increasing numbers of children are now developing type 2 diabetes, partly because today's kid food is laden with sugar, refined carbohydrates, and bad fats. In addition, the children's mothers (and sometimes grandmothers) also ate diets laden with sugar, refined carbohydrates and unhealthy fats, thus modifying their genetic expression. By so doing, they were able to pass the predisposition for diabetes on to following generations, whether they themselves developed diabetes or not.

If for years you eat more sugar than is needed by the muscles for exercise, you strain the pancreas, asking it to make excess insulin constantly to lower your blood sugar level. Eventually, the pancreas cannot make enough insulin, and the blood sugar level remains chronically high. At this point, the patient is diagnosed with diabetes.

Controlling blood sugar is one of the most fundamental requirements of life. When blood sugar levels are too low – less than 80 – that is hypoglycemia. When levels are too high – over 110 – that is hyperglycemia. Insulin is the hormone that "unlocks" the cells of the body, allowing glucose to enter and turn food into energy.

A fasting blood glucose level between 100 and 125 mg/dl signals pre-diabetes. A person with a fasting blood glucose level of 126 mg/dl or higher has diabetes.

So why doesn't everyone develop diabetes? Why can some people eat junk food for years without problems, where others develop diabetes in their youth? Part of it is in your genes. We know that more than 50% of the relatives of diabetics demonstrate insulin resistance decades before they develop overt diabetes.[1]

Type 1 diabetes, previously called insulin-dependent diabetes mellitus or juvenile-onset diabetes:

A malfunction of the pancreas, a progressive autoimmune disease, in which the beta cells that produce insulin in the pancreas are slowly destroyed by the body's own immune system. There is no consensus as to what is the autoimmune trigger. Without insulin to move glucose (blood sugar) into cells, blood glucose levels become excessively high – hyperglycemia. The body cannot utilize the sugar; it spills over into the urine and is lost.

Type 2 diabetes, previously called non-insulin-dependent diabetes mellitus or maturity-onset diabetes:

It begins with insulin resistance – much more insulin is required to move glucose into cells. In time, the pancreas "burns out," it cannot produce enough insulin to overcome resistance. There is usually an abnormal rise in blood sugar after a meal. Eventually, the cycle of elevated glucose further impairs and possibly destroys beta cells, thereby stopping insulin production completely and causing full-blown diabetes.

The Killing Effect of Diabetes

Diabetes can lead to multiple complications including blindness, kidney failure, nerve damage, heart disease, and Alzheimer's.

Diabetics have two times the incidence of acute coronary syndrome (ACS) and two times the mortality rate after ACS compared with patients who do not have diabetes.[2] Diabetes appears to blunt some of the effects of estrogen, which may increase the risk for heart disease. Studies have shown that many diabetics suffer from depression, which sometimes interferes with self-care.[3] Other studies link diabetics to a 65 percent higher risk of developing Alzheimer's disease.[4, 5]

Uric acid is often elevated with metabolic syndrome and diabetes because of the high blood sugar level. Hyperuricemia is presumed to be a consequence of insulin resistance rather than its precursor. Excess uric acid levels can lead to gout, kidney stones, and heart disease.

Too much sugar causes the small blood vessels throughout the body to narrow. That is your body's way of trying to head off damage to organs by minimizing the ability of the excess sugar to reach them. The higher the blood sugar level, the less nitric oxide is available,[6] and the more the small blood vessels narrow. Circulation is impaired. If there is adequate glutathione in the system for dealing with free radicals, the negative circulatory effect does NOT occur. But in the relative absence of glutathione, poor circulation develops, in turn resulting in complications such as: kidney disease, poor wound healing, and foot and eye problems. High sugar levels damage the kidneys so that they can no longer fully cleanse the blood of waste. Sugar imbalance also alters fat metabolism, causing people to gain weight. When sugar sticks to proteins, it changes their structural and functional properties. Wounds do not heal because they have trouble making good collagen, the connective tissue that is the major structural protein in the body.

This is also why sugar is sometimes called "the aging drug."

Insulin Run Amok

A study reported in 2009[7] shed new light on the conventional wisdom that when we eat a calorie-restricted diet, we live longer. But this new study looked deeper and found that the underlying reason for longevity is – less sugar, thus fewer surges of insulin.

Researchers studied 31 patients referred for the treatment of diabetes, cardiovascular disease, excessive weight, fatigue, and other chronic diseases of aging. The group ate a very specific diet for 3 months:

The diet included unlimited amounts of certain fats and oils, a restricted amount of protein, and a very limited amount of carbohydrate. Patients were

217

told to eat when they were hungry. Calories were not explicitly restricted; calorie intake was determined only by levels of hunger. Recommended sources of fat included raw nuts and seeds, avocados, olives and olive oil, flax oil and cod liver oil. The intake of protein was told to be limited to approximately 1.0 grams/kg lean body mass per day (increased for exercise to 1.25 grams/day). As a result, most patients were instructed to eat from 50-80 grams of protein per day. Recommended sources of protein included sardines, fish, eggs, tofu, chicken, turkey, wild meats, low-fat cheeses (cottage, ricotta, swiss), seafood, and veggie burgers. Only non-starchy, fibrous vegetables were acceptable: lettuce, greens, broccoli, cauliflower, cucumbers, mushrooms, onions, peppers, sprouts, asparagus, and seaweed. Though not explicitly stated, the general dietary intake as percent daily caloric intake from macronutrients for most people ended up by history to be approximately 20% carbohydrate, 20% protein, and 60% fat. For drinking, 6-8 eight ounce glasses of water and/or herbal tea were recommended.

Nutritional supplements to support fat metabolism and enhance insulin sensitivity were recommended to all patients to be taken on a daily basis: L-carnitine 2000mg, alpha-lipoic acid 400mg, coenzyme Q10 100 mg, 1 tbsp cod liver oil, magnesium 300mg, potassium 300mg, vitamin C 1000mg, vitamin E 800mg daily, and a multivitamin consisting of all essential B vitamins and minerals.

And what happened on this "high fat, adequate protein, low carbohydrate diet"?

- Patients lost an average of 7 pounds
- Insulin levels dropped almost in half
- Leptin levels dropped almost in half
- Triglyercides and blood pressure levels dropped

These great results were achieved on a high fat diet, the antithesis of what Americans are told to eat. Note there were no refined starchy carbs (corn, potatoes, bread), no grains (rice, wheat, gluten), no modern fats (margarine, vegetable oils) no fried foods, and no sugar. Seaweed served as a natural source of iodine.

This is a clear illustration of the dietary wisdom from centuries ago when natural fats were a much higher percentage of the diet. It has been known for some time that different dietary fats appear to have varying effects on insulin-sensitive tissues.

Less starchy food, less sugar and carbohydrate in the blood lowers triglycerides and fatty acids in the blood by simply not producing them - because these are produced in response to high glucose levels. Less sugar and carbohydrate promotes the break-down of fats (to use as calories, or energy) in the liver, fatty tissue and blood.

The researchers also pointed out that centenarians – people who live to be more than 100 – have lower blood glucose, insulin, leptin, and serum triglycerides than those who do not live to be over one hundred years old.

Reducing sugar consumption can add years to your life.

Metabolic Syndrome

The "civilized" diet has been so full of sugar, refined carbs that rapidly turn into sugar, and trans fats, that many people have become "pre-diabetic." The medical term for this is metabolic syndrome, and it is a disease of the 21st Century.

Twenty-four percent of adults in the United States already qualify for this diagnosis.[8] The syndrome is increasingly diagnosed in children. For the first time in recorded history, it is suggested that, if the current trend in obesity continues into the next generation, our children may have a lower life expectancy than we have ourselves.[9]

Criteria for diagnosis of the metabolic syndrome include at least three of the following five things:

- a waist circumference of more than 40" in men, and more than 35" in women
- elevated triglycerides (>150),
- low HDL cholesterol (<40 in men, <50 in women)
- high blood pressure (>135/85)
- fasting blood sugar levels of 110 mg/dL or greater

So, we see the family practice doctor or internist for our high blood pressure and high cholesterol. We try to lose weight the best we can – by eating egg whites, avoiding fat whenever possible, drinking diet sodas – and still we find that we gain weight. The doctors give us prescription drugs to lower our cholesterol and blood pressure, but we do not feel well.

How many people do we all know who are chubby around the middle? How many of our friends are taking high blood pressure medicine and statin drugs for their "cholesterol"? And these are the folks who consider themselves healthy, because by all insurance-based criteria, they are healthy. Their disease is "well managed."

In fact, they do not have a defined disease. They have diagnostic codes, for which they see multiple specialists, and are given multiple drugs as a "preventative" measure. They are advised to return for follow-up, so that when they get sick enough, they can be given more drugs. As Jeffrey Bland so eloquently put it:

> Somewhere along the line they will develop a 'clean' diagnosis – myocardial infarction, diabetes, stroke, cardiac arrest... In the meantime, they take medicine, eat refined flour, sweets, diet sodas, low-fat manufactured foods... and become more obese, and more ill, until finally their 'diagnosis' becomes apparent.

Insulin is the transporter of glucose across the cell membrane. But it serves other functions as well.

When our bodies think they are under stress, they shift to "storage" mode – to store up fat against the hard times coming, when food is not plentiful and we need every ounce of fat we can store if we are to survive the winter season. Most of us do not have the issue of survival through the winter season any more. But unlike our caveman ancestor who had periodic bouts of stress, we have constant daily stress. We are always fighting the clock, always trying to do more in less time, always shorting ourselves on sleep, always in a hurry... And what does the body do under stress? It stores up fat for the hard times ahead.

To take it one step further – cellular signaling depends on the information coming into the cell, and the state of health of the cell itself. A cell under stress reads somewhat different signals than a healthy cell, and therefore sends out different signals. Not all calories are alike. Is it not possible that meat from animals raised under stressful conditions with hormones and steroids inevitably imparts those stress signals to those of us who eat the meat?[10]

So, one way to treat the metabolic syndrome is to relieve stress. Set realistic goals. Learn to say "no." Read a good book. Get enough sleep. Stop putting chemicals into our bodies. Drink water, not sugar. Eat food, not chemicals.

REDUCING BLOOD SUGAR LEVELS

Besides stress, what else contributes to the body's inability to successfully regulate blood sugar levels?

High Fructose Corn Syrup (HFCS)

HFCS doesn't actually exist in nature. It is a man-made product created by using enzymes to increase the fructose content of corn syrup to about 90%. This super high fructose syrup is then blended "down" with a 100% glucose corn syrup to create various mixes. HFCS 55, for example, which is 55% fructose and 45% glucose is the mix used most commonly in beverages. HFCS 42 is the blend used more commonly in baked goods. Much of the corn is genetically modified. HFCS is a convenient, cheap ingredient, because farm subsidies drastically lower the cost of corn.

Since HFCS's widespread introduction in the 1980's, American obesity rates skyrocketed. The occurrence of new cases of type 2 diabetes has doubled over the past three decades, according to a report in the June 2006 American Heart Association's journal *Circulation*.[11]

221

Fructose is absorbed differently than other sugars, and fructose isolate as found in high fructose corn syrup even more so. It causes major health problems:

- When the liver is asked to handle such large quantities of fructose, there is rapid breakdown of fats and rapid accumulation of triglycerides, which in turn contributes to reduced insulin sensitivity, insulin resistance, and glucose intolerance.
- Unlike glucose, fructose doesn't stimulate insulin production, which means it isn't utilized for energy, but rather is stored in the liver as triglycerides.
- HFCS doesn't increase production of leptin or suppress production of ghrelin, hormones that play a primary role in appetite control. The sweet taste of HFCS encourages you to eat more because it blunts the body's ability to recognize when it is full. And there comes the weight gain and obesity.

Sharon P. Fowler, M.P.H., and colleagues at the University of Texas Health Science Center found that diet sodas actually cause people to gain weight. They looked at eight years of data from 1,550 people aged 25 to 64. "There was a 41 percent increase in risk of being overweight for every can or bottle of diet soft drink a person consumes each day."[12] When you taste something sweet, even "no-calorie" sweetened foods, your brain preps you for an intake of calories. But when they don't arrive, the brain sends out hunger signals, trying to find those calories and that makes it all too easy to down those supersized meals.

Sweet tastes also promote the release of insulin, which blocks the body's ability to burn fat. This is an adaptive response, because for millions of years sweet tastes have meant that blood glucose levels are about to rise, and when there is excess sugar, it ought to be stored for times when food is not readily available. Artificial sweeteners have the same effect on insulin: sweet diet drinks will increase insulin and thus the storage of fat.

Refined carbohydrates

Simply put, "good carbs" are vegetables, "bad carbs" are potatoes, pasta, breads, cereals, cookies, chips, crackers, donuts, instant rice and instant oatmeal. Bad carbs are pure carbohydrates that your body converts to sugar. Bombarding your system with these foods every day makes your pancreas work overtime to produce insulin – and wears it out. So next time you see a hamburger on a bun, envision a beef patty sandwiched between two disks of sugar.

Consumer beware in the marketplace. Products labeled "whole wheat" or "whole grain" in the typical grocery store will probably not meet the criteria for lowering the risk of metabolic syndrome. Increasingly, people have an inflammatory reaction to the gluten in wheat and some other grains. Instant oatmeal is processed and is much higher on the glycemic index than the old fashioned steel cut oats which are much less processed and take 10 minutes or more to cook.

Refined carbohydrates – most or all of the fiber, bran, hull, vitamins, minerals, essential fatty acids, and phytochemicals have been removed during milling or processing.

The process prolongs shelf life, but it also removes important nutrients, such as B vitamins and fiber.

If any of the B vitamins are not available, the conversion of carbohydrates to energy is blocked. Instead, the carbs are converted to fat in the human body.

Plastics

Plastic-derived chemicals like Bisphenol-A (BPA) increase the risk of diabetes and obesity. BPA is an endocrine disrupter that mimics the hormone estrogen. Testing performed by the CDC discovered that about

223

93% of the United States population has BPA in their body at a median concentration of 2.7 ppb.[13]

Repeated exposure to BPA causes insulin resistance at the cell level, which leads to type 2 diabetes. Tissues lose their sensitivity to insulin, causing the pancreas to produce even more insulin, further increasing insulin resistance and diabetes. This leads to a progressive cycle that reinforces itself.[14,15,16]

Trans Fats

Partially hydrogenated oils are a leading cause of type 2 diabetes and heart disease. They change the proteins in our bodies in such a way as to reject insulin. The pancreas makes insulin, but the body can't use it.

"Good" fats such as those from grass-fed animals do not contribute to diabetes. But trans fatty acids in partially hydrogenated vegetable oils cause insulin resistance.[17] When these man-made fats get built into the cell membrane, they interfere with the insulin receptors. Trans fats harden the cell walls, making it harder for nutrition to get in and metabolic waste (toxins) to get out.

Interesterified fats

Some food producers are phasing out partially hydrogenated oils because trans fats have been linked to heart disease and obesity. For certain products, such as baker's shortening and margarine, some companies are turning to interesterified fats.

Interesterified fats are typically created by blending solid fats like fully hydrogenated soybean oil or palm oil with liquid oils (e.g., soybean oil, canola oil) and then using a process to interchange the fats in order to achieve specific attributes in foods such as texture, mouth feel, and structure. Interesterified fats are solid or semi-solid at room temperature. You may find them in margarines, spreads and shortenings, and in confections and baked goods.

Interesterification shuffles the fatty acids that make up each fat molecule. Like partial hydrogenation, interesterification produces molecules that do not appear in nature. In a small study, interesterified fat raised blood-glucose concentrations in the studies and slowed the metabolism of glucose relative to the effects of either of the other fats. Both those changes are associated with increased diabetes risk.[18]

Less sleep

In the United States, the number of people with type 2 diabetes is increasing, while the average amount people sleep is dwindling, according to a sleep study dating from 2005.[19] Those two conditions appear to be linked.

In 2008, researchers found that a mutation called rs1387153, near a gene called MTNR1B, is associated with having an increased average blood sugar level and around a 20 percent elevated risk of developing type 2 diabetes.[20]

MTNR1B forms part of a signaling pathway that controls the action of the hormone melatonin. This hormone regulates the body's circadian rhythm – the internal clock that controls sleeping and eating patterns – by responding to daylight and darkness.

The research places bodily rhythms, including the clock that sets human sleep cycles, squarely in the blood sugar business. Three new genomic studies show that melatonin, a major regulator of the body's sleep clock, is closely linked to increased glucose levels and diabetes.[21]

Too few antioxidants

There is evidence that the ratio of antioxidants to free radicals plays a role in the development of insulin resistance and type 2 diabetes. Antioxidant levels are typically low in overweight people, while research shows that the production of free radicals may increase in bodies that carry too much fat.[22]

225

Too little vitamin E?

$\mathscr{A}$s reported in the journal *Diabetes Care*, the Otago researchers recruited 80 overweight men and women whose ages ranged from 31 to 65. To test the effects of vitamin E on glucose and insulin, as well as ALT levels (a liver enzyme associated with diabetes risk), half the group received 800 IU of vitamin E per day for three months, while the other half took a placebo. At the end of this first phase of the study, the dosage in the vitamin E group was increased to 1,200 IU for an additional three months.

At the end of the first three-month phase, both glucose and insulin levels were considerably reduced, lowering the likelihood of developing the insulin resistance that leads to type 2 diabetes. Unfortunately, the reduction in glucose and insulin levels did not remain steady through the second phase of the study. The researchers note that although vitamin E had a positive impact on oxidative stress, additional studies will be needed in order to clear up the mystery of the fluctuation in glucose and insulin. But throughout the full six months of the study, ALT concentrations had a marked decline.[23] This is significant because elevated ALT indicates the possible onset of diabetes, as well as cancer and other liver diseases.

Too little vitamin D

$\mathscr{T}$hree-quarters of children with type 1 diabetes were found to have insufficient levels of vitamin D, according to a study by researchers at the Joslin Diabetes Center. The study appeared in the January 2009 issue of the *Journal of Pediatrics*. It measured levels of serum 25-hydroxy vitamin D in 128 youths with type 1 diabetes ranging in age from 1.5 to 17.5 years.[24]

Vitamin D, the "sunshine vitamin," is a gene-regulating nutrient. The lack of it sets the stage for autoimmune problems – including damage to the pancreas that can cause type I diabetes.

Mother's diet during pregnancy

$\mathcal{DNA}$ is the primary mechanism of inheritance; kids get half their genes from Mom and half from Dad. However, scientists are just starting to understand additional kinds of inheritance like metabolic programming, which occurs when an insult during a critical period of development, either in the womb or soon after birth, triggers permanent changes in metabolism.

United Kingdom researchers from the Royal Veterinary College, led by Dr. Stéphanie Bayol, found that feeding mother rats junk food during pregnancy and lactation led to an increased preference for fats and sugars in their offspring. Perhaps the biggest surprise here came after birth. Some rat mothers were switched from the junk diet to nutritionally-balanced rat chow and spent their days nursing the rat pups. When weaned, those pups did not have the same strong preference for junk food as the pups whose mothers were still eating the junk diet while lactating. The study's authors conclude that a mother's "nutrition during lactation might play a key role in influencing the long-term appetite of the offspring" for junk food.[25]

When we as physicians work with our patients, we need to realize that we may not be dealing just with the patient sitting before us, but also their children and grandchildren, whether born or yet unborn. This puts a whole new twist on the concept of "family medicine".

Is Diabetes a Medical or Social Issue?

The British medical Journal, *The Lancet*, delivered a stern editorial blast regarding the treatment of diabetes. The cover of the June 26, 2010 issue states:

> *Medicine might be winning the battle of glucose control,*
> *but it is losing the war against diabetes.*

227

The editors explain that although that issue contains various studies that represent great progress in the understanding of how to lower concentrations of blood glucose, there is a glaring absence: no research to report on lifestyle interventions to prevent or reverse diabetes.

> Since 2000, the number of people [worldwide] with diabetes has more than doubled ... even if care was widely accessible, increasing evidence suggests that glucocentric treatment might not result in better overall outcomes... Because type 2 diabetes, which accounts for 90% of diabetes, is largely rooted in reversible social and lifestyle factors, a medical approach alone is unlikely to be the solution. Moreover, medicalisation disempowers individuals and excludes communities, schools, and urban planners who have the potential to reduce diabetes incidence... To lessen the burden of diabetes requires a substantial change in diet and routine, such as that advocated by Michelle Obama's Let's Move campaign... The fact that type 2 diabetes, a largely preventable disorder, has reached epidemic proportion is a public health humiliation.[26]

The majority of doctors in America work in environments where the average patient appointment is about ten minutes long – enough to whip out a prescription, but far too fast to educate patients how to eat fresh, nutrient-dense food instead of processed products with additives in bags and boxes. The national health care reform that passed in 2010 said nothing about the creation of health through nutrition. The conventional medical school curriculum says precious little about nutrition. We have a long way to go.

Perhaps a future editorial will note that a key distinguishing feature between conventional medicine's "Standard of Care" and the Functional Medicine approach is the difference in the emphasis on food as medicine.

---

[1]Beck-Nielsen H, Groop LC. Metabolic and Genetic Characterization of Prediabetic States. *J Clin Invest* 94:1714-21 (1994). 0021-9738/94/11/1714/08

[2]Carlos Sanchez, MD. Diabetes-Related Knowledge, Atherosclerotic Risk Factor Control, and Outcomes in Acute Coronary Syndromes. *The American Journal of Cardiology*, Volume 95, Issue 11, 1 June 2005, Pages 1290-1294

[3]John W. Williams, Jr., MD. MHSc, Wayne Katon, MD, et al. The Effectiveness of Depression Care Management on Diabetes-Related Outcomes in Older Patients. *Annuals of Internal Medicine*, June 15, 2004 | Volume 140 Issue 12, Pages 1015-1024

[4]Zoe Arvanitakis, MD, et al. Diabetes Mellitus and Risk of Alzheimer Disease and Decline in Cognitive Function. *Arch Neurol.* 2004;61:661-666.

[5]A. Ott. et al. Diabetes mellitus and the risk of dementia: The Rotterdam Study, *Neurology*, 1999 Dec 10;53(9):1937-42.

[6]Giugliano D, Marfella R et al. Vascular Effects of Acute Hyperglycemia in Humans Are Reversed by L-Arginine. *Circulation.* 1997;95:1783-1790.

[7]Ron Rosedale, M.D., Eric C. Westman, M.D., M.H.S.,1 and John P. Konhilas, PhD. Clinical Experience of a Diet Designed to Reduce Aging. *J Appl Res.* 2009 January 1; 9(4): 159–165.

[8]Ford ES, Giles W et al. Prevalence of the Metabolic Syndrome Among US Adults. *JAMA* 287;3:356-59 (Jan 16, 2002).

[9]Olshansky SJ, Passaro DJ, et al. A Potential Decline in Life Expectancy in the United States in the 21st Century. *NEJM* 352;11:1138-1145 (March 17, 2005).

[10]Yun AJ, Doux JD. Unhappy meal: How our need to detect stress may have shaped our preferences for taste. *Med Hypotheses.* 2007 Mar 19.

[11]Fox CS, Pencina MJ et al. Trends in the Incidence of Type 2 Diabetes Mellitus From the 1970s to the 1990s. *Circulation.* 2006;113:2914-2918.

[12] Fowler SP, Williams K et al. Fueling the obesity epidemic? Artificially sweetened beverage use and long-term weight gain. Obesity (Silver Spring). 2008 Aug;16(8):1894-900. Epub 2008 Jun 5.

[13] A. M. Calafat, X. Ye, L.-Y. Wong, J. A. Reidy, and L. L. Needham. Exposure of the U.S. population to bisphenol A and 4-tertiary-octylphenol: 2003-2004. *Environmental Health Perspectives.* Available on-line October 24, 2007 at http://dx.doi.org/10.1289/ehp.10753.

[14]Alonso-Magdalena P, Morimoto S, et al. The estrogenic effect of bisphenol A disrupts pancreatic beta-cell function in vivo and induces insulin resistance. *Environmental Health Perspectives*, 2006 Jan;114(1):106-12.

[15]Salmerón J, Hu FB et al. Dietary fat intake and risk of type 2 diabetes in women. *AJCN* 73;6:1019-26 (June 2001).

[16]Ben Harder. Diabetes from a Plastic? Estrogen mimic provokes insulin resistance. *Science News*, January 21st, 2006; Vol.169 #3

[17]Ben Harder. Ingredient Shuffle: A trans fat substitute might have risks too. *Science News*, February 10th, 2007; Vol.171 #6

[18]Sundram K, Karupaiah T, Hayes KC. Stearic acid-rich interesterified fat and trans-rich fat raise the LDL/HDL ratio and plasma glucose relative to palm olein in humans. *Nutrition & Metabolism* 2007, 4:3 (15 January 2007).

[19]Reichmuth KJ, Austin D et al. Association of Sleep Apnea and Type 2 Diabetes. *American Journal of Respiratory and Critical Care Medicine* Vol 172. pp. 1590-1595, (2005).

[20]Valeriya Lyssenko, Cecilia L F Nagorny, et al. Common variant in MTNR1B associated with increased risk of type 2 diabetes and impaired early insulin secretion. *Nature Genetics*, 7 December 2008, doi:10.1038/ng.288

[21]Laura Sanders. Lack of sleep has genetic link with type 2 diabetes – Large genomic studies show body rhythms, melatonin may influence sugar levels in the blood. *Science News*, January 3rd, 2009; Vol.175 #1

[22]Jukka Montonen, MSC, Paul Knekt, PhD, et al. Dietary Antioxidant Intake and Risk of Type 2 Diabetes. *Diabetes Care* 27:362-366, 2004

[23]Wayne H. F. Sutherland, Patrick J. Manning, et al. Vitamin E Supplementation and Plasma 8-Isoprostane and Adiponectin in Overweight Subjects. *Obesity* (2007) 15, 286–391; doi:10.1038/oby.2007.546

[24]Lori Laffel, et al. Overall health in youth with type 1 diabetes. *The Journal of Pediatrics*, January 2009, Joslin Diabetes Center

[25]Mom's Unhealthy Diet May Have Long-Term Impact on Baby. *Washington Post*, Monday, June 30, 2008

[26]Type 2 diabetes—time to change our approach. *The Lancet*, Volume 375, Issue 9733, Page 2193, 26 June 2010

Energy Medicine

*B*ioEnergetic Medicine is a powerful approach to healing based on physics, not chemistry. If chemistry is about the body's components (oxygen, carbon, etc), then physics is about the bigger universe that the body encompasses.

All living things are surrounded by fields of energy and emit visible light in extremely small quantities. Kirlian photography is able to capture these emissions. Other technologies capture some of the body's energetic functions. EKGs are an electronic representation of the activity of the heart, for example. EEGs are an electronic representation of the activity of the brain. Ultrasound machines use high frequency sound energy to create images. The physical plane is simply dense energy and we now have devices that can interface with it, such as MRIs and CT scans.

The field of light and energy that surrounds the body is called a "biophoton field." Eastern medical traditions have operated on this premise for thousands of years. This energetic model for health has influenced Tibetan medicine, traditional Chinese medicine (TCM), and Ayurvedic medicine.

In 1974, Dr. Fritz-Albert Popp proved the existence of the biophoton field. He demonstrated that normal living cells emit a regular stream of photons, or quanta of light radiation. In his book *Biologie des Lichts* (*Biology of Light*) he showed how living cells pass on biological information via photons, through the language of light.

Each of the trillions of cells in the human body undergoes more than 100,000 biochemical reactions per second, all of which are exquisitely timed and sequenced with each other. The DNA sequence contracts and expands several billion times per second, producing a photon of light with each contraction. DNA sends out and receives information on each photon. This all happens with a speed far faster than any computer mankind has devised. Light is fast; it is an efficient carrier of biological information.

So too are the meridians, avenues of electrical energy that flow through the body. In the 1950s, Dr. Reinhold Voll, a German medical doctor, scientifically verified the existence of meridians and acupuncture points, which had been used for thousands of years in Chinese medicine. Dr. Voll created an electronic testing device to pass a tiny electrical current through the human body and measure the amount of resistance encountered at the acupuncture points. He found that the acupuncture points exhibit a different resistance to current than nearby tissues. He also realized the diagnostic abilities of this information. For example, he found that patients with lung cancer had abnormal readings on the acupuncture points referred to as lung points. Dr. Voll made it his life's work to identify and document correlations between disease and changes in the electrical resistance of the various acupuncture points.

To heal with energy is to heal with the body's own essence. Rather than assaulting the body with chemicals, we can encourage our ability to heal through its own inherent mechanisms. It is the body's natural inclination to set itself right again.

> *"Each patient carries his own doctor inside him.*
> *They come to us not knowing that truth.*
> *We are at our best when we give the doctor who resides*
> *within each patient a chance to go to work."*
> ALBERT SCHWEITZER

NES Scan

The NES scan is based on Quantum biology. It is an assessment tool at the energetic level, researched and developed by an Australian physician, Peter Fraser, and a British computer expert, Harry Massey. The scan of the body's quantum electrodynamic (QED) body field allows us to peek into the body's innate wisdom and see where the energy fields are distorted, so that we may determine where physical dysfunction may be occurring before disease sets in.

There is evidence that all plant and animal cells and tissues continuously emit weak light in the visible spectrum (400-800 nm). Experimental evidence shows that DNA is a source of this emission. Electrons and photons are thought to be the carriers of information through the body.

In its external form this human body-field is what some people call the "aura." It has measurable structure, and the NES scan shows us the various components of that field.

The human body field is like the body's energetic mastermind, the operating system which organizes the body's chemical processes.

Chemical reactions are all about making and breaking energetic bonds between molecules. The human body-field provides the information needed for the body to initiate chemical reactions.

The body field has energy pathways that channel information to direct fundamental activities like pumping blood and digesting food. There are 12 such pathways, each representing a band of energy wavelengths and magnetic vectors in the QED field. These compartments are called "energetic integrators" and are folded on one another, such that information must be sequenced in the correct order in order to be correctly interpreted. Chinese Medicine calls these pathways "meridians."

Loss of homeostasis – the break-down of the body's ability to self-correct – is an intricate interplay of a multitude of factors. There is no single "correct" state of being. Most of the body's interactions have considerable flexibility built into them.

In Quantum biology, disease can be thought of as "untunement." This state arises because particles are arranged incorrectly in space, not because they are vibrating at an incorrect frequency.

The human body-field also coordinates with the emotions and the consciousness. It is in constant interaction with its environment.

The NES scan can determine whether any of the information pathways which control the body's metabolic processes have been damaged, distorted or blocked. Remedies can be recommended to correct the distortion of the information pathways, so that the body may have the best chance of returning to full health.

A NES scan can give a broad picture of what is going on inside the body.

BIA Test

A bioimpedance analysis (BIA) energetically measures body the percentage of body fat and lean body mass. This test gives us a reading on many aspects of your body including:

Phase angle: All living substances have a phase angle. Lower phase angles indicate either cell death or a breakdown of the cell membrane. Higher phase angles indicate healthy cells. Phase angle indicates the course of disease. It increases as the result of optimal health based on good nutrition and consistent exercise.

Body Cell Mass: BCM represents the "living cells" such as those found in muscles, organs, blood and immune cells. In the normally nourished individual, muscle tissue accounts for approximately 60% of the body cell mass, organ tissue for 20% of body cell mass, with the remaining 20% made up of red cells and tissue cells, as well as intracellular water – the water inside your trillions of cells.

Extracellular Cell Mass: This is extracellular fluids, the amount of water found outside your cells. ECM includes blood and lymph, plus solids such as bone and cartilage – the primary functions of support and transport.

Lean body mass: The sum of body cell mass and extracellular cell mass.

Fat mass: The amount of fat stored in the body.

Body capacitance: Measures the ability for nutrients to move into the cell and waste to move out. It increases or decreases depending upon the health and the number of cells. Damage to the cell membrane and its functions is as lethal to the cell as direct damage to the nucleus itself. Cells are compartments filled with a concentrated solution of chemicals and salts. Groups of cells perform specialized functions and are linked by an intricate communications system. The cell membrane maintains an electrochemical concentration gradient between the intracellular and extracellular spaces. This gradient creates an electrical potential difference across the membrane which is essential to cell survival. Electrical gradients are necessary to support movement of oxygen, carbon dioxide, and nutrients. Therefore, the cell membrane has electrically insulating qualities, or capacitance.

Basal metabolic rate: Based upon lean body mass, the number of calories your body uses each day, not including the calories burned through exercise, to maintain its weight.

We use the BIA measurements to determine the current state of health of the physical body, as well as for comparison purposes, as treatment progresses.

Evoked Photon Capture
(also known as Gaseous Discharge Visualization, GDV)

Evoked photon capture (EPC) is a tool of quantum medicine. Simply put, it allows us to measure the energy level at which the body is operating.

The EPC technique measures the body's photon and electron emissions. The EPC machine emits a weak electric current that is pulsed and measured in micro-amps. It is safe for the human body because it causes no substantive physiologic effect.

The body has electrical properties. Electrons are generated first from the surface of the skin, and within a short time, electrons from deeper tissues within the body are included in the current flow. The electrons come mainly from the proteins. According to principles of quantum mechanics, these electrons are dispersed among many molecules, and form an "electron

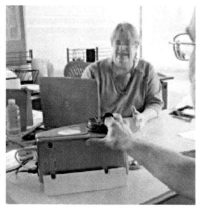

cloud," occupying a specific region in space. Other sources of electrons are the free radicals which form in response to metabolic processes.

When the body is functioning normally, electron clouds are distributed among all systems and organs. The mitochondria inside cells use the mitochondrial electron chain to convert molecules to ATP, packets of energy. When there is imbalance or dysfunction, electrons are not transferred normally to the blood and redistributed to all tissues. This prevents the normal flow of electrons (the basis for energy production), resulting in overall decrease of energy of the system. Accumulation of electrons also allows free radicals to build up in specific organs, resulting in tissue damage. This decrease in energy both to the body as a whole, and to specific organs, is measured by the EPC technique.

Information exchange occurs between the organs and the autonomic nervous system all the time. In a state of health, there is excellent information exchange, the autonomic nervous system can respond to all the needs of the different organs, and the body is in a state of balance (or homeostasis), and is healthy.

When information channels are blocked, by inflammation or tumor or injury, this information transfer is suppressed or completely cut off, and the autonomic nervous system can no longer respond as rapidly or completely. At a given point, the information suppression gets so severe that it may result in insomnia, abdominal pain, fatigue, susceptibility to infection. In conventional allopathic medicine, this is still considered to be a state of health.

Eventually, the body can't compensate enough and you get noticeably sick. You may have organ damage. At this point, allopathic medicine agrees that you are sick and gives you a "diagnosis."

EPC is a means of assessing the energy state of a person, from the point of view of the balance of autonomic nervous system function. It is a unique way of assessing how the body is functioning. The EPC evaluation can be added to other forms of assessment – EKG, ultrasound, blood analysis, etcetera – to give a more complete picture of the state of health of a person's organ systems.

So why is homeopathic medicine not the standard of medicine in this modern age?

*B*y the year 1900, more than 100 homeopathic hospitals operated in the U.S., along with 22 homeopathic medical schools and more than 1,000 homeopathic pharmacies. Interestingly, many students and practitioners were women, and the homeopathic Boston Female Medical College, founded as a school for midwives in 1848, was the first women's medical college in the world. Mark Twain wrote in *Harper's* magazine in 1890, "The introduction of homeopathy forced the old-school doctor to stir around and learn something of a rational nature about his business."[1]

But the allopaths competed for patients. They established the American Medical Association in 1846, two years after the founding of the American Institute of Homeopathy, the nation's first national medical society. Allopaths were called quacks in the 19th century and even before, because they used quicksilver, what we call mercury, also known as quack silver, as medicine. Homeopaths did not support the use of caustic or poisonous pharmaceuticals; homeopathy was the predominant form of medicine at the start of the 20th century. People living on the frontier relied on homeopathic remedies because doctors were few and far between.

As Doctors Paolo Bellavite and Andrea Signorini wrote of that era:

> The rapid initial spread of homeopathy was probably initially due, on the one hand, to the fact that the orthodox medicine of [Hahnemann's] day and age was still extremely backward and lacked truly effective therapeutic remedies, and, on the other to the distinct superiority of homeopathy treating the various epidemics of typhoid fever, cholera, and yellow fever which raged across Europe and America in the 1800s.[2]

In 1855, the AMA incorporated a code of ethics that included expulsion of physicians who even consulted with homeopaths or other "un-scientific" practitioners. Similar events were unfolding in Europe; orthodox physicians in France also banned consultations with homeopaths. Homeopathy was outlawed in Austria.[3]

In 1908 the newly formed American Medical Association's (AMA) Council on Medical Education wrote to Andrew Carnegie to propose a collaboration with the purpose of reforming medical education. The Carnegie Foundation was allied with the Rockefellers, who heavily invested first in oil, then in pharmaceutical companies. It was decided to hire Abraham Flexner to investigate the 155 U. S. and Canadian medical schools.

Flexner was a schoolmaster who knew nothing about the field of medicine but he was well-connected; his brother Simon was director of the Rockefeller Institute for Medical Research.

Flexner's subsequent findings, not surprisingly, heavily favored the medical schools which supported the use of pharmaceutical medicine and "science-based" medicine. Flexner wanted to promote higher status for doctors. He recommended specialization, and recommended that most of the schools for women and blacks be closed, since women showed a "decreasing inclination" to enter the profession, and blacks were a potential source of "infection and contagion." In the report, Flexner called chiropractors "quacks."

Medical journals had mixed reactions. The *Journal of the American Medical Association* announced that "[al]though there may be statements of detail which might be criticized in the Foundation's report, generally speaking the statements made are recognized as the truth by those who are in a position to judge."[4] It was "full of errors," alleged the *Denver Medical Journal*; "a piece of monumental impudence," according to the *American Medical Compound*.[5] Among other failings, the report was produced too fast to for Flexner to visit all the schools. "You don't need to eat a whole sheep to know it's tainted," Flexner later wrote in his autobiography.[6]

The *New York State Journal of Medicine* berated the Carnegie Foundation for attempting to "dictate the policies ... to wipe out institutions with the stroke of a pen" and thereby "threaten the freedom of medical schools."[7]

Despite the clear bias against all forms of medical treatment other than allopathic, the report was widely acclaimed by the allopathic medical community. It sent shock waves through the medical schools of the United States.

The historic Flexner Report[8] dictated that medical schools which would be funded and accredited would be those which trained doctors in the extremes of medicine – emergency and surgical, both of which make extensive use of pharmaceutical drugs. In 1905, 160 medical schools were in operation. By 1927, seventeen years after the Flexner Report, the number had dropped to 80. The homeopathic medical schools were disappearing.

Medicine in America was shifting from its early emphasis on prevention and health to a model of disease management. Influential forces promoted "allopathic" medicine, the suppression of symptoms. And they fought competition fiercely.

Doctors of Chiropractic came to find themselves denied coverage and recognition in all federal and state government agencies. They took the fight all the way to the Supreme Court. The historic 1990 decision[9] found the AMA guilty of an unlawful conspiracy in restraint of trade "to contain and eliminate the chiropractic profession" and, the judge said, that the "AMA had entered into a long history of illegal behavior." Since then, chiropractors have largely been able to continue their practice without medical doctor interference.

George Vithoulkas, a Greek homeopath who is credited for much of homeopathy's revival since the 1960s in Europe, said:

> The immune systems of the western population, through strong chemical drugs and repeated vaccinations, have broken down ... If conventional medicine were really curing chronic diseases, today we would have a population in the West that was healthy, mentally, emotionally and physically.[10]

Americans are beginning to demand more than symptom management. More and more, they want to find out what went wrong and how to fix it at the fundamental level. In 1999, the first homeopathic college to open its doors since the Flexner report did so in Phoenix, Arizona: The American Medical College of Homeopathy under the direction of Dr. Todd Rowe. It currently graduates Homeopathic Medical Assistants, and has plans in the near future to grant the degree of DCH, Doctor of Classical Homeopathy.

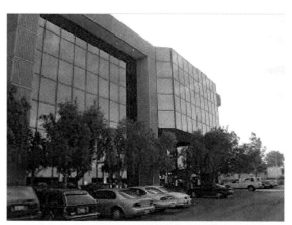

The American Medical College of Homeopathy
Located at 21st Avenue and Camelback Road, Phoenix.
Find out more at http://www.amcofh.org

Where are we headed?

I always envied the doctors in the *Star Trek* programs, with their hand-held scanning and diagnostic devices, and their ability to do surgery – and visualize what they needed to see – without having to use cumbersome and physically dangerous tools. We could be headed in that direction. If we can conceive the device, I am quite certain that someone will build it. Those photons keep popping in and out of existence, showing us the way to a world of infinite possibilities.

And in the meantime, we do our best with what we have available to us. We use those physical tools that are effective, we use pharmaceuticals when we have to, we use nutrition and detoxification to maintain and restore our health, we use supplements to provide that which nutrition does not, and we use the tools of bioenergetic medicine that make sense to us.

And we keep our minds open to new tools, new drugs, new treatments – remembering that ballast is good, to keep the ship stable in the water. But ballast is meant to be jettisoned when the ship needs to move quickly, or the waters become shallow. I read a wonderful little book years ago, talking about how to distinguish true prophets from false. The book's advice:

"You will know them by their fruits."

If use of the tool results in dangerous consequences to the patient, we are well advised to find a different tool. If use of the tool results in accurate assessments or good treatments, then we can use it in good conscience, and with the sure and certain knowledge that something better will come down the pike next year.

[1]Kim Ridley. The Controversial Cure. *Ode Magazine*, January/February 2006

[2]Paolo Bellavite, Andrea Signorini. *The Emerging Science of Homeopathy – Complexity, Biodynamics, and Nanopharmacology*. North Atlantic Books, 2002, p 21.

[3]Kim Ridley. The Controversial Cure. *Ode Magazine*, January/February 2006

[4]Berliner HS. *A System of Scientific Medicine: Philanthropic Foundations in the Flexner Era*. Tavistock Publications; 1985. p. 120-121

[5]Felts JH. Abraham Flexner and medical education in North Carolina. *NC Med J* 1995; 56:534-40. p. 537

[6]Flexner A. *Abraham Flexner: An Autobiography*. Simon & Schuster; 1960.

[7]Berliner HS. *A System of Scientific Medicine: Philanthropic Foundations in the Flexner Era*. Tavistock Publications; 1985. p. 122

[8]Flexner A. Medical Education in the United States and Canada: A Report to the Carnegie Foundation for the Advancement of Teaching; Bulletin No. 4. New York: Carnegie Foundation for the Advancement of Teaching; 1910.

[9]*Wilk v. American Medical Association*, 671 F. Supp. 1465, N.D. Ill. 1987.

[10]Speech to the Swedish Parliament upon acceptance of Right Livelihood Award, 1996. Accessed at http://www.vithoulkas.com/content/view/175/9/lang,en

Erectile Dysfunction

$\mathcal{I}$f you've ever told a doctor you had erectile dysfunction, did the doctor talk to you about cardiovascular disease or diabetes?

Erectile dysfunction, ED, is more than just a bedroom frustration. ED is often an early warning sign of heart disease or undiagnosed diabetes.

Men with erectile dysfunction are 80 percent more likely to develop heart disease compared to men who do not have ED. Men ages 40 to 49 with erectile dysfunction are twice as likely to get heart disease.[1]

Diabetics with erectile dysfunction are perhaps twice as likely as non-diabetic men with diabetes to develop heart disease.[2]

The cause of erectile dysfunction is typically the lack of adequate penile blood supply as a result of damage to inner walls of blood vessels. Sounds like the arterial damage we see in heart disease and diabetes? Yes, because it's the same physiology, the same underlying problem.

- A buildup of plaque blocks arteries around the heart and can also plug the smaller penile arteries, even before we see the effect on heart performance.
- Inflammation causes the blood to become more viscous (thick, sticky) and the red blood cells membranes to become more rigid. These rigid red blood cells then nick the lining of the arteries.
- Arteries may lose elasticity over time, affecting the penis first and the heart later.

The endothelium or inner lining of blood vessels regulates how the heart relaxes and contracts. When there is a problem with blood vessel relaxation, you have bad blood flow and develop heart disease. Endothelial malfunction in the penis causes erectile dysfunction.

243

When the brain gets aroused, it sends a signal to the penis. Nerve cells in the penis start producing nitric oxide, which creates cGMP, an enzyme which tells smooth muscles that line the arteries to relax. Next, blood flow increases and small arteries at the base of the penis dilate. Blood rushing into the penis is shunted into the expandable tissues in the bulk of the penis. These fill under high pressure to compress outlet veins so blood cannot drain back out again.

The small capillaries are the first element that must operate correctly for a successful erection. If the arteries in the penis do not dilate enough, the amount of cGMP produced is not enough to maintain an erection.

More than half of American men age 40 to 70 suffer from erectile dysfunction. That's a lot of men who may be at risk of vascular disease and may not realize it.

Other diseases – kidney disease, chronic alcoholism, and multiple sclerosis – can impact vascular health; such diseases account for about 70 percent of cases of impotence. What if it's not damage to blood vessels which provide blood flow to the penis? Then we look for damage to nerves, medications, chronic inflammation, and and environmental toxicity. In late 2009, it was found that Bisphenol-A (BPA), a chemical found in hard, clear plastic used to make everything from baby bottles to food packaging, caused erectile dysfunction in male factory workers exposed to large amounts of the substance. The men handling BPA were four times as likely to suffer from erectile dysfunction and seven times as likely to have difficulty with ejaculation.[3]

And finally, don't discount psychological factors such as stress. Psychological impotence occurs when erection or penetration fails due to thoughts or feelings.

Erections are triggered by emotional, physical and hormonal signals. The hormone testosterone is important overall but it has no direct impact on blood vessels. Most men who are low on testosterone can blame low adrenal function because of stress.

Statins – The Anti-Viagra

$\mathcal{H}$eart disease is often the result of chronic inflammation. Inflammation increases blood viscosity making it sticky, thicker. The red blood cells get stiff and nick the walls of the arteries. The body uses cholesterol patches to cover the nicks. Although cholesterol does not cause heart disease – it is merely a marker of inflammation – statin drugs were created to reduce the body's production of cholesterol.

Mother Nature knew what she was doing when she made cholesterol. It is a super anti-oxidant, the building block for manufacture of our sex hormones, and a good bandage that can be transported to tissues to repair damage. When you artificially reduce your body's ability to make cholesterol, you also reduce your body's ability to make a whole family of intermediary substances which have important biochemical functions in their own right. Let's highlight Coenzyme Q-10 depletion.

Inside each of the five trillion or so cells in your body are energy factories called mitochondria. They need CoQ-10 as much as a car needs gas. Cardiologist and researcher Dr. Peter Langsjoen says:

> The depletion of the essential nutrient CoQ-10 by the increasingly popular cholesterol lowering drugs, HMG CoA reductase inhibitors (statins), has grown from a level of concern to one of alarm. With ever higher statin potencies and dosages and with a steadily shrinking target LDL cholesterol, the prevalence and severity of CoQ-10 deficiency is increasingly noticeable.[4]

Deaths attributed to heart failure more than doubled from 1989 to 1997.[5] Statins were first given pre-market approval in 1987. Interference with production of CoQ-10 by statin drugs is the most likely explanation because the heart is a muscle which requires high levels of CoQ-10 for healthy functioning.

The most common reported side effect of statins is muscle pain and weakness. So on one hand, statins help heart disease patients by lessening inflammation, but on the other hand, statin drugs can predispose patients to congestive heart failure by lessening heart function and antioxidant activity. Statins are now proven to activate a gene called atrogin-1, a gene that is activated in order to break down skeletal muscle, when the muscle protein is needed for calories (as in diabetes, starvation, and… when taking statin drugs). This explains why patients on statin drugs so often experience muscle pain.[6]

Anecdotal reports have been surfacing for years of impotence, loss of libido, and erectile dysfunction associated with statin drug use. Researchers continue to find a strong relationship between statin drugs and erectile dysfunction. In 2010, an Italian study of 3,484 men found that statin drugs lower testosterone levels and contribute to ED. The authors called upon doctors to be better aware of the association. "Our data suggest that statin therapy, even at low dosage, might induce an overt primary hypogonadism [decreased production of testosterone] and should be considered a possible confounding factor for the evaluation of testosterone levels in patients with erectile dysfunction."[7] Other studies show ED is reversible when men stop taking statins.

Chronic inflammation also can cause prostate enlargement, by the way. That tends to go hand-in-hand with erectile dysfunction, but prostate enlargement does not directly impact the ability to achieve an erection.

The ED Solution

Drugs can enable an erection to be attained and maintained long enough for intercourse, but drugs do not permanently improve the underlying condition.

A healthy artery is a clean, smooth, slick one with flexible walls that can expand to let more blood through when the heart needs to work harder. And what maintains that youthful vigor? Nitric oxide. It is essential for healthy circulation. It helps dilate blood vessels, prevent blood clots, and regulate blood pressure. It also inhibits the accumulation of dangerous arterial plaque.

Drugs can increase the efficacy of nitric oxide temporarily. But drugs come with side effects. The most common side effects of Viagra® are headache, facial flushing, and upset stomach. Less commonly, bluish vision, blurred vision, or sensitivity to light may briefly occur. People taking nitroglycerin need to be especially careful because nitroglycerin works by increasing nitric oxide. The combination of nitroglycerin and ED drugs can lead to major problems maintaining any blood pressure at all. ED drugs can cause a heart attack. As the television commercials say, if you get a painful, long-lasting erection, you have to see a doctor to solve the problem. Treatment involves removal of blood from the penis by needle decompression. Sound painful? You betcha. But so is priapism (painful long-lasting erections). And priapism can cause death of penile tissue – also pretty painful.

Herbal preparations: Many are offered, but effectiveness is questionable. A few have been tested – ginseng, DHEA, propionyl-l-carnitine – but very little research has actually been done with them. Yohimbe, a popular remedy, can cause significant high blood pressure and heart failure.

Acupuncture can be helpful with ED. The placement of acupuncture needles in the back and lower legs support the bladder-kidney meridian. The penis is part of that system. In Chinese medicine, impotence is chiefly due to the deficiency of the kidney's energy, or kidney qi. Acupuncture can 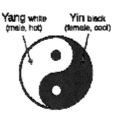 improve the function of the kidney meridian to relieve stagnation, calm the mind, and invigorate the heart and spleen. Relieving stagnation helps to move blood out of the body into the penis. Calming the mind relieves stress, which is a major factor in erectile dysfunction. Invigorating the heart and the spleen gets the blood moving, gets the emotions in a good place, and enhances the entire sexual experience for both men and women.

In the long run, the best way to address ED is not with a pill. Sure, the pill works – but at some considerable cost to the health of the body. If the other health issues are not addressed, you stand the chance of dying in the saddle – not a very nice experience for anyone involved. If emotional issues are addressed, then look at the underlying state of health of the body –

clean up the filters (the liver), make sure the fuel pump is working well (the heart), make sure the fuel lines are clear (the arteries) and make sure that the computer is loaded with the right software (the brain).

---

[1] Martin Miner, MD. Erectile Dysfunction and the "Window of Curability": A Harbinger of Cardiovascular Events. *Mayo Clinic Proceeding*, February 2009, vol. 84 no. 2 102-104

[2] Dr Peter Chun-Yip Tong. *Journal of the American College of Cardiology*, May 2008

[3] Lyndsey Layton. High BPA levels linked to male sexual problems – Study in China is likely to bring further scrutiny of the common chemical. *Washington Post*, November 11, 2009

[4] Langsjoen PH, Langsjoen AM. The clinical use of HMG CoA-reductase inhibitors and the associated depletion of coenzyme Q10. A review of animal and human publications. *Biofactors*. 2003;18(1-4):101-11. http://www.fda.gov/ohrms/dockets/dailys/02/May02/052902/02p-0244-cp00001-02-Exhibit_A-vol1.pdf

[5] Jun-ichi Hanai, Peirang Cao, et al. The muscle-specific ubiquitin ligase atrogin-1/MAFbx mediates statin-induced muscle toxicity. *Journal of Clinical Investigation*, Volume 117, Issue 12 (December 3, 2007)

[6] Rizvi K, Rizvi K, Hampson JP, Harvey JN. Do lipid lowering drugs cause erectile dysfunction? A systematic review. *Family Practice*, 19 (1):95-8, 2002

[7] Corona G, Boddi V, et al. The Effect of Statin Therapy on Testosterone Levels in Subjects Consulting for Erectile Dysfunction. *J Sex Med*. February 5, 2010.)

Heart Disease

$\mathcal{H}$eart attacks were practically unknown in the nineteenth century. Prior to 1925, there was almost no knowledge of the illness that today we call myocardial infarction.[1] By the early 1940s, heart attacks were the leading cause of death among American men, and by 1984, they had become the leading cause of death for American women.

What happened?

It is not nice to fool Mother Nature.

$\mathcal{W}$e began to "manufacture" food. One of the first unnatural ventures was the creation of margarine, patented in 1873. After Word War II, the food processing industry was off and running and its advertising messages were relentless.

Experts writing for the Weston A. Price Foundation explain it:

> Butter consumption at the turn of the century was eighteen pounds per person per year, and the use of vegetable oils almost nonexistent, yet cancer and heart disease were rare. Today vegetable oil consumption has soared – and cancer and heart disease are endemic.
>
> What the research really shows is that both refined carbohydrates and vegetable oils cause imbalances in the blood and at the cellular level that lead to an increased tendency to form blood clots, leading to myocardial infarction. The "artery clogging" fats are not animal fats but vegetable oils.[2]

Margarine represented the introduction of trans-fats. As our consumption of trans-fats rose, so did the number of heart attacks.[3] Trans-fats interfere with the normal function of the cells, and stiffen the walls of the red blood cells, which roughs up the arteries.

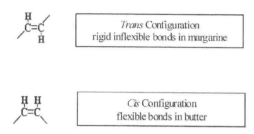

Butter on the other hand, contains nutrients which protect against plaque and heart disease:[4]

- Vitamin A – needed for the health of the thyroid and adrenal glands, both of which play a role in maintaining the proper functioning of the heart and cardiovascular system. Butter is the best and most easily absorbed source of vitamin A.
- Anti-oxidants – protect against the kind of free radical damage that weakens arteries. Vitamins A and E found in butter both play a strong anti-oxidant role. Butter is also a very rich source of selenium, a vital anti-oxidant.

We were persuaded to stop using un-hydrogenated coconut oil which has antiviral and antimicrobial characteristics. Populations that consume natural coconut oil have low rates of heart disease. When coconut oil was fed to patients recovering from heart attacks, the patients had greater improvement compared to untreated patients.[5]

We also began to manufacture meat. Harvard scientists took the first worldwide look at the effects of eating meat and concluded, "The consumption of processed meats, rather than red meats, was associated with increased incidence of coronary heart disease."[6] Things like bacon, sausage, pepperoni, hot dogs, and lunch meat contain chemicals, preservatives, and additives. Often they are smoked, cured, or salted. This landmark study clarified that "natural" meats are indeed healthy; it is manufactured, processed meat that is the problem. When you eat processed meat with additives, you get four times the sodium and twice as many nitrates. Salt drives up your blood pressure. Nitrates cause plaque to build up in your arteries.[7]

Starting in the 1980s, sun screen makers and dermatologists persuaded us to hide from the natural rays of the sun. Big mistake. Vitamin D deficiency is now rampant. Studies have linked vitamin D to the regulation of blood pressure, glucose control, and inflammation, all of which are important risk factors related to heart disease. A 2009 study suggests that inadequate levels of vitamin D increases the risk even among people who've never had heart disease.[8]

Chronic Inflammation

The realization that chronic inflammation plays a big role in heart disease and other chronic diseases gained traction when the Nobel Prize was awarded for the discovery that stress did not, in and of itself, cause stomach ulcers. Rather ulcers were caused by inflammation triggered by the bacterium H. pylori.

"It's hard now to think of a medical specialty that doesn't concern itself in part with the study of inflammation," said Carl Nathan, chairman of the department of microbiology and immunology at the Weill Medical College of Cornell University. "It can go anywhere – lung, heart, blood vessels, brain, wherever."[9]

Inflammation is the body's response to the presence of noxious substances – trans fats, heavy metals, high blood sugar levels, cigarette smoke, toxic chemicals, stress, bacterial infections. Inflammatory stimulants release proteins – cytokines – that trigger an inflammatory cascade. The cytokines make the arterial wall sticky, which attracts immune system cells called monocytes. The monocytes squeeze into the artery wall. Once inside, they can form what is called "vulnerable plaque" with a thin covering.

Dr. Paul Ridker radically changed the thinking about plaque with his hypothesis that small arterial deposits suddenly rupture like popcorn

251

kernels, choking off the blood supply to the heart. About 70% of heart attacks are caused by small obstructions called vulnerable plaque, which narrow the artery by perhaps only a third or so – too small to cause symptoms or to be detected by an X-ray angiogram. Inflammation softens plaque. The softened plaque swells and then may burst, choking off blood flow and causing a heart attack. That would explain why many people suddenly drop dead from heart attacks even though their arteries look fine.[10]

"I think the first thing we have is an epidemic of unhealthy lifestyle," said Peter Libby, a professor of medicine at Harvard Medical School in Boston. "And the way in which the lifestyle is wreaking its havoc is through inflammation."[11]

Infection and Immune System Challenges

Research indicates that infection has an inflammatory role in atherosclerosis. Fingers of blame point to the infectious bacterium Chlamydia pneumoniae; it may travel from the lungs to the heart via immune system cells.[12] The herpes simplex virus has also been proposed as an inflammatory infectious agent in atherosclerosis.[13]

Studies of arteries taken from people who died of coronary heart disease reveal evidence of some form of infection.[14] People with high levels of inflammatory cells are more likely to develop heart disease.

Dental root canals are often a focus of chronic infection, which can affect the entire system, just as water dripping every day from a leaky pipe eventually fills the bucket. Dr. Weston Price, a former Director of Research for the American Dental Association, observed that the removal of root canal teeth from patients with kidney or heart disease would typically lead to an improvement. When he inserted a removed root canal tooth under the skin of a rabbit, the rabbit would die within two days. When he implanted normal teeth there was no adverse health effect, the rabbit survived.[15]

Homocysteine

Homocysteine levels are more valuable than cholesterol levels in providing an accurate assessment of cardiovascular health. Elevated homocysteine is considered an independent risk factor for heart disease.[16] Levels must be kept low to help prevent plaque buildup on blood vessel walls. High levels may make blood clot more easily than it should.

Homocysteine is an amino acid used in the body's detoxification cycle, involving methylation and sulfation, the body's way of getting rid of toxins. Supplementation of vitamins B6, B12 and folic acid, together with betaine, are an excellent way to decrease homocysteine levels and decrease the risk of developing heart disease.

C-Reactive Protein

Forget cholesterol. Cholesterol screening fails to identify 50 percent of the people who have heart attacks in the United States each year, because their total cholesterol is either normal or only moderately elevated.[17] The better measurement is for cardiovascular disease is C-reactive protein (CRP). This marker is produced by the liver as a response to injury or infection and is a sign of inflammation in the body. Research correlates high levels of CRP with an increased risk of heart attack and stroke. Elevated levels of CRP could mean that some part of the cardiovascular system is inflamed, which can lead to stroke or heart attack.

Dr. Paul Ridker and his colleagues had shown that healthy middle-aged men with the highest CRP levels were three times as likely to suffer a heart attack in the next six years as were those with the lowest CRP levels.[18]

CRP can enhance destruction of arterial lining cells, activate adhesion molecules and blood clotting factors, and interfere with substances that increase circulation to the heart.

Cholesterol in Perspective

"For nearly four decades I was a staunch advocate of the anti-cholesterol crusade. I talked the merits of margarine at schools and libraries. I lectured at men's clubs about the evils of eggs. Despite my diet of whole milk, rich butter and daily eggs as a farm boy, I raised my family on skim milk, and almost complete absence of eggs and margarine. So great was my brainwashing during my 23 years of duty as a family doctor that I counseled thousands of my often-bewildered patients about the heretofore unknown evils of eggs, milk and butter.

"Often times I could see skepticism in their eyes but I was the doctor, parroting what the pharmaceutical industry, AMA and AHA told me. How could I be wrong? I wrote thousands of prescriptions for whatever cholesterol buster was in vogue at the time. I regarded the first statin as a boon to mankind. I now am humbled at my colossal ignorance, never suspecting that all this time I had been led astray by my naivety, my unfailing allegiance and faith in 'those in charge'. It never occurred to me to challenge.

"Now we find that cholesterol seemingly has little to nothing to do with cardiovascular disease. It is the most important biochemical in our bodies. Inflammation it now appears is the true cause of cardiovascular disease, according to many researchers."

—Duane Graveline, M.D., MPH*
Former USAF Flight Surgeon
Former NASA Astronaut

* http://www.spacedoc.net/statins_inflammation_heart_disease.html

---

Insulin and Leptin Resistance

Research has linked insulin resistance and more recently leptin resistance to cardiovascular disease much more strongly than cholesterol, and they are in fact at least partially responsible for cholesterol abnormalities.[19] Insulin and leptin resistance result in "small dense" LDL particles and a greater number of particles.

This is much more important than the total cholesterol number. Because of particle size shift to small and dense, the total LDL cholesterol could still be low even though the number of particles and the density of the particles is greater. Small, dense LDL particles can squeeze between the cells lining the inside of the arteries, the "gap junction" of the endothelium, where they can get stuck and potentially turn rancid (i.e. oxidize), and cause inflammation of the lining of the arteries and plaque formation.

Hypertension

Chronically elevated high blood pressure, hypertension, forces the heart to work far beyond its capacity and hardens artery walls, increasing the risk of heart disease and stroke. It's an early warning sign that bigger troubles are on the way.

The top number of a blood pressure reading, the systolic pressure, represents the force of blood in the arteries as the heart beats. The bottom number, diastolic pressure, is the force of blood in the arteries as the heart relaxes between beats. A blood pressure level of 140 over 90 mm Hg (millimeters of mercury) or higher is considered high.

Medical books say that 90 percent of the cause of hypertension is idiopathic, meaning they don't know what causes it. But research points the finger to several culprits: sugar (as insulin levels rise, blood pressure goes up[20]), vitamin D (normalizing vitamin D levels can have a powerful effect on normalizing blood pressure[21]), and refined salt (when you eat more than your kidneys can handle, sodium accumulates in your blood, attracts water, increases blood volume which makes your heart work harder to move more blood through your blood vessels, increasing pressure in your arteries). An increased body burden of heavy metals has also been shown to cause high blood pressure.[22]

Fibrin

Fibrin is a protein produced by the body in response to infectious illnesses. Fibrin gets plastered up against the blood vessel walls and restricts the movement of oxygen into the tissues. The tissues become oxygen-starved, and start producing lactic acid. If unchecked, over-production of lactic acid leads to death of the myocardial cells.

Also, bacteria and viruses hide very well in fibrin coatings, adding to your load of low-grade, chronic infections. In fact, these micro-organisms may produce the fibrin coating, for a shield against the cells of our immune system.

NO – Nitric Oxide

*N*itric oxide may do more good than any prescription drug to prevent a heart attack. Nitric oxide is essential for healthy circulation. It helps dilate blood vessels, prevent blood clots, and regulate blood pressure. It also inhibits the accumulation of dangerous arterial plaque.[23] It is an antioxidant that inhibits the passage of monocytes, a type of immune cell, into the artery wall. This reduces the underlying inflammation that promotes plaque.

Healthy coronary arteries are clean, smooth, and slick. The artery walls are flexible and can expand to let more blood through when the heart needs to work harder, thanks to nitric oxide. The disease process in arteries begins with an injury to the linings and walls of the arteries. Unfortunately, beginning in early adulthood, nitric oxide levels gradually decline, most often due to damage to the endothelial cells caused by such factors as an inflammatory diet and a sedentary lifestyle.

Mercury

A 14-year study of 1,871 men found those with the highest levels of mercury in their hair had a 60 percent increased risk of an acute coronary event and a nearly 70 percent increased risk of cardiovascular death compared with men with lower mercury levels.[24]

The study also found that high mercury concentrations in the body reduced the heart-protective effects of the fatty acids in fish oils. Researchers hypothesized that mercury promotes formation of free radicals in the body, which can harm cell membranes and tissues, and at the same time reduce the body's ability to protect itself from theses free radicals, increasing the vulnerability to heart attack and death.

Herbert Needleman, the scientist who did more than any other to document the toxicity of lead to developing brains, wrote, "Sensitivity to mercury toxicity may have a genetic basis." Variations in a gene called coproporphyrinogen oxidase (CPOX4) "altered the impact of mercury on cognitive and mood scores."[25] Approximately 1 out 4 people in the U.S. has the sensitive-to-mercury gene.

Besides fish and coal-fired power plants, a common exposure is "silver" fillings. More than half of an amalgam filling is made up of mercury, a metal more poisonous than lead. It is now accepted that fillings constantly emit mercury vapor, which then makes its way into the bloodstream and organs.[26]

Study after study has shown that mercury negatively affects the heart. Here's a sampling of the findings:

- Mercury causes hypertension by contracting smooth muscle in arterial walls.[27, 28]
- Mercury affected the ability of heart muscle to contract, accumulating in both heart muscle and valves. Damage was evident from ECG changes and through histological studies.[29]
- Various mercury compounds in low concentrations accelerated blood clotting.[30]
- Subjects with amalgam fillings had significantly higher blood pressure, lower heart rate and lower hemoglobin counts. They also had a greater incidence of chest pains, tachycardia, anemia and fatigue, and became tired easily and awoke feeling tired.[31]

Chinese Medicine tells us another reason why mercury fillings trigger heart attacks: Every tooth has a separate acupuncture meridian running though major organs in the body. The heart meridian runs right through the wisdom teeth sites; many people have fillings in their molars. A metallic filling of any sort, including gold, usually exhibits some form of battery-like action, generating microvoltages in each filled tooth that can interfere with the body's natural electronic field. Conventional acupuncture theory recognizes that teeth are significant points along recognized acupuncture meridians and that any foreign voltages generated on these meridians can disturb the body's natural state of health.

Emotions

The Chinese call the heart the Emperor organ. All emotions are perceived by the heart. Emotions may not be expressed, but they are all perceived by the heart. If we grow up in a family where heart disease is an issue, it may be that on a subconscious level we learned that any emotional imbalance may express itself as heart disease.

Solutions

The allopathic medical world relies on drugs and surgery. Studies published in the *New England Journal of Medicine*, including the COURAGE and FAME studies, suggest surgical procedures are not working all that well. People with clogged heart arteries are being overtreated with stents. Fewer deaths, heart attacks, and repeat procedures occurred when doctors implanted fewer of these tiny artery props, and when doctors used the blood-flow test to decide when they were truly needed.[32, 33]

An angioplasty procedure pushes a balloon into a blood vessel to flatten the blockage, leaving a stent to prop the artery open. A stent is a foreign object in the body; it incites an immune/inflammatory response. This may cause scar tissue to grow rapidly over the stent. Also, there is a strong tendency for clots to form at the site where the stent damages the arterial wall.

Stents and bypass surgeries don't address the causes of heart disease. Statins are anti-inflammatory, and that is a help. But they also come with side effects because they suppress the body's normal production of cholesterol which is not good – cholesterol is a powerhouse anti-oxidant.

Blood tends to get more viscous (sticky, thick) thanks to inflammatory foods, inflammatory heavy metals like mercury, chronic infections, lack of nutrients (especially B vitamins, folic acid, vitamin C and vitamin D, and omega-3s), and lack of exercise. Thick blood roughs up the arterial walls.

As a result of disease in the small vessels, heart cells suffer from inadequate oxygen and nutrient supply. Lactic acid begins to collect in the tissues. Because the heart, unlike your leg muscles, cannot rest, the acidosis can lead to actual death of the myocardial cells. If it's just a couple of cells, we may not feel it. If it's a whole section of the heart, it hurts a lot and we call it a heart attack.

Chelation is Fundamental

Chelation has long been a successful, non-invasive treatment for heart disease. A common misperception is that it works like Drano to "rotor rooter" the arteries, get rid of the calcified plaques. Wrong. Plaque reversal is not the primary mechanism of action with chelation therapy.

It is established that 70% to 85% of sudden heart attack and stroke deaths are due to the rupture of vulnerable, non-calcified arterial plaque and subsequent clot formation – what Dr. Ridker calls popcorn kernel-like ruptures.[34, 35] Researchers are realizing that many people who have heart attacks do not have arteries severely narrowed by plaque. Scientists at the Texas Heart Institute have discovered that vulnerable plaque has a low pH (is more acidic) and that such acidic plaques are more likely to rupture.[36]

Chelation goes after the primary sources of inflammation. Chelating agents are often combined with vitamin C and other supplementation. The treatments are typically given in a series of IVs delivered once a week for perhaps 30 weeks.

Chelation works because:

- It removes heavy metals which trigger chronic inflammation.
- The removal of toxic metals restores the ability of the cells which line arteries to produce nitric oxide, keeping arteries dilated and fending off free radicals. Lead interferes with all zinc-mediated enzymes which include those used in the synthesis of nitric oxide, so lower lead leads to improved conversion of dietary arginine to nitric oxide.
- Blood flow is increased.
- Viscosity is lowered, meaning thick blood becomes thinner and less sticky.
- It is anti-viral so it reduces chronic infections – this is one of the reasons chelation is also a vital part of the treatment of autistic children.
- It increases production of nitric oxide which dilates arteries.
- Vitamin D is often part of the supplementation, and vitamin D is an anti-calcifying agent.

Because chelation is not approved by the American Heart Association, insurance companies do not cover it. Many practitioners feel the AHA is protecting the economic interests of the pharmaceutical industry.[37] In 2003, the National Institutes of Health launched the first large scale study of chelation for patients with coronary artery disease. Hundreds of medical clinics across the country are participating in this five year, placebo-controlled, double-blind study. This study was long resisted by the holistic community because many view double-blind studies as unethical; they require withholding treatments from participants who receive just a placebo.

The study has completed enrollment of patients. Participants will be followed through 2011, and the results will be analyzed in 2012.[38]

Nutritional Therapy

𝒟n the 1950s, the Shute brothers documented the use of vitamin E to prevent and treat heart disease. Data also indicated that intravenous magnesium could reduce deaths from heart attacks. It makes sense – the closer we stay to the natural elements designed by nature, the healthier we are. Magnesium helps the blood vessels to relax, providing better circulation to heart cells.

Many of us who practice chelation combine it with nutritional supplementation. Depending upon the cardiac patient, here are a few examples:

- D-ribose, a naturally occurring sugar that feeds the heart muscle. Adenosine triphosphate (ATP) exists in all our cells; it is the primary energy source for many metabolic processes. Our body needs ribose to make ATP.

- CoQ-10 is also absolutely essential to the ATP production process. It supplies the cellular energy necessary for the heart to pump well and reduces LDL oxidation.

- Vitamin K2 because it regulates mineralization of bone and prevents calcification of blood vessels. Arteries without atherosclerosis (plaque) have a 20-50 fold increase in vitamin K2 concentration compared with plaque-filled arteries in the same human body.[39] Arteries with vitamin K2 were found to be more flexible and elastic than other arteries.

- Proteolytic enzymes to attack the fibrin that forms from inflammation. Fibrin is a great place for infectious bacteria to hide. Enzymes break down the protein coating on the surface of the bug so the immune system can see it and get rid of it.

- Fish oils and "baby aspirin" to decrease the viscosity (thickness) of the blood and lessen the stickiness of platelets, thus reducing the odds of having a blood clot in the coronary arteries.

- Magnesium is greatly beneficial to the heart. It reduces platelet adhesion, is a vasodilator, and is a potent antiarrhythmic agent.

- Garlic and ginkgo and vitamin E each play a role in making a healthier heart.

Removal of mercury fillings and root canals by a biological dentist is well worth the trouble. Colonics are a good way to detoxify. And, because nutritional deficiencies and sedentary lifestyle is where this whole subject began, some changes in habit will be good for your heart.

[1] A.G. Gibbon. Ischemic necrosis of the heart. *The Lancet*, 1925, i, pp. 1270-9.

[2] Sally Fallon. Ancient Dietary Wisdom for Tomorrow's Children, Weston A. Price Foundation website.

[3] Enig, MG. *Trans Fatty Acids in the Food Supply: A Comprehensive Report Covering 60 Years of Research*, 2nd Edition, Enig Associates, Inc, Silver Spring, MD, pages 93-96, 1995

[4] Sally Fallon and Mary Enig. Why Butter is Better. 1999, accessed at http://www.westonaprice.org/foodfeatures/butter.html

[5] Marvin L. Bierenbaum; Donald P. Green; Alvin Florin; Alan I. Fleischman; Anne B. Caldwell. Modified-Fat Dietary Management of the Young Male With Coronary Disease: A Five-Year Report. *JAMA.* 1967;202(13):1119-1123.

[6] Renata Micha, Sarah K. Wallace, Dariush Mozaffarian. Red and Processed Meat Consumption and Risk of Incident Coronary Heart Disease, Stroke, and Diabetes Mellitus: A Systematic Review and Meta-Analysis. *Circulation*, online May 17, 2010.

[7] Paikabc, DC., Wendel, TD., Freeman, HP. "Cured meat consumption and hypertension: an analysis from NHANES III (1988-94)." *Nutrition Research*, 2005; 25(12):1049-1060.

[8] News release: New study links vitamin D deficiency to cardiovascular disease and death – Study finds inadequate levels of vitamin D may significantly increase risk of stroke, heart disease and death. Intermountain Medical Center, Murray, Utah. November 16, 2009

[9] Rob Stein. Body's First Defense May Be Root of Diseases. *The Washington Post*, February 16, 2003; Page A01

[10] Ron Winslow. Heart-Disease Sleuths Identify Prime Suspect: Inflammation of Artery. The Body's Efforts to Repair Irritated Lining of Vessel Can Backfire Disastrously Plaques Burst Like Popcorn. *The Wall Street Journal.* October 7, 1999

[11] ibid

[12] Giovambattista Desideri, Achille Gaspardone, Marco Gentile, Anna Santucci, Pier Agostino Gioffrè, and Claudio Ferri. Endothelial Activation in Patients With Cardiac Syndrome X. *Circulation.* 2000;102:2359-2364

[13] American Heart Association fact sheet, Inflammation, Heart Disease and Stroke: The Role of C-Reactive Protein

[14] Stephan J. Ott, Nour Eddine, El Mokhtari, et al. Detection of Diverse Bacterial Signatures in Atherosclerotic Lesions of Patients With Coronary Heart Disease. *Circulation*, 2006;113:929-937

[15] George E. Meinig. *Root Canal Cover-Up*. Bion Publishing, 1994

[16]McCarty MF, Thomas CA. The Vascular Toxicity of Homocysteine and How to Control It. Downloaded January 23, 2009 from the Linus Pauling website, http://lpi.oregonstate.edu/f-w99/vascular.html

[17]Dr. Eric S. Rawson of the University of Massachusetts Medical School, *Medicine & Science in Sports & Exercise*, July, 2003.

[18]P.M. Ridker, et al. Inflammation, aspirin, and the risk of cardiovascular-disease in apparently healthy men. *New Engl. J. Med.*, 336(14): 973-9, 1997

[19]Martin SS, Oasim A, Reilly MP. Leptin resistance: a possible interface of inflammation and metabolism in obesity-related cardiovascular disease. *Journal of American College of Cardiology*, 2008 Oct 7;52(15):1201-10

[20]AS Krolewski, M Canessa, et al. Predisposition to hypertension and susceptibility to renal disease in insulin-dependent diabetes mellitus. *New England Journal of Medicine*, January 21, 1988, Volume 318:140-145

[21]Li YC et al. 1,25 dihydroxy D3 is a negative endocrine regulator of the renin angiotensin system. *J Clin Invest* 2002:1,229-238

[22]Navas-Acien A, Guallar E et al. Lead Exposure and Cardiovascular Disease – A Systematic Review. *EHP* 2007 March; 115(3):472-82.

[23]Martinet W. Croons V. Nitric oxide selectively depletes macrophages in atherosclerotic plaques via induction of endoplasmic reticulum stress. *British Journal of Pharmacology* (2007) 152, 493–500; doi:10.1038/sj.bjp.0707426.

[24]Press release: Presentation to the American Heart Association's Asia Pacific Scientific Forum in Honolulu, Hawaii. April 24, 2002. Accessed at http://news.bio-medicine.org/medicine-news-2/Mercury-ups-heart-disease-risk-8269-1/

[25]Needleman. Mercury in Dental Amalgam a Risk-a Neurotoxic Risk? editorial in *Journal of the American Medical Association*, April 19, 2006 ;296(12):1462-1463.

[26]International Academy of Oral Medicine and Toxicity. "Smoking Teeth" video at http://www.iaomt.org/videos

[27]Proc Soc Exper Biol Med, 1965; 120: 805-8; Proc Soc Exper Biol Med, 1967; 124: 485-90; *Am J Physiol*, 1970; 219: 755-61; *Am J Physiol*, 1971; 220: 808-11

[28]HS Solomon and NK Hollenberg. Catecholamine release: mechanism of mercury-induced vascular smooth muscle contraction. *Am J Physiol* 229: 8-12, 1975

[29]Cardiotoxic Effects of Mercury. DHEW (NIH) Publication No 74-473, 1974, pp 109-34, 199-210

[30] Wierzbicki R, Michalska M, Cierniewski CS. Interaction of fibrinogen with mercury. *Thromb Res.* 1983 Jun 15;30(6):579-85.

[31] Robert L. Siblerud. The relationship between mercury from dental amalgam and the cardiovascular system. *Science of The Total Environment*, 1190;99:23-25

[32]Mike Mitka. Cardiologists Get Wake-up Call on Stents. *JAMA*. May 2007;297(18):1967-1968.

[33]Many with clogged arteries may not need stents. *Associated Press*. January 14, 2009

[34]Ridker PM, Hennekens CH, Buring JE, Rifai N. C-reactive protein and other markers of inflammation in the prediction of cardiovascular disease in women. *N Eng J Med.* March 23, 2000:836.

[35]Morteza Naghavi, MD; Peter Libby, MD; et al. From Vulnerable Plaque to Vulnerable Patient-A Call for New Definitions and Risk Assessment Strategies. *Circulation*. 2003;108:1664-1672

[36]Morteza Naghavia, Reji John, et al. pH Heterogeneity of human and rabbit atherosclerotic plaques; a new insight into detection of vulnerable plaque. *Athlerosclerosis*, September 2002,164;1:27-35

[37]Stephen T. Sinatra, James C. Roberts. *Reverse Heart Disease Now*, Wiley Publishing, 2006, p 164

[38]http://nccam.nih.gov/health/chelation/

[39]Cees Vermeer, Lavienja Braam. Vitamin K supplementation: A simple way to bone and cardiovascular health. *AgroFOOD industry hi-tech*, Nov/Dec 2003, 17-20.

Lyme Disease

$\mathcal{L}$yme disease gives rise to the growing school of thought that we can never get rid of all the bugs that do harm; it's about learning to minimize them and live with them.

Ixodes ticks, the principal vector for Lyme disease, were present in Massachusetts in the 1920s and 1930s. Ticks from Long Island, New York, collected in the late 1940s/early 1950s, were infected with Lyme. Then in 1975, a cluster of cases brought formal recognition of the disease. A number of children and some adults in the town of Lyme, Connecticut, mysteriously showed up with what looked like rheumatoid arthritis. The disease was named after the town. Eventually Lyme disease spread from the East coast across the country.[1]

The spirochete responsible for Lyme disease was identified in 1981 by Dr. Willy Burgdorfer, and named Borrelia burgdorferi (B. burgdorferi), after its discoverer.[2] It is similar in shape to the spirochete Treponema pallidum which causes syphilis.

Mankind's earlier experience with a disease caused by a spirochete was syphilis, the scourge of Europe for hundreds of years. Syphilis was called "the Great Imitator" because its symptoms mimicked so many other diseases. The same is true with Lyme.

Lyme is now the fastest growing infectious disease, faster than AIDS.

Lyme disease presents a host of challenges. Once the corkscrew-shaped spirochetes enter the bloodstream, they can cause a wide range of physical and mental symptoms.

B. burgdorferi's spiral shape aggressively embeds itself, usually first in the joints – when the cluster of Lyme cases showed up in Connecticut, most people described arthritis-like symptoms. Then the spirochetes typically go to the muscles and tendons, and can go into the heart and brain. Lyme spirochetes are also pleomorphic, meaning they can change shape, making it hard for the immune system to detect them, and hard for anything you throw at them to destroy them. The strength of one's immune system often dictates the severity of symptoms. The longer symptoms go untreated, the more intractable they can become.

Diagnosing Lyme

Some victims see a classic "bulls eye" rash from a tick bite, but more than half do not, according to ILADS, the International Lyme and Associated Diseases Society.

Recent studies reveal Lyme disease is now transmitted by human-to-human transmission, including from mother to fetus. Spirochetes have been found in semen,[3] vaginal fluid,[4] tear ducts, sweat, and mothers' breast milk.[5] The CDC found Lyme bacteria live in blood that has been purified for donation. Blood banks do not screen for Lyme, but if you have Lyme, you will be told not to donate your blood.[6] Researchers at the University of Wisconsin found dairy cattle infected with the Bb bacterium, which raises the question of whether milk or other products in our food chain may be a danger.[7]

According to ILADS:

> After a tick bite, serologic tests (ELISA, IFA, western blots, etc.) are not expected to become positive until several weeks have passed. Therefore, if [a bulls eye rash] is present, treatment must begin immediately, and one should not wait for results of Borrelia tests. You should not miss the chance to treat early disease, for this is when the success rate is the highest. Indeed, many knowledgeable clinicians will not even order a Borrelia test in this circumstance.[8]

A good test to determine whether you have Lyme can be hard to come by. The Lyme spirochete can hide in the human body and fool the immune system into thinking it isn't there by hiding behind a protein wall called "biofilm." So, antibodies are not produced, resulting in negative tests. The spirochetes can also morph into a different form, a cyst, which the immune system does not recognize.

The Western Blot test essentially makes a map of the different antibodies the immune system produces to the bacteria. It used to be that virtually every lab had accepted bands 22, 23, 25, 31, and 34 kDa as specific and significant, and reported them as positive for exposure to Borrelia burgdorferi. Then in 1994, the Association of State and Territorial Public Health Laboratory Directors set nationwide standards for Western Blot reporting and disqualified those bands as even being reportable. Currently among Lyme literate doctors, significance is associated with 41 kDa band, which appears the earliest but can cross-react with other spirochetes. In addition, there should be at least one of the following: 18 kDa, 23-25 (Osp C), 31 kDa (Osp A), 34 kDa (Osp B), 37 kDa, 39 kDa, 83 kDa and the 93 kDa are all species-specific, but may or may not appear during the course of the disease. 55 kDa, 60 kDa, 66 kDa, and 73 kDa are nonspecific and nondiagnostic.[9] The 58kDa band is considered both specific and diagnostic in Scotland and other European laboratories.[10]

The ELISA Test (Enzyme-Linked Immunosorbant Serum Assay) is automated. Many different patient samples can be performed by a single machine simultaneously. It may be convenient for the lab, but many consider the ELISA not sensitive enough to serve as an adequate screen, and there are many patients with Lyme who test negative by ELISA yet have fully diagnostic western blots.

A 2005 Johns Hopkins study, published in the *Journal of Clinical Microbiology*, claims that the CDC's two-tiered testing procedure, use of both ELISA and Western Blot, misses 75% of positive Lyme cases.[11]

Proving a persistent infection requires that you locate something in the blood. Since spirochetes leave the blood for body tissue, and tissue samples are something best collected at an autopsy, finding evidence can be tough.

Lyme-literate physicians generally prefer to use the IGeneX or Central Florida Research labs because their accuracy rates are better. But again, they are not perfect. Other tools can be helpful:

- measurement of the CD57 natural killer cell level, an immunologic marker that can be used to monitor treatment in chronic Lyme
- if neurologic symptoms are severe, a single-photon emission CT SPECT brain scan to see how much inflammation is present in the brain

Clinical diagnosis is key; even the CDC calls for objective physical findings.

The Great Imitator

"*O*bjective physical findings", however, run smack into The Great Imitator. That term was first used with syphilis because spirochetes affect people in so many different ways – their symptoms are all over the map. One Lyme patient can look like a case of rheumatoid arthritis, another like fibromyalgia or multiple sclerosis, and yet another can look okay physically but obviously has cognitive issues. Lyme-induced psychiatric illness is sometimes indistinguishable from other psychiatric diagnoses.

In July 2005, football fans were stunned by newspaper stories that police found Florida State University quarterback Wyatt Sexton doing push-ups in the street and reportedly saying he was the "son of God." Medical exams later found that Sexton was suffering from advanced Lyme disease. His physician, S. Chandra Swami, reported that the infection caused both neuropsychiatric and cardiovascular defects.[12]

In March 2009, Reverend Fred Winters was confronted outside his Illinois church by a 27-year-old man. After fatally shooting Winters, the man pulled out a knife and stabbed himself repeatedly. The killer's mother explained that her son got Lyme 10 years earlier and it had triggered a series of erratic behaviors and mental difficulties.[13]

New York pathologist Dr. Alan MacDonald found B. burgdorferi DNA in 1986 in seven out of ten autopsy samples from the brains of people with Alzheimer's.[14, 15] MacDonald was also the first to document B.

burgdorferi in fetal tissue, meaning the infection passes from mother to child in the womb.

Infection with B. burgdorferi for a long time allows the bacteria to replicate and wreak havoc throughout the entire body. The bacteria hide inside nerve cells and destroy them from within. B. burgdorferi also burrows into tendons and ligaments causing inflammation in the tissues and the nearby bone. B. burgdorferi infects the brain causing swelling and interruption of blood flow. In some patients, the bacteria invade the heart, resulting in heart block and myocarditis, life-threatening cardiac abnormalities. That is why it is called a multi-system illness.

Lyme can be mistaken for an estimated 350 conditions, including:

- Alzheimer's disease
- amyotrophic lateral sclerosis (ALS)
- chronic fatigue syndrome
- fibromyalgia
- irritable bowel syndrome
- lupus
- Bell's Palsy
- memory loss
- meningitis
- rheumatoid arthritis
- scleroderma
- multiple sclerosis (MS)
- Parkinson's disease
- autism
- encephalitis
- vertigo
- tremors

Often, chronic Lyme patients get a diagnosis that actually hinders meaningful treatment when Lyme is the root problem. For example, when Lyme attacks the joints and a person receives a diagnosis of rheumatoid arthritis, typically they are given a prescription for anti-inflammatory steroids. However, steroids suppress the immune system – exactly what you would NOT want to do if you knew you had Lyme. Also, we know that B. burgdorferi can induce secretion of aggrecanase, an enzyme that breaks down cartilage.[16] Steroids do nothing for that.

Let's look a little more closely at another diagnosis on the list: autism.

"The epidemics of Lyme and autism have gone from mild ripples in the water to roaring, all-consuming tidal waves, destroying thousands of lives and tearing apart countless families," said Bryan Rosner and Tami Duncan, co-authors of the book, *The Lyme-Autism Connection*.

Duncan founded the Lyme-Induced Autism (LIA) Foundation in California. The LIA Foundation estimates the majority of children with autism may be also infected with Lyme disease. Informal studies put the number at about 30 percent; clinicians are reporting up to 90% of the children with autism testing positive for B. burgdorferi. At the LIA Foundation's June 2008 conference, several experts suggested that at least 70% of the population has Lyme, and that it is being passed to children through congenital transmission, possibly through DNA. Dr. Dietrich Kinghardt said, "Most autistic kids have Lyme disease because most docs do not treat for Lyme first to knock it down enough that the white blood count can mount an attack and give you something to measure; that is why it is unknown."[17]

The Polymorphic Spirochete

Lyme disease starts with an attack of spirochetes. The tip of a spirochete can spin and twirl until it stimulates the cell's own enzymes to digest a part of the membrane, allowing entry. Once inside, the spirochete can lie dormant, protected from both the immune system and the action of antibiotics.

The cell division time of B. burgdorferi is very long compared to other bacteria. Strep and staph cells, for example, divide in less than 20 minutes. B. burgdorferi takes 12-24 hours to divide and this is a key reason Lyme is so hard to knock out. Most antibiotics are effective at the moment when bacteria are dividing because antibiotics inhibit the creation of a new cell wall.

When Lyme spirochetes encounter antibiotics, they can go into cyst form immediately. Most feel the cyst form is impervious to antibiotics, although some physicians have had success with metronidazle (Flagyl) and tinidazole and the non-drug, grapefruit seed extract.[18]

Cysts are small sacs containing immature spirochetes. Eventually the sacs might lodge in tissue or travel the blood stream where white blood cells sense their foreign presence but have little ammunition to kill them.

Spirochetes have the ability to burrow into or between cells and hide, gaining protection from the immune system. Both B. burgdorferi and Treponema pallidum have highly unusual outer membranes; the molecular architecture of these membranes is responsible for their ability to cause persistent infection.

---

3 polymorphic forms of Borrelia burgdorferi:

Spirochete – spiral-shaped bacterium responsible for the initial, rapid spread of the infection throughout the body and various organs thanks to its highly-mobile, drill-capable shape.
Cyst form – a symptomless, protective, survival-oriented form that is elusive, difficult to identify in laboratories, and nearly impossible to kill. It often lies in wait for a stressful event to trigger it back to the spirochete form.
CWD or cell-wall-deficient form – can hide inside cells, including immune system cells, to avoid detection. Over time, the population of cell-wall-deficient bacteria tends to increase. This accounts for many of the most severe symptoms and organ dysfunctions associated with Lyme disease. CWD is sometimes called L-form.

Each of these forms is able to convert to another form under the right conditions. Think of it as three different suits of armor.
Cysts convert to spirochetes usually in spring and fall as a proliferation tactic, to spread the disease to other tissues. The CWD (cell-wall-deficient) form is used to survive treatments including cell wall inhibiting antibiotics.

The Co-infections

Ticks harbor more infections than just B. burgdorferi. Some of the most common are Bartonella, Babesia, Ehrlichia, Mycoplasma, Chlamydia, Anaplasma, and Rocky Mountain Spotted Fever. Sometimes, these co-infections are more common and more debilitating than B. burgdorferi.

A 2004 New Jersey study examined the prevalence of coinfections in *Ixodes* ticks that transmit Lyme disease and found the prevalence of B. burgdorferi infection was 33.6%, but the prevalence of Bartonella infection was 34.5%. Thus, Bartonella species were found more often in that geographical area than the Lyme spirochete in these ticks.[19]

Dr. Garth Nicolson, Ph.D., well known in the Lyme community for his study of chronic intracellular infections, identified a variety of infections present in common chronic conditions:

Condition identified by Symptoms	Infections Commonly Observed
Amyotrophic Lateral Sclerosis (ALS)	Mycoplasma fermentans (and other species), Borrelia burgdorferi, HHV6, Chlamydia pneumoniae
Multiple Sclerosis (MS)	Chlamydia pneumoniae, Mycoplasma species, Borrelia burgdorferi, HHV6 and other Herpes viruses
Alzheimer's Disease	Chlamydia pneumoniae, Borrelia burgdorferi, HSV1 and other Herpes viruses
Parkinson's Disease	Helicobacter pylori, coronavirus, Mycoplasma species
Autism Spectrum Disorders	Mycoplasma fermentans (and other species), Chlamydia pneumoniae, HHV6, Borrelia burgdorferi
Chronic Fatigue Syndrome	Mycoplasma pneumoniae (and other species), Chlamydia pneumoniae, Borrelia burgdorferi

Singer Daryl Hall of the rock group Hall & Oats had to cancel tour dates in 2005 because of unexplained fevers and tremors. At his girlfriend's advice, he got tested for Lyme and found four co-infections. He went public with his story because he feels chronic Lyme disease needs to be acknowledged as a serious health issue.

"There are two very, very strong-feeling camps. One camp is really sure that if you're bitten by a tick you get tests, medicine. But with the chronic disease, that won't put a dent in it. It manifests in so many ways. It can lead to heart disease, depression. It can be so serious that people have died. It's a battle," said Hall.[20]

Co-infections present their own set of challenges for physicians and patients. Agents used to kill B. burgdorferi may not even touch the co-infections. "Many an 'incurable' Lyme patient has discovered the existence of a second, lurking disease – ehlichiosis or anaplasmosis – only to be treated with doxycycline and, finally, get well," author and Lyme patient Pamela Weintraub documented in *Cure Unknown–Inside the Lyme Epidemic.* [21]

Biofilms – a Cloaking Disguise

One of the great advances in understanding Lyme will come from understanding biofilms, a cloaking device bacteria use to survive in adverse conditions. Drs. Eva Sapi and Alan MacDonald did the first clear work on a Lyme biofilm in early 2008. Lyme bacteria are capable of forming a slimy matrix over themselves that shields pathogenic bacteria from antibodies and white blood cells, the sentinels of the immune system. Biofilms producing bacteria are also notorious for their ability to withstand extraordinarily high concentrations of antibiotics that are otherwise lethal in smaller doses to their planktonic counterparts. Biofilms are well described with other bacteria such as dental bacteria, Pseudomonas and E. coli. Biofilms have been seen in brain tissue. This may be why neuroborreliosis, or "neuro Lyme," is so hard to cure and why it causes dementia.

Biofilm is comprised, in part, of heavy metals. Heavy metals are perhaps the most troublesome toxins because they have been found to feed and make up the biofilm that surrounds B. burgdorferi. Combining systemic enzymes like serapeptase with heavy metal chelators is one strategy for "punching holes" in the biofilm. Garlic extract and heparin may help to break up the biofilm, as well. Once this is done, then anti-microbials can attack bacteria, yeast, and other bugs.

The Battle Over Treatment

𝓛yme disease causes incredibly deep-seated controversies, pitting patients against their insurance companies, and members of the medical establishment against each other. The 8,000-member Infectious Diseases Society of America (IDSA) maintains that Lyme is hard to catch and easy to treat:

> Treatment usually involves 10-28 days of oral antibiotics and is highly effective. When Lyme disease is diagnosed and treated quickly, 95 percent of people are cured within a few weeks of treatment ... There is no convincing biologic evidence to support a diagnosis of chronic Lyme disease after completion of the recommended treatment.[22]

The International Lyme and Associated Diseases Society (ILADS) describes itself as:

> ... a group of forward-thinking doctors who understand the complexities of Lyme disease ... Undertreated infections will inevitably resurface, usually as chronic Lyme, with its tremendous problems of morbidity and difficulty with diagnosis and treatment and high cost in every sense of the word.[23]

ILADS contends that "persistent symptoms have been noted in 25%-80% of patients with Lyme disease after 2-4 weeks of antibiotic therapy."[24]

Key points of contention between the two groups are whether chronic Lyme exists, and whether antibiotics should be used long term. Some doctors have been brought before their state medical boards for prescribing long-term antibiotics for Lyme patients. But no one has been brought before a medical board for prescribing months and months of antibiotics for tuberculosis.

The Lyme patient advocacy movement gained momentum in 2006, when IDSA updated its written guidelines for identifying and treating Lyme disease. Patients complained they were written primarily to spare insurance companies from having to pay for the long-term treatment of chronic Lyme. Connecticut Attorney General Richard Blumenthal launched an antitrust investigation into IDSA. In May, 2008, Blumenthal stated that:

> My office uncovered undisclosed financial interests held by several of the most powerful IDSA panelists. The IDSA's guideline panel improperly ignored or minimized consideration of alternative medical opinion and evidence regarding chronic Lyme disease, potentially raising serious questions about whether the recommendations reflected all relevant science.[25]

IDSA agreed to create a new review panel. In April, 2010, IDSA decreed that its controversial guidelines on Lyme disease will stand unchanged. The review panel agreed that all of the 69 original recommendations were "medically and scientifically justified" in the light of the evidence. The panel made a number of new recommendations that would revise the guidelines, but voted that the new revisions need not be considered until the next time the Guidelines are updated by IDSA.

Tina Garcia of Lyme Education Awareness Program, a non-profit organization in Mesa, Arizona, testified that the IDSA Practice Guidelines actually prevent patients in the United States, Canada, and Europe from receiving diagnosis and treatment:

> The truth about the IDSA Guidelines is that they accommodate some of the Guideline authors' collaboration with the CDC in the development of a Lyme disease vaccine. It would take years and years for vaccine clinical trials to be conducted if those developing the vaccines acknowledged persistent Lyme infection. That is an inconvenient truth for these vaccine developers. It would be great if a safe and effective Lyme vaccine was developed. However, it is inhumane to sweep so many suffering patients under the carpet and deny them treatment in order to bring a vaccine to market.[26]

On the one hand, the CDC endorses IDSA's guidelines. On the other hand, there is no rule that doctors must follow them. The problem is, as Blumenthal wrote:

The IDSA guidelines have sweeping and significant impacts on Lyme disease medical care. They are commonly applied by insurance companies in restricting coverage for long-term antibiotic treatment or other medical care and also strongly influence physician treatment decisions.

Meanwhile, many argue whether antibiotics should even be used extensively in cases of chronic Lyme. The first generation of Lyme literate medical doctors (LLMDs) primarily used long-term antibiotics. In recent years, others have focused less on pharmaceutical agents.

The battle lines have been drawn; both patients and doctors get caught in the crossfire.

Treatment Approaches

*A*ntibiotics: There is much agreement that if you have just been infected, a course of penicillin and/or tetracycline family of antibiotics for at least six weeks is the best treatment. The idea here is to knock it out before it can mutate and burrow in to too many tissues. After initial infection, B. burgdorferi travels rapidly via the bloodstream, and can be found within the central nervous system as soon as twelve hours after entering the bloodstream.[27] Early infections require full dose antibiotic therapy with an agent capable of penetrating all tissues in concentrations known to be bactericidal to the organism.

But it is often months or years after the initial infection that people suspect or confirm they have Lyme. The pleomorphic qualities of Lyme mean that when you throw an antibiotic at a spirochete, the organism can simply morph into its cyst or cell wall deficient (CWD) form, and hide itself in a biofilm, to escape destruction. When the cyst or CWD form no longer senses the stress of antibiotics, it can morph again into the spirochete form and continue burrowing into new tissues.

Lyme patients report that B. burgdorferi is also able to outsmart many of the herbal remedies.

Vitamin D avoidance, pulsed antibiotics: Some people infected with chronic, subclinical infections do not handle vitamin D the way Nature intended. Their bodies convert too much of it to a type of secosteroid known as 1,25 dihydroxy vitamin D. That triggers a production of macrophages – soldiers with inflammatory ammunition to overwhelm the bacteria. But the soldiers cannot see the bacteria because the bugs are hiding behind a wall of biofilm. The host is left with lots of inflammation – an army dressed for battle who can't find the enemy. Since soldiers will do battle, they attack whatever moves; it happens not to be the enemy. Whoops.

So how do we find the hidden enemy? Can we give the soldiers better glasses? That would be years and years of antibiotics. Or, we perhaps we can destroy the enemy's camouflage. That would be the biofilm.

When sickness takes hold, the body sometimes loses the ability to regulate levels of various things. For example, abnormally high serum copper levels have been observed in cancer patients with progressive tumors. Copper plays a big role in the formation of blood vessels. By depriving tumors of the copper supply they need to form new blood vessels, the growth of cancer can be slowed. In the case of Lyme disease, part of the problem may be abnormally high levels of vitamin D, causing excessive production of macrophages and their native inflammatory proteins. Researcher Trevor Marshall, Ph.D., developed a protocol to handle patients who bodies make too much vitamin D.

First, patients avoid the sun and foods with vitamin D. Herxheimer (also called Herx) reactions may pop up as the immune system rights itself and begins to attack the infection and kill bacteria.

Jarisch-Herxheimer reaction – a transient, short-term immunologic reaction commonly seen following antibiotic treatment of syphilis and less often in other diseases, such as borreliosis, brucellosis, typhoid fever, and trichinellosis. Manifestations include fever, chills, headache, myalgias, and exacerbation of cutaneous lesions. The reaction has been attributed to liberation of endotoxin-like substances or antigens from the killed or dying microorganisms, but its exact pathogenesis is unclear. Called also *Herxheimer reaction.*

—*Dorland's Medical Dictionary*

Second, if there is a great deal of inflammation, we use fairly large doses of an angiotensin receptor blocker (ARB) called Benicar® (olmesartan) to bring the inflammation under reasonable control. Then we pulse small amounts of various antibiotics, each of which inhibits the formation of the biofilm proteins in a different way. Marshall found that after vitamin D levels are balanced and the inflammation is somewhat controlled, the immune system is then able to detect the foreign bacteria and deal with them.

Herbs and homeopathic remedies are also used extensively in Lyme treatments. Carnivora® for example appears to work through the immune system and acts as an antimicrobial and virucidal, with great safety. Intravenous vitamin C can be very useful for detoxification. Chlorella's many benefits include the ability to bind toxic metals, increase glutathione production, bind neurotoxins, and serve as an overall super-nutrient. Zeolite can be helpful in removing toxins from the body. TAO-free cat's claw, olive leaf extract, and colloidal silver are used like non-pharmaceutical antibiotics.

Energetic approaches: Homeopathy teaches us that everything in the world carries frequencies which are unique identifiers. Science teaches us that we can discover some of these frequencies by using measurement equipment like mass spectrometers. The treatment of physical ailments using energetic frequencies has been known for centuries. Some frequencies are beneficial, some are harmful – an infra-red sauna is good for most people, but an electromagnetic field can be bad. Certain frequencies are damaging to specific types of organisms, but not damaging to our own bodies – these frequencies can be used to good therapeutic effect.

One of the real challenges for the patient is that often the agents employed to knock down Lyme and co-infections lose their efficacy over time. There may be an initial beneficial impact, inducing Herx reactions and improvement, but eventually the bacteria learn how to outsmart them. So, depending upon the severity of the case, many different approaches are used.

When treating Lyme, *there is no perfect remedy for everyone.* But the better shape you are in when you start treatment, the better the outcome will likely be. The shape you are in is determined in large measure by the integrity of your inner terrain.

Infections From the Toxic Load

The predominant focus in many treatment programs is the elimination of infection. Patients take antibiotics and other anti-microbial agents, but a holistic approach considers what factors set the stage for illness in the first place – what is the condition of the inner terrain.

The average person today has a high total body burden of pathogens. There are 10 times as many microbes within us as there are cells in our body. Some of those microbes play a good role, like bacteria which help digest food, but many are pathogenic, meaning they harm us.

The more toxic we become, the more pathogens are able take over. Various studies have shown that we all have a toxic body burden of heavy metals – lead, mercury, aluminum, and cadmium for example. Pathogens bind to and tightly hold heavy metals. Fungi such as Candida have an affinity for binding heavy metals. Stored toxins suppress the immune system, creating an environment where chronic infections flourish. An immune system weakened by toxins enables pathogens to take hold. To make things worse, the pathogenic microbes themselves are a producer of toxins in the body.

However, as heavy metals, fungi, and environmental toxins are removed, blood flow is enhanced. The molds, fungi, and other micro-organisms that may be making us unwell are less likely to survive in a body with adequate blood flow and optimal distribution of oxygen. The microbes lose their playground and our health recovers.

Beyond the damage that B. burgdorferi and co-infections themselves create, they prompt the body to create fibrin which protects the organisms from the reach of many therapeutic interventions by making the blood more viscous (thick, sticky) and providing the pathogens with a place to hide. Viscous blood reduces the body's ability to get nutrients in and toxins out of tissues.

Fortunately, the reverse is also true. The more we can do to reduce our toxic load, the more capable our bodies will be to manage chronic infections which are universally present. An excellent way to begin to relieve the toxic body burden is with colon hydrotherapy. Chelation of heavy metals is a time-honored, useful therapy for reducing chronic inflammation. Amalgam dental fillings and root canals are an ongoing and significant source of mercury toxicity and infection, respectively; partnering with a biological dentist is crucial in order to remove mercury fillings and root canals.

The connection between mold and Lyme disease increasingly pops up in the literature. Mold mycotoxins can form 36-48 hours after water intrusion into drywall, insulation, carpeting or cellulose-filled materials; EPA reports 30% of USA structures have indoor mold. Mold spores contain potent nerve toxins or neurotoxins. When these spores are inhaled, about three out of four people can produce antibodies to the toxins and quickly eliminate them. But one out of four has a genetic makeup that does not identify the toxins as invaders and does not eliminate them effectively. The liver can send them to the digestive tract via the bile, but they are quickly reabsorbed back into the blood. Continual or repeated exposure to mold toxins results in an ever increasing amount of these toxins in the body. When Lyme is also present, Lyme toxins build up in the body the same way. Mold and Lyme toxins attach to fat cells and cause the fat cells to continually release inflammatory cytokines. The result is chronic inflammation, often with symptoms such as fatigue, pain, brain fog and out-of-control weight gain.[28]

Keeping the Genie in the Bottle

The disease can be controlled, but it can almost never be eradicated. It waits, like a genie in a bottle, for the right moment to pop out. Although some still want to dispute the concept of chronic Lyme, the abilities of bacteria to go dormant, only to reappear years later, are well documented with other infections. People who had a childhood case of chicken pox can have a case of shingles, for example, much later in life. Shingles is a reactivation of the virus that has been in the body in a dormant form. The testimony of thousands of Lyme patients is that the genie comes out of the bottle when life delivers a major stress such as a death in the family, a surgery, or the loss of a career.

Most people with chronic Lyme seem to wrestle with it for the rest of their lives. The most successful learn to control it by avoiding foods which feed Lyme and its co-infections – foods such as sugar, refined carbs, alcohol, gluten, and caffeine. They also use chelation to lessen the chronic inflammatory burden of metals and infections, and systemic enzymes to lessen fibrin and thin the blood. Cutting edge research is looking into the effects that genetically modified foods and EMF from cell phones and microwave towers may have on Lyme and its co-infections.

Resources

Under Our Skin – an eye-opening documentary that walks you through Lyme's biology, and its political and economic dimensions. The film consists in large part of interviews with people who have suffered from chronic Lyme disease. You can order the CD on line.

Public Health Alert – A monthly newspaper of the Lyme community, available by subscription. Past issues available on line at http://www.publichealthalert.org

For specific information about various co-infections, see
ilads.org/burrascano_1102.htm
lymedisease.org/lyme101/coinfections/coinfection.html

BOOKS

Cure Unknown – Inside the Lyme Epidemic
by Pamela Weintraub, 2008

The Lyme-Autism Connection: Unveiling the Shocking Link Between Lyme Disease and Childhood Developmental Disorders
by Bryan Rosner, Tami Duncan, 2008

The Baker's Dozen & the Lunatic Fringe: Has Junk Science Shifted the Lyme Disease Paradigm?
by P. J. Langhoff, 2008

The Top 10 Lyme Disease Treatments: Defeat Lyme Disease With The Best Of Conventional And Alternative Medicine
by Bryan Rosner, 2007

---

[1] Kirby C. Stafford III. *The Tick Management Handbook*, Fall 2007

[2] *Science* 216:1317, 1982

[3] Dr. Alan MacDonald. Gestational Lyme borreliosis. Implications for the fetus. *Rheum Dis Clin North Am* 89; 15(4):657-77

[4] Dr. Gregory Bach. *Recovery of Lyme Spirochetes by PCR in Semen Samples of Previously Diagnosed Lyme Patients*, presented by Dr. Bach at the International Scientific Conference on Lyme Disease, April, 2001.

[5] David Williams. The New Great Impostor. *Alternatives Newsletter*, December 2004

[6] http://www.cdc.gov/ncidod/dvbid/LYME/ld_transmission.htm

[7] Ji B; Collins MT. Seroepidemiologic survey of Borrelia burgdorferi exposure of dairy cattle in Wisconsin. *Am J Vet Res*. 1994 Sep;55(9):1228-31.

[8] Dr. J Burrascano. *Diagnostic Hints and Treatment Guidelines for Lyme and Other Tick Born Illnesses.* November 2002, accessed at http://www.ilads.org/burrascano_1102.htm#bkintro

[9] Burrascano J. *Advanced Topics in Lyme Disease.* 16th edition. Downloaded June 7, 2009 from the International Lyme and Associated Diseases website, http://www.ilads.org/ .

[10] Evans R, Mavins S et al. Audit of the Laboratory Diagnosis of Lyme in Scotland. *Journal of Medical Microbiology* (2005), 54, 1139–1141. DOI 10.1099/jmm.0.46003-0.

[11] P Coulter, C Lema, et al. Two-Year Evaluation of Borrelia burgdorferi Culture and Supplemental Tests for Definitive Diagnosis of Lyme Disease. *Journal of Clinical Microbiology*, October 2005, p. 5080-5084, Vol. 43, No. 10.

[12] Lyme Disease Benches FSU Football Quarterback, *Fox News*, July 11, 2005

[13] *CBS News,* Edwardsville, Il. Lyme Disease Linked To Illinois Church Shootin–Preacher Shot To Death During Sunday Sermon. March 9, 2009

[14] Alan B. MacDonald. Plaques of Alzheimer's disease originate from cysts of Borrelia burgdorferi, the Lyme disease spirochete. *Medical Hypothesis*, May 2006, Volume 67, Issue 3, Pages 592-600

[15] Alan B. MacDonald. Alzheimer's neuroborreliosis with trans-synaptic spread of infection and neurofibrillary tangles derived from intraneuronal spirochetes. *Medical Hypotheses*, 2006 Oct 19

[16] Behera AK, Hildebrand E, Szafranski J, et al. Role of aggrecanase 1 in Lyme arthritis. *Arthritis Rheum* 2006; 54:3319–29.

[17] M Budinger. Pasteur's Legacy Feeds the Epidemics of Lyme and Autism. *Townsend Newsletter*, November 2008

[18] Brorson, O. Grapefruit seed extract is a powerful in vitro agent against motile and cystic forms of Borrelia burgdorferi sensu lato. *Infection*, June 2007; 35 (3): 206-8

[19] Adelson ME, Rao RV, Tilton RC, et al. Prevalence of Borrelia burgdorferi, Bartonella spp., Babesia microti, and Anaplasma phagocytophila in Ixodes scapularis ticks collected in Northern New Jersey. *J Clin Microbiol* 2004; 42:2799–801.

[20] R Forest. Daryl Hall speaks out on his battle with Lyme disease. Seacoast Media Group, June 12, 2008

[21] Pamela Weintraub. *Cure Unknown-Inside the Lyme Epidemic.* St. Martin's Press, 2008, p.169

[22] http://www.idsociety.org/lymediseasefacts.htm, accessed May, 2009

[23] http://www.ilads.org/index.html, accessed May, 2009

[24] Raphael B. Stricker. Counterpoint: Long-Term Antibiotic Therapy Improves Persistent Symptoms Associated with Lyme Disease. *Antibiotic Therapy and Lyme Disease* CID 2007:45 (15 July) 149

[25] http://www.ct.gov/ag/cwp/view.asp?a=2795&q=414284

[26] *Public Health Alert,* July 2010

[27] Gary Wormser, MD; Donna McKenna, NP et al. Brief Communication: Hematogenous Dissemination in Early Lyme Disease. *Annuals of Internal Medicine*, Volume 142, Issue 9, Pages 751-755; May 3, 2005

[28] Richard Loyd. Mold and Lyme Toxins. 2008 Lyme Disease Annual Report, accessed at http://lymebook.com/blog/the-recovery-process/mold-and-lyme-toxins/

Multiple Chemical Sensitivity

$\mathcal{I}$t is estimated that 74 million Americans have some form of a chemical sensitivity. For some this might be something as simple as an occasional, temporary headache from the odor of a perfume or fresh paint, but about 10 million are so severely affected by chemicals that they must totally change their lifestyle and no longer can live in a normal manner.

Doris Rapp, M.D., author of *Our Toxic World*

$\mathcal{T}$his phenomenon was first described in the early1950s by Dr. Theron G. Randolph, then a professor at Northwestern University. He noted several of his patients had a "petrochemical problem" in that they became ill when passing through the heavily industrialized areas of northwest Indiana and South Chicago. Dr. Randolph suggested that human failure to adapt to modern-day synthetic chemicals had resulted in a new form of sensitivity to these substances.

Randolph was a new breed of "clinical ecologist" who believed chemical antigens are not always eliminated from the body and can lodge in fatty tissue and act as continual irritants to the immune system. Once a person is sensitized to a substance, future exposures can lead to increasingly severe and debilitating reactivity.

Chemicals and Health

$\mathcal{M}$ultiple Chemical Sensitivity (MCS) is generally defined by clinical ecologists as an adverse reaction to potentially toxic chemicals in air, food or water, at concentrations generally accepted as harmless to the bulk of the population.[1]

Others describe MCS as "the ultimate 20th century illness" and people who have succumbed are sometimes referred to as "the modern-day canaries in the mine." Researcher and author Pamela Reed Gibson, Ph.D., suggests:

> MCS is an illness that is caused by industrialism, it is an indictment of industrial culture because it directly points to chemicals as a cause of disability, and it is totally incongruent with industrial culture. We are a culture that does "risk assessment" of each of our chemicals allowing a certain number of people to get sick or die from exposure to each chemical.[2]

There are an estimated 80,000 chemicals in use today in our environment, most of which have not been tested either individually or in combination for their effects on human health. A person with MCS typically reacts most often to those chemicals which are members of the petrochemical family.

People with MCS often have great difficulty when they encounter:

- pesticides sprayed outdoors and in buildings
- perfumes and fragrances
- cigarette smoke
- scented soap
- dry cleaning residues
- air fresheners
- strong smells in the detergent aisle at the grocery store
- clothing washed in detergents and fabric softeners that leave a smell
- common household cleansers
- new carpet or flooring
- common building paints with VOCs (volatile organic compounds)
- solvents
- chlorine in municipal water supplies
- pressed wood or plywood, especially that which contains formaldehyde
- moldy carpets
- newsprint

- natural gas
- plastic with strong smells as in new cars and products made of soft, pliable plastics
- computers, printers, and copiers — often toner is the culprit

People at particular risk are workers in heavy industry, occupants of "sick" buildings, Gulf War veterans, and residents of communities exposed to toxic waste dumps, aerial pesticide spraying, groundwater contamination, or industrial pollution.

It appears that people with MCS have detoxification mechanisms that have been seriously compromised, most likely from a combination of environmental insults superimposed on inefficient genetic detoxification pathways.

What triggers MCS? Some people report its onset after one significant exposure, such as being in the driveway of their home and sprayed from above with pesticides. Others report that it manifested after prolonged exposure to a small but significant dose of chemicals, such as when they moved into a new home, or went to work in a newly built or newly remodeled office.

Once the excessive reactivity develops, then it can "spread" so that the body now either reacts to a wider range of chemicals over time or develops dysfunction in more organ systems.

MCS – Real or Imagined?

Unlike chronic fatigue, which now receives some recognition and study from the medical profession, MCS remains a condition surrounded by medical controversy. There is also uncertainty regarding its definition, causes, and indicated treatments.

Many recognized medical groups, including the American Medical Association (AMA), the American Academy of Allergy, Asthma and Immunology (AAAAI), and the Centers for Disease Control (CDC) do not consider MCS to be a distinct physical disorder. According to the Office of Safety and Health Administration (OSHA), for example, MCS is merely a "theory":

> ...in theory, an adverse physical reaction to low levels of many common chemicals. Chemical sensitivity is generally accepted as a reaction to chemicals but debate continues as to whether MCS is classifiable as an illness. There are a number of synonyms for MCS, including 20th century disease, environmental illness, total allergy syndrome, idiopathic environmental illness, and chemical AIDS.

Proposed theories to explain the cause of MCS include allergy, dysfunction of the immune system, neurobiological sensitization, and various psychological theories. There is insufficient scientific evidence to confirm a relationship between any of these possible causes and symptoms.[3]

Patients often have a difficult time requesting medical help. Many allopathic physicians are unfamiliar with or do not believe in MCS. Some doctors still tell patients that "it's all in your head." Many doctors' offices are loaded with offending chemicals (which the doctors themselves may not be able to smell) that MCS patients simply cannot tolerate.

Meanwhile, physicians frequently are baffled when they face a patient with multiple complaints that do not fit into a known diagnostic disease category. It doesn't help that regular laboratory tests (e.g. CBC, liver function tests, sedimentation rate, urinalysis) often appear to be completely normal.

People with MCS have physical *and mental* symptoms that are far ranging – fatigue, concentration or memory difficulties, irritability, nervous tension, depression, daytime drowsiness, food cravings, insomnia, headaches, nasal congestion, muscle and joint aches, ringing in the ears, gastrointestinal distress, palpitations... the list goes on...

Few allopathically-trained doctors know to look for demonstrated physical effects such as enzyme deficiencies, chemical messenger changes,[4] airway changes, improvement with nasal lavage, or restricted blood flow to the brain during chemical exposure.

MCS, for many, defies classification as a disease.

"I have seen nothing to demonstrate that [MCS] exists ...
[it is] an 'irrational fear of man-made chemicals.'"

Dr. William Waddell,

former chair of pharmacology and toxicology at the
University of Louisville School of Medicine[5] and consultant to industry

MCS is commonly either misdiagnosed or under-diagnosed by physicians.[6] The National Academy of Sciences estimates that up to 15% of the American public could be experiencing a heightened sensitivity to common chemical products; this was confirmed in a 1999 study on hypersensitivity to low levels of common chemicals.[7] Household population studies have found prevalence rates for MCS that range from 12.6% to 33% of the population.[8]

Connecting the Dots

- MCS occurs in all races, usually developing after age 30; it also strikes many more women than men.
- Symptoms range from mild to disabling and even to life-threatening.
- Chronic fatigue syndrome, irritable bowel syndrome, fibromyalgia and Candida overgrowth are frequently found in people with MCS. It is not yet clear whether these are separate diseases or different manifestations of the same underlying problem.
- The avoidance of pollutants/toxicants is the best protection, albeit extremely hard to achieve.
- One's genetic makeup is key; one can inherit a predisposition to MCS.

Let's look at that last factor. It explains why nobody in the elevator has a problem with the guy who steps in reeking of aftershave – except the person with MCS.

289

All day long, your liver is detoxifying all manner of substances which you encounter as you move through the world. The liver sorts out the good from the bad and breaks almost everything down into parts that can be excreted primarily in urine, feces, and sweat. The liver uses special proteins called enzymes to break things down and other special compounds called conjugating molecules to attach the waste products to. This is called the process of detoxification.

However, if the supply of enzymes or nutrients is depleted or damaged, as appears to be the case in people with MCS, the liver is unable to break down toxic substances efficiently.

Suppose your friends invite you to dinner and they've lit candles to provide a pleasant ambiance. The scent the candles exude is actually a petro-chemical that you have now inhaled. If your liver is in great condition and your diet gives your body everything it needs to break down and excrete those chemicals, you will be fine. (You are also a very rare person these days.) If your liver is in so-so condition, you will have problems breaking down the petrochemical fragrance and, unbeknown to you, the fragrance molecules are probably stored in the soft tissues of your body. If you have MCS, you will quickly feel ill and likely need to leave that house within a few minutes.

One reason pesticides cause so much trouble for the human body in general, and those with MCS in particular, is that the manufacturer often adds an enzyme blocker to the formulation so that the poison cannot be metabolized properly. This means that the chemical remains in the body (of insect or human) longer, making it even more toxic. That may be desirable if we are talking about killing cockroaches. It is definitely not good for human beings who share the same air and end up inhaling the same toxic chemicals or absorbing them through their skin.

Women are more prone to MCS because of their "enzyme inventory." There is an enzyme called alcohol dehydrogenase that detoxifies carbohydrates, sugar, alcohol, and chemicals. Men have much more of this enzyme than do women.[9]

What's more, levels of butylcholinesterases, which scavenge chemicals, are lower in females (over the age of ten) than in males, and decline further in women over the age of thirty.[10]

Additionally,

- Women have a greater total percentage of body fat, which stores chemicals.
- Women's immune systems are more complicated because they need to protect and accept a "foreign" fetus in the womb.
- Women use more fragrances, hair coloring, hair sprays, lipstick and other makeup with known toxic ingredients.
- Women typically do the house cleaning, and are exposed daily to toxic products.
- Women are more likely to use diet foods with synthetic content, such as aspartame (Nutrasweet®), sorbitol, etc.
- The past or present use of antibiotics and/or birth control pills is an additional risk factor.

Many clinical ecologists believe that the immune system has a threshold which, once reached, will precipitate a variety of other symptoms in response to toxicity. The body's threshold is not fixed – it can be lowered by stress, infections, lack of sleep, lack of exercise, as well as exposure to chemical substances.

If a person has a high body burden of lead, mercury, or other heavy metals, those heavy metals are thought to contribute to the development or aggravation of MCS.

Over time, people with MCS may react to a widening array of things in their everyday world – foods, pet dander, house dust mites, pollen, mold, synthetic fabrics, and electromagnetic fields.

Patients with a history of chemical injury may develop chronic fatigue headaches and fibromyalgia.

Canaries in the Mineshaft

 To many, it makes sense that humans would become weaker – physically and mentally – in the face of increased environmental contamination. This is the canary-in-the-mineshaft theory.

Claudia Miller from Texas Health Science Center, and a national expert on MCS, believes that the loss of ability to tolerate poisons is the mechanism for the development of many modern diseases. She postulated in 1997 that the shift to understand toxins as causes of illness may be as important as it once was for science to understand germ theory.

Miller and Iris Bell, of the Department of Psychiatry at the University of Arizona Health Sciences Center, shed light on why MCS has both physical and mental components. There are rich neural connections between the olfactory system and the limbic and temporal regions in the brain's cerebral hemispheres, which, in part, regulate mood and autonomic functioning. The pair suggested a decade ago that many environmental chemicals gain access to the central nervous system via the olfactory and limbic pathways, inducing lasting changes and altering a broad spectrum of behavioral and physiological functions to produce clinical MCS syndromes.[11, 12, 13, 14]

Desert Storm Veterans

"Many of these veterans are suffering from the same kind of symptoms seen in people with multiple chemical sensitivity," said Claudia Miller, of the Texas Health Science Center. "We have to look to MCS as a working hypothesis."

An estimated 4,000 Persian Gulf veterans returned from the first Gulf war complaining of widespread health problems such as fatigue, depression, irritability, memory and concentration difficulties, muscle aches, shortness of breath, diarrhea, and a host of other problems which they attribute to exposures in the Gulf. Such exposures include combustion products from oil-well fires, paints, fuels, pesticides, solvents and vaccines. Some reports raised the specter of possible chemical or biological warfare.[15]

There is a direct pathway from the nose into the central part of the "old" animal brain, or limbic system, which is involved in governing sleep, mood, eating, aggression, and other very basic survival behaviors. Limbic "kindling" refers to the process of sensitizing nerve tissue. For example, if you put a frog's nerve in a Petri dish, and stimulate it with electrical impulses that individually are too mild to fire the nerve, eventually the nerve will fire due to repeated stimulation. Some individuals are thought to have "kindled" to low-level chemicals. In this way, very small amounts of chemicals can induce abnormal reactions. Because the limbic system is involved in regulating so many body systems, its disruption could easily cause many of the symptoms reported by people with MCS.

Dr. Gunnar Heuser and Dr. William Ross have found that brain scans can identify damage in people with MCS. Though MRIs may show normal results, the use of PET and SPECT scans have found areas of decreased blood flow or metabolism in areas of the brain that correlate with the symptoms expressed by the patients.[16]

Biochemist Martin Pall suggests that a vicious chemical cycle may be to blame.

Pall cites many studies that suggest that the initial chemical exposure creates a hypersensitivity in the neurons in the brain, which react by creating the two chemicals that cause further hypersensitivity. Pall believes that organic solvents activate N-methyl-D-aspartate (NMDA) receptors in the brain, stimulating a feedback loop in which both peroxynitrite and nitric oxide are elevated. As the NMDA receptors become more sensitive, cytochrome P450 is inhibited by the nitric oxide, and the blood brain barrier made more permeable by the peroxynitrite. Pall sees organophosphate and carbamate pesticides and organic solvents as the primary sensitizers in MCS. His theories are congruent with the self-reported sensitization histories of those with MCS.[17]

"The MCS response is produced," said Pall, "when chemical exposure produces excessive responses over large regions of the brain. In this way, normal and important mechanisms may act to generate this chronic illness. Thus, not only is the brain constantly inundated by chemicals to which it is normally somewhat sensitive, but the brain of a person suffering from MCS becomes abnormally sensitive to the chemicals – from 100 to 1,000 times more sensitive than in an unaffected person." MCS overlaps with other medical conditions of uncertain mechanism including chronic fatigue syndrome, fibromyalgia, posttraumatic stress disorder, and Gulf War syndrome. Pall has proposed similar mechanisms for all of these conditions. "The notion that a biochemical vicious cycle may underlie all four is very exciting and, if correct, suggests that this is a major new paradigm of human disease."[18,19]

The general public accepts that some people are unable to tolerate many chemicals. The popular television show "Northern Exposure" featured a chemically sensitive attorney who lived in a dome in Alaska, isolated from the toxins of industrialization and mainstream society.

Segments of the federal government seem to be several steps ahead of the mainstream medical community in their willingness to accept chemical sensitivity. In 1990, the Americans with Disabilities Act included MCS as a recognized condition, and by mid-1992, the Department of Housing and Urban Development established disability status for the disorder.

The EPA got an unintended, up-close look at MCS in 1987 when it installed new carpet in its Waterside Mall headquarters in Washington, D.C. The agency received more than 1,100 health complaints from employees, but waited two years to remove the toxic carpet. Some employees, who said they had become chemically sensitized, sued the EPA and initially won the jury trial. But the court overturned the verdict saying that it was not convinced.

Typical wall-to-wall carpet includes chemical adhesives to bind fiber to backing, more glues or adhesive strips to attach carpet to floor, and chemical surface treatments to stainproof and mothproof. Tufted fibers are usually affixed to the carpet with an adhesive that contains 4-phenyl-cyclohexene (4-PC), which irritates the eyes and respiratory tract.

Resistance Gives Way

𝓜ainstream medical resistance remains robust. Just ask the esteemed Dr. William J. Rea of Dallas, one of the earliest medical professionals to recognize MCS. He has been a target of the medical establishment for the last 25 years. He has been threatened with disciplinary action that could lead to revocation of his medical license. In August of 2007, the Texas Medical Board challenged his recognition and treatment of MCS.

Many parties have a vested interest in keeping all manner of chemicals a large part of the world economy. It is sobering to know that in 1990 for example, the Chemical Manufacturers Association vowed to work with state medical associations to block the recognition of MCS.[20]

It appears that such interests, however, are losing their ability to manage the public perception that we always "live better through chemistry." Just as global warming is receiving more serious consideration, so too is the potential danger that is inherent in the links between chemicals and human health.

The evidence that MCS is a real – and a growing problem – is becoming irrefutable. In November of 2007, the California Medical Association adopted a Resolution on a "Chemicals Policy for California" that says, in part:

> The state, national, and global scale of industrial chemical production is immense and is expected to grow four-fold by 2050 ...
>
> Ever-expanding research confirms that many chemicals are ... known to be hazardous to human biology and health, particularly in utero and in developing children.
>
> Numerous other nations including Canada and the European Union are adopting more proactive health-oriented chemicals policies, based upon scientific knowledge, assessment, and accepted public health principles ...
> Problems include the projected appearance of 600 new hazardous waste sites each month in the U.S. over the next 25 years and the development of chronic diseases caused by chemical exposures on the job among 23,000 California workers each year ... Therefore, be it resolved that the CMA calls upon the State of California and United States to implement a modern,

comprehensive chemicals policy in line with current scientific knowledge on human health, and which requires a full evaluation of the health impacts of both newly developed and existing industrial chemicals now in use... [21]

Treatment Options

℘here are no easy tests to confirm a diagnosis of MCS. A knowledgeable doctor will rule out allergies and other physical or mental health disorders as the cause of the symptoms, and conduct a complete medical history and physical examination.

To treat, we identify and eliminate as many toxins as possible. These may include toxic foods, cleaning chemicals, heavy metals, pesticides... the list goes on. You want to identify toxins in the home or workplace, and create a safe environment in your own home. Nutrition is important – using both organic foods and supplements to improve physical status. Test for heavy metals. Many people with MCS report that colon hydrotherapy to flush the toxic burden from the colon and help rebalance beneficial flora in the gut is very beneficial. Test for allergies and sensitivities, and use immunotherapy to treat these sensitivities. The goal is to desensitize your body, so you can eventually return to the world fully functional.

Most commercial office buildings present barriers to those with chemical sensitivities. Fortunately, the green movement is teaching the construction industry how to build and furnish with less toxic materials.

The U.S. Green Building Council has developed a certification program for environmentally responsible construction and building maintenance. More information on LEED ("Leadership in Energy and Environmental Design")
Certification is found at http://www.usgbc.org.

RESOURCES

The James Madison University MCS Research Team, Harrisonburg, Virginia. http://www.mcsresearch.net

The Chemical Sensitivity Foundation in Maine (207-725-8570) has numerous resources about MCS produced by CSF chair, Alison Johnson. www.ChemicalSensitivityFoundation.org

Chemical Injury Information Network (CIIN), A non-profit support and advocacy organization dealing with Multiple Chemical Sensitivities. It is run by the chemically injured for the benefit of the chemically injured. http://www.ciin.org/

Fragranced Products Information Network www.fpinva.org

BOOKS

They're Poisoning Us!: From the Gulf War to the Gulf of Mexico – An Investigative Report by Arnold Mann, 2011

Strategies for Surviving Chemical Sensitivity: The Basics
by Robert S. Mayer, 2010

Amputated Lives – Coping with Chemical Sensitivity
by Alison Johnson, 2008

Multiple Chemical Sensitivity – A Survival Guide
by Pamela R. Gibson, Ph.D., of James Madison University, 2006
available only at www.earthrivebooks.com

Our Toxic World
by Dr. Doris Rapp, 2003

Living with Multiple Chemical Sensitivity
by Gail McCormick, 2000

[1]Dr. William J Rea, et al. Confirmation of chemical sensitivity by means of double-blind inhalant challenge of toxic volatile chemicals. *Clinical Ecology*, Volume VI, number 3.

[2]Pamela Reed Gibson. Understanding & Accommodating People with Multiple Chemical Sensitivity in Independent Living. James Madison University, 2002

[3]http://www.osha.gov/SLTC/multiplechemicalsensitivities/index.html. Accessed November, 2007

[4]Millqvist E, Ternesten-Hasséus E et al. Changes in Levels of Nerve Growth Factor in Nasal Secretions after Capsaicin Inhalation in Patients with Airway Symptoms from Scents and Chemicals. *Environmental Health Perspectives*, 113: 7 (July 2005).

[5]William Waddell. Better Data Needed on Sensitivity Syndrome. *Science*, Vol 251, p 1558

[6]Kutsogiannis, DJ., & Davidoff, A.L. (2001). A multiple center study of multiple chemical sensitivity syndrome, page 19. Retrieved June 22, 2004, from http://www.findarticles.eom/p/art icles/mi_m0907/is_3_56/ai_77276221

[7]Caress, S.M., & Steinemann, A.C. (2003). A review of a two-phase population study of multiple chemical sensitivities. Retrieved June 22, 2004, from http://www.emagazine.com/septembero\ctober_1998/ 0998feat2.html

[8]ibid

[9]National Institute on Alcohol Abuse and Alcoholism No. 10 PH 290 October 1990

[10]Cynthia Wilson. Chemical Injury As A Women's Health Issue. *Our Toxic Times*, 8(9):1,3, 1997

[11]Buskila, D. Fibromyalgia, Chronic Fatigue Syndrome, and Myofascial Pain Syndrome. *Current Opinion in Rheumatology*, 11:119-126. 1999

[12]Dunstan, R.H.; Donohoe, M.; Taylor, W.; Roberts, T.K.; Murdoch, R.N.; Watkins, J.A.; McGregor, N.R. A Preliminary Investigation of Chlorinated Hydrocarbons and Chronic Fatigue Syndrome. *Med. J Australia*, 163: 294-297. 1995.

[13]Heuser, G.: Chemical Exposure as a Cause of Chronic Fatigue. Fourth Annual Conference on Medical Neurobiology of Chronic Fatigue Syndrome and Fibromyalgia, Los Angeles, California, May 7-9, 1993.

[14]Tirelli, U.; Chierichetti, F.; Tavio, M.; Simonelli, C.; Bianchin, G.; Zanco, P.; Ferlin, G. Brain Positron Emission Tomography (PET) in Chronic Fatigue Syndrome: Preliminary Data. *Am. J. Med.* 105: 54S-58S. 1998.

[15]Claudia S. Miller. Toxicant-induced Loss of Tolerance. *Journal of Nutritional and Environmental Medicine.* January 2001, vol 96, issue 1

[16]Heuser, G., Wu, J.C. Deep Subcortical (Including Limbic) Hypermetabolism in Patients with Chemical Intolerance: Human PET Studies. *Annals of the New York Academy of Sciences* 933 (March 2001):319-322.

[17]http://www.mcsresearch.net/causes.htm

[18]Progress in MCS Research: Washington State Univ. Biochemist Provides Theory & Evidence that a Vicious Chemical Cycle May Cause Multiple Chemical Sensitivity, *Mold Reporter*, 2002, Vol 2, No 5

[19] Pall, Martin L. NMDA sensitization and stimulation by peroxynitrite, nitric oxide, and organic solvents as the mechanism of chemical sensitivity in multiple chemical sensitivity. *The FASEB Journal.* 2002;16:1407-1417

[20]The Chemical Manufacturers Association. The Chemical Manufacturers Association Environmental Illness Briefing Paper. *The Reactor Fall* 1990;V(4):1,2,9-13.

[21] http://www.healthandenvironment.org/articles/doc/2616

Negative Emotions

Fear is a poison produced by the mind, and courage is the antidote stored always ready in the soul.

Dean Koontz, *One Door Away from Heaven*, Chapter 16

$\mathcal{N}$egative emotions make us ill. This has been a tenet of Eastern philosophy for millennia, and is a firm principle of all sorts of energy medicine in the 21st century. Allopathic medicine is less convinced about this principle, although there are articles in the literature relating personality type to the development of various cancers. We are now able to demonstrate how this actually manifests in the body.[1]

Experiments in the 1960s showed that when young animals were exposed to a series of electrical shocks over which they had no control, they never learned to escape from similar stressful environments as adults. They stayed put and developed ulcers. This exemplifies the behavior known as "learned helplessness." It sounds a lot like people in abusive relationships – being abused as children seems to predispose them to find and stay in abusive relationships as adults.

On the other hand, young animals who were exposed to shocks over which they had some control were able to learn to escape their environment, and did not develop learned helplessness.

So, control over one's situation would appear to be crucial – definitely for animals and likely for humans too. Is it really control over the situation? Or is it perhaps control over our own reactions to the situation? It's a subtle but very real distinction. We have very few options when we are infants and small children. We are completely dependent upon the adults around us for our very lives. If our environment is one of uncertainty, or fear, or abuse, then we are likely to seek out similar environments when we grow up. We don't know any better. This explains why so many abused children grow up to be abusers. And why so many children of alcoholics grow up to be alcoholics themselves. It is learned behavior.

However, humans are not mice. We have free will. We can learn. Learned helplessness is just that – learned. It can be unlearned. It just takes a lot of work. And first, we must realize that there is a problem. First, we have to see that there is a box. Then we can learn to see the walls of the box (our mindset, those assumptions which we do not even question). Then we can figure out how to get outside the box – we can realize that there might be a door in places where we might not normally look, like the ceiling. We can escape the boundaries of what we learned as small children.

How does this relate to medical issues?

The Biological Answer

$\mathcal{N}$egative or painful emotions generate a chemical neurotransmitter called glutamate. In the brain, glutamate causes gateways in nerve cells to stay open, triggering a process called apoptosis, which results in cell death by suicide. If enough cells die, function is lost, and we become dys-functional, or ill. Chronic stress, for example, increases glutamate levels in the brain.[2]

Glutamate creates lasting memories in the brain by changing the connections between nerves (synaptic connections).[3] It helps us learn things – both the pleasurable and the painful. Glutamate is involved with addiction – if the receptors are blocked, there is no development of addiction. Glutamate keeps receptors open, allowing continuous or prolonged nerve stimulation and possibly production of dopamine, the "feel-good" neurotransmitter. Dopamine is released in huge amounts when an addiction is satisfied – whether gambling, cocaine, sex, alcohol, whatever... If we block the glutamate receptors, no massive dopamine release, no addictive behavior.

The Lifestyle Answer

$\mathcal{I}$f, for example, we learn that we have developed breast cancer, that sets off a whole cascade of thoughts, emotions, and neurotransmitters. After the initial discovery, we have the option to continue to dwell in those thoughts and emotions – generating the negative neurotransmitter glutamate – or to turn our sights in a different direction.

This is an area where I find the standard medical advice to undergo chemotherapy and/or radiation to be particularly disempowering. Eventually, most people discover the statistics are somewhat rigged – if your cancer does not come back within the first five years, you go down in the statistic books as a cancer survivor. If your cancer comes back in five years and five days, the statistics are not changed to reflect that. Radiation and chemotherapy are, by any measure, harsh therapies that solve some problems (the immediate reduction in size of the tumor) while creating others (massive damage to the immune system, the bone marrow, the GI tract, the hair follicles). One of the well-known side effects is appetite loss and impaired digestion. Radiation, like antibiotics, creates an imbalance in gut flora. Thus the body starts to become depleted of vitamins, minerals, and essential fatty acids. And new information is coming to light that the chemotherapy drugs can actually cause additional cases of cancer. A recent UCLA study has shown that chemotherapy can change the blood flow and metabolism of the brain in ways that can linger for 10 years or more after treatment.[4]

If we truly believe that cancer is a death sentence rather than a wake-up call, we will likely dwell in the negative emotions of fear, helplessness, and anger. The negative mental state can allow the harsh therapies to do even more extensive damage due to the underlying mental stress. Extensive rodent and human research has shown that the hippocampus in the brain is crucially involved in memory formation and is also highly sensitive to stress. By altering brain cell properties, stress can disturb cognitive processes such as learning and memory, and consequently limit the quality of human life.[5]

301

A different way to look at the whole cancer diagnosis issue is to realize we do have some control over the factors that influence our health. We can stop smoking, stop drinking sodas, stop showering in chlorinated water, stop dousing our environments in pesticides, and stop eating heated vegetable oils and processed foods. We can choose non-toxic paints and carpets when remodeling our home. We can choose toothpaste without fluoride. We can choose organic meats without hormones and antibiotics. When vaccinating our children, we can choose to avoid vaccines which contain mercury (thimerosal) or aluminum preservatives. We can choose a dentist who does not use mercury (silver amalgam) fillings. We can choose to take jobs which are less stressful and more enjoyable. We can choose whether to see a doctor who spends five minutes with us, or one who spends an hour. We can choose whether to allow our insurance company to dictate our health care, or whether to go outside that system, pay for our care, and get the care which is actually appropriate to this paradigm – that which will help us keep our bodies and minds in good shape.

Even if we are faced with a diagnosis of cancer, it is never too late to institute healthy lifestyle changes. The treatment, as toxic as it may be – whatever route we choose – will be more effective if the underlying body is not full of additional toxins.

Truth is, we have cancer cells in us all the time. A healthy immune system, combined with the right nourishment and an absence of toxicities, is able to keep the cancer cells from ever reaching critical mass. We need only look at our children to see the effects of the modern world at work: Cancer is now the leading cause of disease-related death among children and adults in the U.S. Simply put, our children live in a world full of pollution and eat a diet far, far removed from what has nurtured the human race for tens of thousands of years. Our bodies simply cannot adapt to this much change, this quickly. Our bodies break down.

Erosion of Health or Aging?

*H*ere is another very disempowering notion: Most people have been told that chronic illness is an inevitable consequence of aging, and that there is nothing we can do to prevent it – it's all in the genes. Thus we think "health" is simply the "absence of disease." No reason to do anything until you notice something and a doctor gives you a diagnosis.

An alternative and healthier approach is to realize that illness is NOT merely an inevitable consequence of aging or genetics. The fuel we put into our body and the amount of environmental challenges - heavy metals, organic pollutants, stressful situations – can and do have a great effect on our health. Sickness usually is years in the making. It is a slow decline away from health.

However, if we accept that we actually do have control over many of the factors that lead to sickness, then we can see that we do have power to control outcomes. All the time without exception? No. A saying comes to mind:

"We cannot direct the wind but we can adjust our sails."

And now we can explain biochemically why choice is a good thing. We can take control by "reprogramming" our thoughts, and breaking old habits to enable us to make different daily choices.

---

[1]Stewart JC. Negative Emotions and 3-year Progression of Subclinical Atherosclerosis. *Arch Gen Psychiatry* 2007;64: 225-233

[2]Lowy MT, Gault L, Yamamoto BK (1993). Adrenalectomy attenuates stress-induced elevations in extracellular glutamate concentrations in the hippocampus. *J Neurochem* 61:1957–1960

[3]Amat J, Baratta MV. Medial prefrontal cortex determines how stressor controllability affects behavior and dorsal raphe nucleus. *Nature Neuroscience* 2005 Mar;8(3):365-71. Epub 2005 Feb 6.

[4]Daniel H. S. Silverman. Altered frontocortical, cerebellar, and basal ganglia activity in adjuvant-treated breast cancer survivors 5–10 years after chemotherapy. *Breast Cancer Research and Treatment*, September 29, 2006; also
http://springerlink.metapress.com/content/mq53511v473u2253/?p=82c66698ef224115a10256c6feec5225&pi=1

[5]Jeansok J. Kim & David M. Diamond. The Stressed Hippocampus, synaptic plasticity and lost memories. *Nat Rev Neurosci.* 2002 Jun;3(6):453-62.

Osteoporosis

*B*one is living, active tissue. The body is constantly breaking down old bone and rebuilding new bone. The process is called remodeling. When bone is built faster than it is removed, bone mass increases and bones get stronger. When bone is broken down faster than new bone is made, you are losing bone mass. Optimum bone density is a dynamic balance between bone removal and the deposit of new tissue.

Approximately 20 percent of bone tissue in the body is replaced each year by this process on a cyclical basis throughout the skeleton.

Are you breaking down bone faster than you are building it? A simple urine test will tell you.

The Bone Resorption Assay detects biochemical markers, called collagen cross links, which reflect the amount of bone turn-over. Collagen is a fibrous protein which provides the bone with strength and flexibility. When the urinary level of collagen cross links is high, this indicates that bone is being removed faster than it is replaced. This indicates osteoporosis in the making.

Osteoporosis is caused by more bone cells being resorbed than being deposited. This imbalance results in a progressive loss of bone density and a thinning of bone tissue. Osteoporotic bones are more porous and therefore more vulnerable to fracture.

Osteoporosis is Preventable

*I*n many people today, the total amount of bone that is grown peaks around age 30. The rate in which bone mass is lost increases during the first five to ten years when women become postmenopausal.

Osteoporosis affects more women than it does men, but men are not immune to it. The National Osteoporosis Foundation says that despite the large number of men affected, osteoporosis in men remains under-diagnosed and underreported.

Knowing what causes osteoporosis can mean all the difference in helping protect yourself from it.

Osteoporosis Is Not A Calcium Deficiency

Osteoporosis is due in great measure to a proportional decrease in a range of minerals. Bones are made of at least 12 minerals, including calcium.

Dr. Robert Thompson's book, *The Calcium Lie*, draws attention to the misleading focus on just one mineral:

> Expecting to keep bones strong by giving someone calcium supplements is like expecting that you can make a loaf of bread from yeast alone. It simply won't work and, in the case of calcium supplements, it can do great harm as crystallized excess calcium concretions make their way into arteries and joints and force the adrenals to compensate for calcium excess to their own detriment.
>
> If you get too much calcium, through food sources or by taking supplements, you set yourself up for an array of negative health consequences, including obesity, Type 2 diabetes, Type 2 hypothyroidism, hypertension, depression, problem pregnancies and more.

Thompson makes the case for supplementation with trace minerals to make up for what we do not get from food grown in today's mineral depleted soils.

Amino Acids Are Part Of The Bone Matrix

Amino acids are the building blocks of protein. So eating high quality protein like eggs and grass-fed beef is good. What? You've read that eating meat and a high-protein diet weakens bones?

306

The protein theory was first presented in 1968[1] and followed up in 1972 with a study comparing bone density of vegetarians and meat eaters.[2] But the studies were not well done. Dr. Herta Spencer, of the Veterans Administration Hospital in Hines, Illinois, notes that the studies used isolated, fractionated amino acids from milk or eggs.[3] Her follow up studies show that when protein is given as natural meat, subjects do not show any increase in calcium excreted, or any significant change in serum calcium, even over a long period.[4]

The textbooks tell us that the body needs vitamin D for calcium utilization, and vitamin A for both calcium and protein assimilation. Protein powders usually lack these fat-soluble co-factors that the body can use to build and maintain healthy bones.[5]

The "acid-ash" of meat is given as the reason high meat diets cause bone loss. But meats also supply phosphorus, which counteracts this acidity. Phosphorus is needed for the phosphate component of bone matter. Meats are also excellent sources of vitamin B12, which plays a little understood role in maintaining the integrity of the bones.

The type of saturated fats found in tropical oils, butter and other animal fats, plays an important role in bone modeling. This may explain why population groups in tropical areas, where coconut and palm oils form a major component of the diet, have very little osteoporosis.

Omega 3 Fatty Acids

Omega 3 fats prevent excessive bone turnover. Many studies show that adding omega 3 fatty acids to the diet preserves bone density. The phenomenon of losing bone density in older people, or at the beginning of menopause for women, is thought to be related to inflammation. Omega 3 oils have an anti-inflammatory effect.

The standard American diet is too low in omega-3s, and too high in omega 6s. Investigators at Purdue University found that high levels of free radicals from omega 6 linoleic acid (found principally in corn, soy and safflower oils) interfered with bone formation.[6]

Vitamin K

Vitamin K is best known for its role in blood clotting. However, vitamin K is also absolutely essential to build strong bones and prevent heart disease. It acts as the biological "glue" that helps plug calcium into the bone matrix.

It also functions as a cofactor in the process that replaces old bone.

Vitamin K is commonly found in fermented foods, like natto (Japanese fermented soybeans), and dark green leafy vegetables like collard greens and spinach.

Vitamin D

It is well established that calcium needs 1,25-dihydroxy-vitamin D for transport. Insufficient vitamin D leads to less calcium absorption, elevated blood concentrations of parathyroid hormone, and increased rates of bone resorption, which may eventually lead to osteoporosis and bone fracture. Several studies found that older people who experience a hip fracture have lower serum concentrations of 25-hydroxy vitamin D than do those without a fracture.[7]

Some 25 percent to 50 percent of the elderly are thought to have vitamin D deficiency, which can lead to loss of muscle strength and an increased likelihood of falling that, in turn, increases the risk of hip fracture. Very often when people "fall and break a hip," the bone in the hip actually breaks first, and then the person falls down.

Synthetic vitamin D, however, can cause hypercalcemia, a disturbance of calcium equilibrium leading to excessive blood calcium and calcification of soft tissues.[8] Synthetic vitamin D added to commercial milk does not have the same beneficial effect as vitamin D from sunshine or fermented cod liver oil in preventing rickets and strengthening the bones.

Forget the Milk Moustache

Milk is often thought to decrease osteoporotic bone loss and fracture risk since it is promoted as a primary source of calcium and vitamin D. But the form of vitamin D that is typically added to grocery store milk is not natural.

A 2003 Harvard Medical School study found that neither milk nor calcium supplementation reduces the risk of osteoporotic hip fractures in postmenopausal women.[9] Researchers found no association in other groups of people between calcium intake and fracture risk.[10]

Celiac Disease Decreases Bone Density

People with osteoporosis are more likely than the general population to also have celiac disease, an intestinal disorder caused by intolerance to wheat flour – gluten. Celiac disease renders people unable to absorb certain nutrients, including calcium and vitamin D.

A classic 1998 study found that children and adolescents with low bone mineral density due to celiac disease who follow a gluten free diet experience a rapid increase of bone mineral density that leads to a complete recovery of bone mineralization.[11] In adults, however, no spontaneous recovery has been documented.

Fluoride and Iodine

Sodium fluoride added to municipal drinking water is one of a number of substances that is harmful to our bones. It causes an apparent increase in bone mass, but the bone structure is abnormal and weak.[12] As fluoride accumulates in your bones, they become more brittle and prone to fracture. Recent studies indicate that hip fractures are more common in areas where water is fluoridated.[13]

Iodine found in natural sea salt, sea foods and butter helps maintain healthy ovaries and thyroid gland, both of which play a role in maintaining bone integrity.

Sugar, Caffeine, Soda, Alcohol

The renowned dentist Dr. Melvin Page demonstrated that sugar consumption upsets the natural homeostasis of calcium and phosphorus in the blood. Normally, these minerals exist in a precise ratio of ten to four. Sugar consumption causes serum phosphorus to decrease and calcium to rise.[14] The excess serum calcium, which comes from the bones and teeth, cannot be fully utilized because phosphorus levels are too low. It is excreted in the urine or stored in abnormal deposits such as kidney stones and gallstones.

Caffeine also upsets the natural balance of calcium and phosphorus, and causes increased calcium to be excreted in the urine. Phosphoric acid in soft drinks is a major cause of calcium deficiency in children and osteoporosis in adults.[15] Aluminum from antacids, cans, and pollution also contributes to bone loss.[16]

Osteoporosis is often associated with excess consumption of alcohol.[17] This is the likely explanation of bone loss in Eskimos, who are highly prone to alcoholism. In a healthy person, the tearing down and building up of bone is in balance so there is no net loss of bone. However, chronic and heavy drinking can disrupt the balance by suppressing new bone formation. The empty space created by normal bone-removing activity is inadequately filled by newly formed bone. This process continues at other skeletal sites during the next remodeling cycle. The cumulative effect of this process during several remodeling cycles is manifested as measurable bone loss over a period of just a few years.[18]

Take a Pill for Osteoporosis?

The Food and Drug Administration (FDA) has approved several antiresorptive medications to treat osteoporosis; these medications are in a class of drugs called bisphosphonates.

Bisfosphonate drugs kill the osteoclasts in your bones – these are the cells which destroy bone as part of the natural bone regeneration process. Osteoclasts replace old bone by releasing acids and enzymes to remove minerals and collagen. Once the osteoclasts have done their job, protein-secreting cells called osteoblasts deposit new tissue, thus building bone. When the osteoclasts are destroyed, the osteoblasts do indeed continue to function. So you get thicker bone that is denser, but not necessarily stronger, because they have not undergone the normal remodeling process. Your bones can become denser but more brittle, increasing your long-term risk of developing a fracture.

The constant remodeling of bone requires both osteoblasts and osteclasts to remove old bone and rebuild new bone.

Bone Resorption: The process by which osteoclasts break down bone and release the minerals, resulting in a transfer of calcium from bone fluid to the blood.

Bone resorption can also be the result of disuse and the lack of stimulus for bone maintenance. Astronauts, for example, undergo a certain amount of bone resorption due to the lack of gravity providing the proper stimulus for bone maintenance.

Now What?

You have choices. You could assess the state of your bones with a standard dual energy X-ray absorptiometry, or DEXA, the most common method to measure bone mass density. The DEXA bone scan involves ionizing radiation at two different frequencies to get an idea of the amount of calcium contained in a bone. The scan can roughly measure bone density, but cannot tell you if you are headed in the right direction – if you are gaining or losing density except by repeating the scan and exposing yourself to ionizing radiation.

Or, you can assess the state of your bone health with a simple urine test that detects biochemical markers which reflect present remodeling activity.

Type I bone collagen contains unique cross linked protein structures that give greater stability. Active bone resorption requires a breakdown of this protein structure; the peptide fragments from this breakdown are excreted in urine. Since bone resorption is a relatively constant process, the amount of specific peptides found in the urine provides an accurate measure of the rate of bone loss.

The Bone Resorption Assay urine test measures the deoxypyridinoline fragment of Type I collagen breakdown from a single urine specimen. This is the fragment that contains the cross linking point and has been demonstrated to be more specific to bone resorption than breakdown fragments measured in some earlier assays.

If your bone density is declining, the good news is: osteoporosis is a preventable condition.

[1] A Wachman and D S Bernstein. "Diet and osteoporosis." *The Lancet* 1968 1:958

[2] Frey R Ellis, et al. "Incidence of osteoporosis in vegetarians and omnivores." *American Journal of Clinical Nutrition*, June 1972, 25:555-558

[3] Herta Spencer and Lois Kramer. "Factors contributing to osteoporosis." *Journal of Nutrition*, 1986 116:316-319

[4] Herta Spencer and Lois Kramer. "Further studies of the effect of a high protein diet as meat on calcium metabolism." *American Journal of Clinical Nutrition*, June 1983 37 (6):924-929

[5] M E Melton and M L Kochman. Reversal of severe osteoporosis with vitamin B12 and etidronate therapy in a patient with pernicious anemia. *Metabolism: Clinical & Experimental*, 1994 43 (4) 468-9

[6] BA Watkins et al. "Importance of Vitamin E in Bone Formation and in Chondrocyte Function." *American Oil Chemists Society Proceedings*, 1996, at Purdue University

[7] J A Cauley, A Z LaCroix, et al. Serum 25-Hydroxyvitamin D Concentrations and Risk for Hip Fractures. *Annals of Internal Medicine*, August 19, 2008 vol. 149 no. 4 242-250. Accessed at http://www.annals.org/content/149/4/242.abstract

[8] Judith A DeCava. *The Real Truth About Vitamins and Antioxidants*. Brentwood Academic Press, Columbus Georgia, pp 102-113.

[9] D Feskanich, WC Willett, GA Colditz. Calcium, vitamin D, milk consumption, and hip fractures: a prospective study among postmenopausal women. *Am J Clin Nutr*. 2003 Feb;77(2):504-11. Accessed at http://www.ncbi.nlm.nih.gov/pubmed/12540414?dopt=Abstract

[10] Bischoff-Ferrari HA, Dawson-Hughes B, Baron JA, et al. Calcium intake and hip fracture risk in men and women: a meta-analysis of prospective cohort studies and randomized controlled trials. *Am J Clin Nutr*. 2007; 86:1780–90. summary accessed at http://www.hsph.harvard.edu/nutritionsource/what-should-you-eat/calcium-full-story/index.html

[11] S Mora, G Barera, et al. Reversal of low bone density with a gluten-free diet in children and adolescents with celiac disease. *Amer J of Clinical Nutrition*, 1998. Accessed at http://www.ajcn.org/cgi/reprint/67/3/477.pdf

[12] Yiamouyiannis, John. *Fluoride. The Aging Factor*. Health Action Press, 1986

[13] C Cooper et al. Water fluoridation and hip fracture. *Journal of the American Medical Association*, July 1991, 19(32):513-514

[14] Melvin E Page. Degeneration, Regeneration 1949. Available from the Price Pottenger Nutrition Foundation, San Diego, CA

[15] E Mazariegos-Ramos, et al. Consumption of soft drinks with phosphoric acid as a risk factor for the development of hypocalcemia in children: A case control study. *Journal of Pediatrics* 1995 126:940-942

[16] Herta Spencer and Lois Kramer. Osteoporosis: Calcium, Fluoride and Aluminum Interactions. *Journal of the American College of Nutrition* 1985 4:121-128

[17] Herta Spencer, et al. Chronic Alcoholism: Frequently Overlooked Cause of Osteoporosis in Men. *The American Journal of Medicine*. March 1986 80:393-397

[18] Dennis A. Chakkalakal. Alcohol-induced bone disease; Alcohol can inhibit the formation of new bone cells called osteoblasts, thereby decreasing bone formation. Omaha Veterans Affairs Medical Center, December 14, 2005. Accessed at http://www.eurekalert.org/pub_releases/2005-12/ace-abd120705.php

The Prostate

$\mathcal{T}$he prostate gland completely surrounds the urethra, making it the single most troublesome gland of the male reproductive system. When the prostate becomes enlarged, as it tends to do as early as age 30, it presses on the urethra, causing obstruction of flow of urine, diminished urinary stream, and sometimes complete urinary obstruction.

Obstruction may well eventually require insertion of a catheter to allow the urine to drain, and sometimes even a surgical operation which, while it relieves the symptoms of prostatic hypertrophy, may also relieve the symptoms of erection by destroying the nerve supply – a not uncommon complication of surgery.

By the age of 80, approximately 85% of men have so-called BPH, benign prostatic hypertrophy – enlargement of the prostate without any evidence of cancer.[1]

The only requirement for developing BPH is age and functioning testes. There may be a genetic form of BPH also, but it accounts for less than 10% of BPH.

So, what's a guy to do? He can't help getting older. He finds himself getting up two or three times during the night to urinate, he feels as though his bladder does not empty completely, perhaps he gets a bladder infection which requires treatment with antibiotic. His doctor starts talking about urologists…

So your prostate is enlarging. Now, how do you tell if the situation is benign or cancerous?

Since the lifetime risk of developing prostate cancer is about 16% but the mortality rate is only 3%, it would be good to find a test which could detect the variety of prostate cancer that is liable to kill you without subjecting 97% of you to unnecessary surgery, radiation and chemotherapy.

Unreliable PSA Tests

*C*ancer screening is controversial. Diagnostic tests to differentiate BPH from cancer of the prostate can be unreliable. The PSA test measures the prostate specific antigen, or PSA. This antigen is elevated with any enlargement of the prostate – be it benign or cancerous. If this level goes up rapidly, over the space of a few months, this may be more suggestive of rapidly growing prostate, hence more suggestive of cancer. About 50% of men with a PSA over 10 have cancer when their prostates are biopsied, and about 25% of those whose PSA is over four.

Even when screening does detect a cancer, it is hard to know how dangerous the cancer is. Doctors can't be sure which men need treatment and which would be fine without any. And men who are told they have prostate cancer may have a hard time just doing nothing, even if the cancer is unlikely to cause them harm.

The American Cancer Society revised the PSA screening guidelines in 2010 because of too many false positives – about 30 percent of patients are misdiagnosed as having an aggressive form of cancer. And many prostate cancers develop so slowly that they never cause problems during the man's lifetime. Better to leave them alone than to engage in invasive procedures that detract from quality of life.

The new guidelines stress that men should talk to their doctors about taking the test instead of automatically taking it:[2]

- The discussion should begin at age 50 for men with an average prostate cancer risk and at age 45 for men at higher risk, including African-Americans and men with a close relative diagnosed with the disease before age 65. For men at the highest risk, including those with a strong family history of the disease, the discussion should begin at age 40.
- Men who are tested and have an initial PSA of less than 2.5 ng/mL can be retested every two years.

- Yearly screening is warranted for men with PSA levels of 2.5 ng/mL or higher.
- Men without prostate cancer symptoms who are not expected to live for at least 10 years are not likely to benefit from screening and should not be tested.
- APSA of 4.0 ng/mL or higher remains a "reasonable threshold" for recommending a biopsy.

The guidelines were revised in the wake of two studies that were less than a ringing endorsement for screening. The American study involved more than 76,000 men. One group received "usual care;" the other group had annual PSA tests for six years and digital rectal examinations (DRE) every year for four years. The researchers found little difference in prostate cancer death rates between the two groups at seven years and again at 10 years of follow-up.[3] The European trial randomly assigned 182,000 men from seven different countries to either a control group or a screening group. Men in the screening group had PSA tests on average every four years and a DRE twice over that period of time. After about nine years, the researchers found that screening reduced the rate of prostate cancer death by 20%. But they also found that 48 men would need to be treated to prevent one death from prostate cancer.[4]

In 2010, researchers found a potential marker for prostate cancer that could be the starting point for less invasive testing and improved diagnosis of the disease. They found one compound that is present in cancerous prostate tissue but not in healthy prostate tissue – cholesterol sulfate. It's a fat. Researchers will next try to figure out the how and why of this compound's presence in cancerous tissue.[5]

There is no known link between BPH and prostate cancer.

Shrinking the Prostate

Doxazocin (Cardura) and terazocin (Hytrin) are alpha-adrenergic blockers commonly used to decrease the adrenergic tone of the prostate, relaxing the gland itself, and its grip on the urethra. Saw palmetto is an herb used for the same purpose.

Levels of testosterone in young men are quite high, levels of DHT are low. DHT is a metabolite of testosterone. The enzyme responsible for the conversion of testosterone to DHT, 5-alpha reductase, becomes more active with age. Thus the levels of testosterone decrease while the levels of DHT increase. So pharmaceutical companies focused on blocking the conversion of testosterone to DHT. Finasteride (Propecia) and dutasteride (Avodart) are used for this.

The alpha-adrenergic drugs have side effects of dizziness and fatigue, where the 5alpha-reductase drugs cause, in about 5% of men, reduced erections or ejaculations.

Standard allopathic therapy uses the techniques of burning, slashing and poisoning to treat the enemy – in this case, the enlarged prostate, the urinary obstruction, and the inability to urinate.

The idea of surgery on the prostate is not so exciting. Three varieties of surgical treatment are available. TURP stands for "trans-urethral prostatic resection," removal of prostatic tissue through the urethra. TUMT, "trans-urethral microwave thermotherapy," coagulates prostatic tissue and reduces its size by cooking it with microwaves. TUNA, "trans-urethral needle ablation," uses radio frequency waves sent into prostatic tissue through needles placed directly into the prostate. TUMT and TUNA both are less invasive than TURP, but they do not reduce the size of the gland as much either.

Is there no therapy for enlarged prostate which does not treat the gland like an enemy to be destroyed?

Answers within the Gland

Look at what the functions of the prostate gland tell us. The prostate provides about 20% of the volume of seminal fluid, that fluid which is ejaculated by the male at sexual climax. Since the gland wraps itself around the urethra, it is ideally suited to help regulate the flow of urine, by contracting its muscle fibers. This is probably why the -2 blockers (saw palmetto, Hytrin, etc) are effective in reducing symptoms of enlargement of the prostate (BPH, or benign prostatic hypertrophy).

The prostate also contains large numbers of receptors for thyroid hormone. We know that a woman's breasts also contain large numbers of these same thyroid hormone receptors. The woman's breasts and the man's prostate are the two largest accessory sexual organs of their bodies. It is not unreasonable to suspect that thyroid hormone plays some role in their function.

We know that iodine deficiency is linked with fibrocystic breast disease and breast cancer. When a woman with fibrocystic breasts is treated with iodine, the fibrocystic breasts soften and turn into normal breasts. It would not be unreasonable to conclude that the same thing could happen when men with enlarged prostates are treated with iodine. Nature tends to be fairly conservative, and does not invent new processes when the old ones are perfectly adequate to the task. Iodine deficiency is associated with increased risk of several different cancers, including breast, thyroid and stomach, all of which have thyroid hormone receptors.[6]

The prostate also contains thyroid hormone receptors.[7] Thyroid hormone requires iodine for its synthesis. Therefore the prostate must also require iodine, since it has the receptors for thyroid hormone, and nature really does not create useless redundancies. This could explain why therapy with iodine or iodide could help to shrink the size of the prostate. It is known that iodine deficiency in adolescents results in enlargement of the testes, just as it results in enlargement of the thyroid gland without concomitant production of androgenic hormones and virilization.

Prostate cancer has been associated with decreased total body levels of vitamin D3 (cholecalciferol),[8] vitamin E,[9] selenium[10] and other micro-nutrient deficiency.[11]

And if there is cancer – or even if there isn't – how can we treat, to decrease the chances of cancer? There are as yet no studies on iodine and prostate cancer, but there are studies on iodine and breast cancer. Iodine induces apoptosis (cellular suicide in a "clean" way, that does not create a lot of inflammatory debris) in breast cancer cells at concentrations which are healthy for the body as a whole.[12] These concentrations can be attained by ingesting 50 mg per day of iodine and/or iodide.

We know that the American population at large is iodine deficient. We know that the incidence of prostate cancer is rising – one out of every three American men have it. How could it hurt, to ingest sufficient iodine, until the studies are in?

[1]http:///www.nlm.nih.gov/medlineplus/ency/article/00381.htm#Causes.%20incidence.%20and%20rish%20factors

[2]American Cancer Society."Guideline for the Early Detection of Prostate Cancer: Update 2010," CA: *A Cancer Journal for Clinicians*, published online March 3, 2010.

[3]Prostate, Lung, Colorectal, and Ovarian Cancer Screening Trial. The National Cancer Institute.

[4]European Randomized Study of Screening for Prostate Cancer. ERSPC.

[5]Potential Prostate Cancer Marker Discovered. *Science Daily*, August 6, 2010

[6]Venturi S, Donati FM. Role of iodine in evolution and carcinogenesis of thyroid, breast and stomach. *Adv Clin Path*. 2000 Jan;4(1):11-7.

[7]Jannini EA, Crescenzi A et al. Ontogenetic Pattern of Thyroid Hormone Receptor Expression in the Human Testis. *J Clin Endocrin* Met 85;9:3453-57.

[8]Zhuang SH, Burnstein KL. Antiproliferative Effect of 1 ,25-Dihydroxyvitamin D3 in Human Prostate Cancer Cell Line LNCaP Involves Reduction of Cyclin-Dependent Kinase 2 Activity and Persistent G1 Accumulation. *Endocrinology* 139;2:1197-1207.

[9]Heinonen OP, Albanes D, Virtamo J, et al. Prostate cancer and supplementation with alpha-tocopherol and beta-carotene: incidence and mortality in a controlled trial. *J Natl Cancer Inst* 1998; 90: 440-446. MEDLINE

[10]Clark LC, Dalkin B, Krongrad A, et al. Decreased incidence of prostate cancer with selenium supplementation: results of a double-blind cancer prevention trial. *Br J Urol* 1998; 81: 730-734. MEDLINE

[11]Ames BN. DNA damage from micronutrient deficiencies is likely to be a major cause of cancer. *Mut Res* 475;7-20. (2001).

[12]Shrivastava A, Tiwari M et al. Molecular iodine induces caspase-independent apoptosis in human breast carcinoma cells involving the mitochondria-mediated pathway. *J Biol Chem*. 2006 Jul 14;281(28):19762-71.

Vitamin D, Sun, Skin Cancer

℘enturies ago, when Vikings and other European seafarers took to the high seas for years at a time, they pioneered new trade routes and they mostly died of skin cancer. Native American Indians, living mostly outdoors, also mostly died of skin cancer.

What?

You never heard that? Right. *Because it didn't happen.*

Here are a few things that really did happen:

- In the 1980s, dermatologists began warning about the dangers of sunlight. Their advertisements were heavily funded by the cosmetics and sun screen industry.
- In the 1980s, the current triple childhood epidemics of asthma, diabetes, and autism quietly began. Rates of cancer and other chronic illnesses began to escalate.[1]
- In 1989, the American Medical Association's Council on Scientific Affairs warned about the dangers of sun-exposure, advising mothers and children to "stay out of the sun as much as possible."
- In 1999, the American Academy of Pediatrics warned mothers to always keep infants out of direct sunlight, use sun-protective clothes, sun block, and make sure children's activities in general minimize sunlight exposure.
- In 2000, it was documented that rickets – vitamin D deficiency – is making a comeback in American children who drink less milk and more juice and sodas.[2]

Today, we have escalating rates of cancer and chronic disease. Many say hiding from the sun's rays, and living with the subsequent low levels of vitamin D, was one of the tickets to that train wreck.

Let There Be Light

*M*ankind was designed to bask in the rays of the sun.

About 90 percent of the vitamin D in your body is made when your skin is exposed to sunlight. Only about 10 percent comes from food – butter, egg yolk, fish oil, and human milk.

Because people have been told to fear the sun, there is a widespread vitamin D deficiency today. Boston University researcher Michael Holick estimates that approximately 1 billion people worldwide are vitamin D deficient.[3]

If you've been avoiding the sun, have you been getting enough vitamin D in your daily multi-vitamin? Probably not. Just 15-20 minutes in the summer sun produces a blast of 10,000-20,000 international units. Ancient humans spent all their time outdoors and got such doses. By contrast, the U.S. government recommends a mere 200 to 600 IU a day, depending on age – what you might get in two to six cups of "fortified" milk.

The government's recommendation is based on the effects of vitamin D on bone health and calcium absorption. It does not reflect the other vital biological functions of vitamin D – its roles in cancer prevention, regulation of blood pressure, insulin production, mental health, and regulation of immune function and cell growth.

Sunlight is the most efficient way to get vitamin D. And ancestry really makes a difference here. The figure of 10,000-20,000 units of vitamin D from being outdoors applies to fair skinned adults sunbathing in the summer. Dark-skinned people require 10 times that exposure to make an equivalent amount. And considering how important vitamin D is to a baby's brain development, what happens to pregnant women who avoid the sun? They would have to drink 200 glasses of milk or take 50 prenatal multivitamins to equal 20 minutes in the sun. An autistic boy who plays inside the house, instead of outside, would have to take several thousand units of vitamin D to make up for what his skin would have produced had he played outside that day.[4]

Ultraviolet A (UVA): wavelength 315–400 nm. UVA penetrates deep into the skin and can cause damage like wrinkles and discoloration. UVA's intensity is more constant than UVB, as it does not vary with time of day or year. No UVA is blocked by the ozone layer nor is it filtered by glass.

Ultraviolet B (UVB): wavelength 280–315 nm. UVB can cause sunburn yet is also what enables vitamin D production in the skin. Depending upon the angle at which the sun's rays reach the earth, optimal UVB exposure is between 10:00 am–2:00 pm in the summer (70% of a person's yearly dose is received in summer). UVB does not penetrate glass and most is blocked by the ozone layer.

When it comes to getting vitamin D from a pill, the most useful form is the D3 – the form found in animal foods. Beware that many vitamin D and multivitamin supplements use the D2 form which the body has a harder time assimilating.

Vitamin D's Connection to Chronic Disease

Doctors have observed that where there is less sun, we see more cancer, flu, and even autism. And, there are more of these diseases in winter, which has less sunlight. There are also more of these diseases the further you get from the equator – the further you move away, the less sunlight there is.

1. The Diabetes Connection
Blood sugar is closely associated with your vitamin D level. Researchers in Australia added to the growing evidence that sun avoidance may have caused the epidemic of type 2 diabetes. The Australians' findings were straightforward and powerful. The higher your vitamin D level, the lower your blood glucose.[5]

2. The Breast Cancer Connection

In 2007, researchers at the Moores Cancer Center at University of California, San Diego (UCSD), published research findings that women with higher levels of vitamin D had lower levels of breast cancer. The researchers estimated that possibly half the cases of breast cancer and two-thirds of the cases of colorectal cancer in the United States could be prevented with higher levels of Vitamin D:[6]

> For the first time, we are saying that 600,000 cases of breast and colorectal cancer could be prevented each year worldwide, including nearly 150,000 in the United States alone. —study co-author Cedric F. Garland

3. The Overall Cancer Connection

The UCSD research team also reported links between low vitamin D levels and endometrial cancer (Feb 2007), ovarian cancer (Oct 2006), and kidney cancer (Sept 2006).[7]

In 2009, the UCSD team proposed a new model of cancer development that hinges on a loss of cancer cells' ability to stick together. The model differs substantially from the current model which suggests genetic mutations are the earliest driving forces behind cancer.

"The first event in cancer is loss of communication among cells due to, among other things, low vitamin D and calcium levels," said epidemiologist Cedric Garland, who led the work. "In this new model, we propose that this loss may play a key role in cancer by disrupting the communication between cells that is essential to healthy cell turnover, allowing more aggressive cancer cells to take over."[8]

A Norwegian study found that vitamin D levels, calculated on sun exposure, were linked to survival rates for cancer patients. Those who lived in sunnier, southern latitudes, and had higher vitamin D levels, were less likely to die from cancer than people in northern latitudes.[9]

The Creighton University School of Medicine studied 1,179 postmenopausal, cancer-free women between 2000 and 2005 who took nearly three times the Recommended Daily Amount of vitamin D3.

Participants showed a dramatic 60 percent or greater reduction in cancer risk compared with women who did not get the vitamin.[10]

"The findings are very exciting. They confirm what a number of vitamin D proponents have suspected for some time but that, until now, have not been substantiated through clinical trial," said principal investigator Joan Lappe, Ph.D., R.N., Creighton Professor of Medicine. "Vitamin D is a critical tool in fighting cancer as well as many other diseases."

It's known that vitamin D stimulates white blood cells to produce a powerful natural antibiotic called cathelicidin. Vitamin D has the capacity to turn on powerful antimicrobial genes.

Some of these genes make proteins that halt cancer by inducing apoptosis (programmed cell death), which destroys aberrant cells before they become cancerous, like adenoma cells in the colon and rectum. Other genes rein in out-of-control growth of cancer cells like those in the prostate. Vitamin D-expressed genes inhibit angiogenesis, the formation of new blood vessels that malignant tumors need to grow, as studies on lung and breast cancers show. Other genes inhibit metastases, preventing cancer that arises in one organ from spreading its cells to other parts of the body, such as in breast and prostate cancers.[11]

4. Growing Healthy Children

In 2007, the Canadian Cancer Society made big news as it announced a national program to prevent cancer using vitamin D. The society now advises all Canadians to take 1000 IU of vitamin D daily. The Canadian Pediatric Society now recommends that pregnant women take 2,000 IU of vitamin D per day (10 times more than the 200 IU/day the National Institutes of Health recommends for pregnant women in the USA). According to the Canadian press, the Canadian Pediatric Society acted "to protect babies from a litany of illnesses later in life."

Others feel that even 4,000 IU/day is not enough for breast-feeding mothers to maintain adequate levels of vitamin D in their breast milk; that would take about 6,000 IU/ day.[12]

5. The Autism Connection

Dr. John Jacob Cannell of the Vitamin D Council believes that falling levels of vitamin D in the last 20 years parallel the rise of the autism epidemic:

> The theory that vitamin D deficiency causes autism...has a plausible mechanism of action ... The very different effects estrogen and testosterone have on vitamin D metabolism may explain why boys are much more likely to get it than girls are. Lower vitamin D levels in blacks may explain their higher rates of autism ...
>
> Professor John McGrath and Dr. Darryl Eyles of the University of Queensland in Australia have repeatedly warned us that normal brain development depends on adequate amounts of activated vitamin D to orchestrate the cellular architecture of the brain ... Abnormal inflammation is associated with both autism and vitamin D deficiency. For example, autistic individuals show increases in cytokines (inflammatory mediators) that show a striking similarity to the immune processes regulated by vitamin D ...
>
> Vitamin D's role in increasing glutathione levels may explain the link between mercury and other heavy metals, oxidative stress, and autism.[13]

Glutathione is the body's main detoxifing agent. It helps the liver remove chemicals that are foreign to the body, such as drugs and pollutants. Dr. Cannell makes a fascinating observation: If vitamin D levels are low, glutathione levels also may be low, thus children may not be able to detoxify the mercury, aluminum, formaldehyde and other ingredients in vaccines.

6. Keeping Our Brains Healthy

Renowned UCLA researcher Bruce Ames, Ph.D., noted the wide distribution of vitamin D receptors throughout the brain, and underscored the role of the vitamin in maintaining brain health.

He emphasized that vitamin D appears to affect brain proteins responsible for learning and memory, motor control, and behavior. Although the evidence remains inconclusive, results of previous human and animal studies indicate that inadequate vitamin D levels may impair cognition and give rise to behavior problems.

"We conclude there is ample biological evidence to suggest an important role for vitamin D in brain development and function," Ames said.[14]

Why the Rise in Skin Cancer?

$\mathcal{A}$ number of researchers would point first to the imbalance of omega 3 and omega 6 fatty acids in our diet – our grandparents ate cod liver oil high in omega 3s, and we eat French fries high in omega 6s. The research is piling up that omega 3 deficiencies are a far more significant risk factor for deadly skin cancers than sun exposure.

Studies, particularly a comprehensive review from the National Academy of Sciences, show that omega 3 fatty acids, including docosahexaenoic acid (DHA) and eicosapentaenoic acid (EPA), can reduce the risk of skin cancer whereas omega 6 fatty acids such as arachidonic acid (AA) increase the risk.[15,16]

Processed foods tend to be full of partially hydrogenated oils – trans fatty acids – which stiffen your body's cells and block the flow of nutrition coming in and toxins passing out. Dr. Johanna Budwig, a seven-time Nobel Prize nominee, demonstrated that certain wavelengths of sunlight vibrate at the same frequency as chemical bonds in trans fats. Dr. Budwig believed this leads to early mutations that can become skin cancers. After studying thousands of blood samples, she discovered a key difference between the healthy and the ill was that healthy people had a higher content of omega 3 oils.[17]

The National Academy of Sciences published a comprehensive review which showed that the omega 6:3 ratio is key to preventing the development of skin cancer; DHA was a more efficient inhibitor than EPA.[18] An earlier Australian study showed a 40% reduction in melanoma for people who eat fish regularly. And this was without paying any attention to lowering the omega-6 fats which encourage cancer.[19]

Nutritional deficiencies related to sunshine and health are not limited to omega 3s and vitamin D. One of the first signs of a niacin (B3) deficiency is photosensitivity. The term "redneck" originally described the bright red necks of eighteenth-and nineteenth-century niacin-deficient fieldworkers who got sunburned easily, and did not develop a protective tan. As author Dr. Eldon Haas writes:

> The American Indians processed corn using potash (which is highly alkaline) that makes the B vitamins in corn available for assimilation during digestion. But the American settlers, not understanding how to prepare corn (and too arrogant to follow the food preparation ways of the Indian 'savages'), would simply grind up their corn and consume it as corn flour (corn meal). By the way, that's how most people eat corn today: as ground up cornmeal ingredients in chips and foods. It's no wonder so many modern Americans remain so deficient in B vitamins.[20]

Perhaps that explains why the Melanoma Research Foundation reports that tanning bed use among people under the age of 30 can increase the risk of developing melanoma by up to 75 percent. Grab a fast food burger, fries, and soda – then hit the tanning booth. Intense sun exposure without enough vitamins and antioxidants on board is a prescription for trouble.

Sunscreens are another factor increasingly implicated in skin cancer because they promote vitamin D deficiencies – remember, vitamin D fights cancer. The rise in skin cancers over the last 25 years parallels the rise in use of sunscreen lotions, which block vitamin D-producing UVB rays. And many sunscreens contain potentially harmful ingredients that absorbed through the skin.

Working indoors where light is artificial may also account for the rise in skin cancer. A U.S. Navy study found that the most malignant melanoma was found not in people who worked in the sun, but with people who worked indoors under artificial light. They found that most of these skin cancers occur on areas of the body not even exposed to the sun.[21] A study published in *The Lancet* found that it was not sunlight that caused melanoma but rather fluorescent light that caused more than twice the melanoma risk. The study found that long exposure to sunlight actually "immunized" people from the later development of melanoma.[22]

Not All Skin Cancers Are the Same

Skin cancer is responsible for perhaps less than two percent of all cancer deaths, accounting for about 11,000 of the 565,000 American cancer deaths recorded in 2006.

Nearly all skin cancer deaths stem from relatively rare malignant melanomas, which constitute about nine percent of all skin-cancer cases.

Basal cell carcinoma is the most common form of cancer, with about a million new cases estimated in the U.S. each year. Basal cells line the deepest layer of the epidermis. Basal cell carcinomas are malignant growths – tumors – that arise in this layer.

Basal cell carcinoma can usually be diagnosed with a simple biopsy and is fairly easy to treat when detected early. This cancer has an extremely low rate of metastasis, and although it can result in scars and disfigurement, it is not usually life threatening.

Doctors have noted that basal cell carcinomas often occur behind the ears, an area not generally affected by sunlight. President Richard Nixon had an inch-long basal cell carcinoma removed from behind his left ear.

Squamous cell carcinoma is the second most common form of skin cancer, with some 250,000 new cases per year estimated in the United States. It arises in the squamous cells that compose most of the upper layer of the skin.

Pre-cancerous patches of rough or scaly skin known as actinic keratoses are patches of damaged skin. If not addressed, some of this can develop into squamous cell skin cancer. Squamous cell cancer appears on the skin as small lumps or sore spots that don't heal properly. This is a superficial cancer, and non-life-threatening unless allowed to progress over many years. By treating keratoses, however, you may be able to head off squamous cells before they develop. Glycoalkaloids, natural compounds found in an Australian botanical known as the devil's apple plant, and in other nightshade family plants like tomatoes, peppers, eggplant and potatoes, can be used for this. Historically, the use of glycoalkaloid-rich plants in addressing skin conditions goes back to the second century A.D.

Glycoalkaloids are thought to work by exploiting structural differences between healthy and damaged skin cells. As skin cells become damaged, the cell walls become more permeable, allowing glycoalkoloids to penetrate abnormal cells. Once inside the cell walls, glycoalkaloids release enzymes that break down the cells from the inside out. As the abnormal cells die, they're replaced by healthy skin cells, which don't absorb the glycoalkaloids, thus avoiding their destructive effects.

Melanoma, however, cannot be reversed with glycoalkaloids. Melanoma is the most dangerous form of skin cancer. It is not the most common skin cancer, but it causes the most deaths. If recognized and treated early, it is nearly 100 percent curable. When not caught early, a melanoma spot the size of a dime can spread to other parts of the body where it becomes hard to treat.

The basic facts simply do not add up that simple sun exposure leads to melanoma:

1. In 1900, about 75% of the U.S. population worked outdoors. Melanoma was rare. But since the 1970s, the incidence of melanoma has been steadily rising. It is rising at a time when sun exposure is decreasing, when vitamin D deficiencies are becoming epidemic.

2. Melanoma is more common in indoor workers than outdoor. It is not a disease of farmers; it is a disease of office workers.

3. Melanoma is more common on regions of the body that are not exposed to the sun.

4. It was not until about 1990 that professional opinion began to suggest that melanoma was caused by exposure to the sun. A meta-analysis reported in 2005 found that studies undertaken before 1990 generally found no association between sun exposure and melanoma, but later studies did find an

association. The research team suggests that these later studies were influenced by biased recall of participants who knew from wide publicity that experts believed skin cancer was caused by sun exposure.[23]

5. Melanoma is the second leading cause of cancer death for people age 15 to 30, and the rate is increasing.[24]

A number of people connect these dots and come up with an important factor that has drastically changed since 1970, one that would also account for melanoma striking younger people: diet. Other connect different dots and come up with EMF – electromagnetic fields.

Something in the Air Causing Skin Cancer?

Some experts looked at the expanding communication technology in the last several decades and found a striking association between the increase in certain cancers, including melanoma. They point to the ever-increasing electronic bombardment by radio and TV signals.

The first to raise the issue were researchers Dr. Olle Johansson and colleague Örjan Hallberg at the Karolinska Institute in Sweden. They found a strong association between the increase in certain cancers during the 20th century and exposure to electromagnetic fields as measured by radio and TV broadcasts. They reported that there is a common environmental stress that accelerates several forms of cancer – colon cancer, lung cancer, breast cancer, bladder cancer, and melanoma. They site the introduction of AM radio (1920s), radar (1940s), FM radio and TV (1950s), computers (1970s), mobile phones (1980s), and wireless technologies and compact fluorescent lighting (2000s), and conclude that artificially created EMR is the most likely environmental stress to account for the rise in cancers.[25,26,27]

We know that our brains, hearts, and cells use electromagnetic signals – we measure the electrical output of the heart for example with an EKG. Much study is underway to determine exactly how the body's electrical

331

signalling can be affected by external electromagnetic fields. The 2004 Reflex study out of Europe determined that radio waves from mobile phones harm body cells and damage DNA in laboratory conditions.[28]

Think Twice Before Slathering That Sunscreen

The active ingredients of sunscreen are many times less efficient than melanin, our own skin pigment, at dissipating the sun's rays into nonreactive forms of energy. Sunscreens block your skin from producing the pigment melanin. This prevents your body from employing its natural defense against overexposure to sunlight – a tan. Sunscreens primarily block UVB waves, the wavelength that stimulates the skin's vitamin D production. Sunscreen with a sun protection factor (SPF) of 8 inhibits more than 95% of vitamin D production.[29]

A team of researchers from the University of California-Riverside found sunscreen can do more harm than good once it soaks into the skin.[30]

The research team found that three commonly used ultraviolet (UV) filters – octylmethoxycinnamate, benzophenone 3, and octocrylene – eventually soak into the deeper layers of the skin after application, leaving the top skin layers vulnerable to sun damage. UV rays absorbed by the skin can also generate harmful compounds called reactive oxygen species (ROS), which can cause skin cancer and premature aging. The researchers found that once sunscreen filters soak into the lower layers of skin, the filters react with UV light to create more damaging ROS.

The UC-Riverside team's research is the first to indicate that sunscreen filters – intended to protect the skin from UV damage – apparently end up promoting such damage instead.

In June, 2007, the Environmental Working Group (EWG) released an in-depth analysis of the safety and effectiveness of more than 700 name-brand sunscreens:

Our review of the technical literature shows that some sunscreen ingredients absorb into the blood, and some are linked to toxic effects. Some release skin-damaging free radicals in sunlight, some act like estrogen and could disrupt hormone systems, several are strongly linked to allergic reactions, and still others may build up in the body or the environment. FDA has not established rigorous safety standards for sunscreen ingredients.[31]

A March, 2008 study by the U.S. Centers for Disease Control (CDC) revealed that 97% of Americans are contaminated with a widely-used sunscreen ingredient called oxybenzone that has been linked to allergies, hormone disruption, and cell damage. A companion study from the Mt. Sinai School of Medicine revealed that this chemical is linked to low birth weight in baby girls whose mothers are exposed during pregnancy.[32] Oxybenzone is also a penetration enhancer, a chemical that helps other chemicals penetrate the skin. EWG's analysis of ingredient labels found oxybenzone in nearly 600 sunscreens and in lip balm, lipstick, moisturizers, and fragrance for women.

The FDA recently proposed to disallow manufacturer claims on bottles that using sunscreens prevents cancer. This came on the heels of a 2006 class action lawsuit filed in Los Angeles alleging that five of the leading U.S. makers of sunscreen lotions – including Coppertone, Banana Boat, Hawaiian Tropic – deceptively promote their products as protection from harmful sun rays. "Sunscreen is the snake oil of the 21st century," said attorney Samuel Rudman.[33,34]

Old News, New News

"Up until now we looked at vitamin D the way we look at an iceberg. Eighty-five percent of its function has been hidden, and we had no idea until two or three years ago," Robert Heaney, an endocrinologist at Creighton University in Nebraska told *Forbes* in 2008. "The field has just exploded."[35]

Current research indicates vitamin D deficiency plays a role in causing some 17 kinds of cancer as well as heart disease, stroke, hypertension, autoimmune diseases, diabetes, depression, chronic pain, osteoarthritis, osteoporosis, muscle weakness, muscle wasting, birth defects, and periodontal disease. Vitamin D regulates cells, systems, and organs throughout the body.

A 2008 study showed that adults in sunny southern Arizona are commonly deficient in vitamin D; more than a quarter of the adults tested had dangerously low blood levels of vitamin D. Those who had higher vitamin D levels developed fewer colorectal polyps.[36]

In the largest study of possible links between vitamin D and respiratory infections, researchers reported in 2009 that people with the lowest blood vitamin D levels had significantly more recent colds or cases of the flu. The risks were even higher for those with chronic respiratory disorders, such as asthma and emphysema.[37]

Once you realize the many connections that vitamin D makes to keep people healthy, you'd want to patent it to make bundles of $$$. If it were a drug, it would be a mega-blockbuster outselling all others. But it's a nutrient that cannot be patented. Your body makes it for free. Of course the pharmaceutical companies have made a vitamin D "analog" called Calcitriol – an unnatural substance that looks kind of like vitamin D and is converted to active vitamin D in the body – if you have the right genetics to make the conversion.

In February, 2008, the *New York Times* pointed out the lackluster response from the mainstream medical community:

> The so-called sunshine vitamin is poised to become the nutrient of the decade, if a host of recent findings are to be believed. Vitamin D seems to dampen an overactive immune system. The incidence of autoimmune diseases like Type 1 diabetes and multiple sclerosis have been linked to low levels of vitamin D.
>
> The federal committee that establishes daily recommended levels of nutrients has resisted all efforts to increase vitamin D intake significantly, partly because the members are not convinced of assertions for its health-promoting potential and partly because of time-worn fears of toxicity.[38]

As Dr. John Cannell of the vitamin D Council put it:

> A child has never gotten into a vitamin D cabinet and gotten poisoned. That happened hundreds of thousands of times though with Tylenol or aspirin or other things ... This whole thing when you think about it is patently absurd. They refuse to change, they refuse to even look at the science.[39]

The current RDAs for vitamin D are 400 IU for adults aged 51 to 70 and 600 IU for people over 70. And the RDA for all persons younger than 51 is a scant 200 IU. Studies show that much more than that is needed to prevent falls and fractures. In double-blind, randomized controlled trials involving 2,426 older people, daily supplemental doses of vitamin D between 700 and 1,000 IU reduced the risk of falling by 19 percent, while doses below 700 IU per day showed no benefits.[40] Researchers noted that muscle weakness is both an important risk factor for falls and a proven, prominent symptom of vitamin D deficiency.[41] Vitamin D stimulates synthesis of protein, the building material for muscle.

The American Academy of Pediatrics broke ranks in 2008 and recommended that infants and adolescents take 400 IU daily. It didn't get much response. A 2010 study said most babies should take a daily vitamin D supplement.[42] That would be a big change for most parents and pediatricians. Even breast-fed and formula-fed babies don't get enough vitamin D, studies show. Although taking prenatal vitamins helped, more than 30% of moms who took them were still deficient. Getting lots of sunlight helped raise vitamin D levels in moms, but not in their newborns.

The CDC found that only 5 to 13 percent of breast-fed infants were receiving at least 400 IU of vitamin D per day.[43] Vitamin D is available in inexpensive drops. Problem is, the AAP's recommendations are still in the Old News category amongst the rest of their information: sunlight is a hazard so keep infants out of direct sunlight and make sure they wear protective clothing and sunscreen.[44]

Let the Sun Shine

*In the early 1900s, most Americans lived a rural lifestyle and spent a lot of time outdoors. Today, most people simply aren't getting enough mid-day summer sun to make an adequate amount of vitamin D. Strike a balance. Remember: never get sunburned, that is key. If you have lots of omegas and antioxidants on board, you will not burn nearly as easily.

Sunscreen? It is certainly useful for preventing sunburn, which may be responsible for a small percentage of the relatively small number of fatal skin cancers that occur. But read up on toxic ingredients before you buy. And clothing is a time-honored way of covering up. It's less messy than sunscreen, too.

Almost everyone is deficient in D3. Supplement appropriately, since vitamin D is so important in so many different functions in the body - kind of like the chicken soup vitamin. Michael Holick feels that we should all have levels that measure greater than 50 in order to function properly. Most of us fall in the 20-30 range – which is considered "normal" in allopathic medicine. Remember that bell-shaped curve? Ninety-five percent of us have those distressingly low levels of Vitamin D. No wonder we get so sick all the time.

Of course, if you want to spend hours and hours in the sun, it will turn your skin dark and leathery, and you'll wind up looking like an Arizona lizard. But in moderation, vitamin D from the sun is excellent for your health.

Remember: Intense sun exposure without enough vitamins and antioxidants on board is a prescription for trouble.

RESOURCES

Subscribe to the newsletter of the Vitamin D Council,
www.vitamindcouncil.org

BOOKS

The UV Advantage
by Michael Holick, Ph.D., M.D. and Mark Jenkins, 2004

[1] *The Vitamin D Newsletter*. The Vitamin D Council. November 2007

[2] Linda B. White. Vitamin D: Sunshine and So Much More. *Mother Earth News*, February/March 2008

[3] Michael Holick. Vitamin D Deficiency. *New England Journal of Medicine*, July 19, 2007

[4] Autism and Vitamin D, The Role of Sunshine; The Vitamin D Council

[5] Need AG, O'Loughlin PD, Horowitz M, Nordin BE. Relationship between fasting serum glucose, age, body mass index and serum 25 hydroxyvitamin D in postmenopausal women. *Clin Endocrinol* (Oxf). 2005 Jun;62(6):738-41.

[6] Garland, Cedric; Gorham, Edward; et al. Vitamin D and prevention of breast cancer: pooled analysis. *The Journal of steroid biochemistry and molecular biology*, 103 (3-5), p.708-711, Mar 2007

[7] November 14, 2007; News Release from University of California, San Diego, Medical Center

[8] http://www.eurekalert.org/pub_releases/2009-05/uoc--nms052009.php

[9] Johan Moan, Alina C Porojnicu, et al. Addressing the health benefits and risks, involving vitamin D or skin cancer, of increased sun exposure. *Proceedings of the National Academy of Sciences*, January 7, 2008.

[10] *American Journal of Clinical Nutrition*, June 8, 2007

[11] Dr. Donald Miller, Jr. Vitamin D in a New Light. September 10, 2007, accessed January 2008 at www.donaldmiller.com

[12] Basile LA, et al. The effect of high-dose vitamin D supplementation on serum vitamin D levels and milk calcium concentration in lactating women and their infants. *Breastfeed Med.* 2006 Spring;1(1):27-35.

[13] John Jacob Cannell, MD. What is Autism? accessed at http://www.vitamindcouncil.org/health/autism/what-is-autism.shtml

[14] Joyce C. McCann, Bruce N. Ames. Is there convincing biological or behavioral evidence linking vitamin D deficiency to brain dysfunction? *The FASEB Journal*. 2008;22:982-1001

[15] Guangming Liu, Douglas M. Bibus, et al. Omega 3 but not omega 6 fatty acids inhibit AP-1 activity and cell transformation in JB6 cells. *Proceedings of the National Academy of Sciences*, June 19, 2001, vol. 98, no. 13, 7510-7515

[16] Anthony P. Albino, Gloria Juan, et al. Cell Cycle Arrest and Apoptosis of Melanoma Cells by Docosahexaenoic Acid: Association with Decreased pRb Phosphorylation. *Cancer Research*, 60, 4139-4145, August 1, 2000

[17] Johanna Budwig. *Flax Oil as a True Aid Against Arthritis, Heart Infarction, Cancer and Other Diseases.* Apple Tree Pub Co Ltd, Vancouver, British Columbia, Canada, 1994

[18] Guangming Liu, Douglas M. Bibus, et al. Omega 3 but not omega 6 fatty acids inhibit AP-1 activity and cell transformation in JB6 cells. *PNAS*, June 19, 2001 vol. 98 no. 13 7510-7515

[19] Bain C, Green A, et al. Diet and melanoma. An exploratory case-control study. *Ann Epidemiol.* 1993 May;3(3):235-8.

[21] Eldon Haas, MD. *Staying Healthy with Nutrition: The Complete Guide to Diet and Nutritional Medicine.* Celestial Arts, November, 1995, page 118

[22] Garland FC, White MR et al. Occupational sunlight exposure and melanoma in the U.S. Navy. *Arch Environ Health.* 1990 Sep-Oct;45(5):261-7.

[23]Beral V, Shaw H et al. Malignant Melanoma and Exposure to Fluorescent Lighting at Work. *The Lancet* 320;8293:290-293.

[24]Gandini, S et al. Meta-analysis of risk factors for cutaneous melanoma: II Sun exposure. *European Journal of Cancer*, 2005.

[25]Melanoma Research Foundation

[26]Hallberg, Örjan and Olle Johansson. Cancer Trends During the 20th Century. *Journal of the Autralasian College of Nutrition and Environmental Medicine*. 2002a. 21(1): 3-8

[27]Hallberg, Örjan and Olle Johansson. Melanoma Incidence and Frequency Modulation (FM) Broadcasting. *Archives of Environmental Health*. 2002b. 57(1): 32-40

[28]Hallberg, Örjan and Olle Johansson. FM Broadcasting Exposure Time and Malignant Melanoma Incidence. *Electromagnetic Biology and Medicine*. 2005. 24: 1-8.

[29]http://www.worldhealth.net/news/mobile_phone_radiation_harms_dna_new_stu

[30]Linda B. White. Vitamin D: Sunshine and So Much More. *Mother Earth News*, February/March 2008

[31]Sunscreens Can Damage Skin, Researchers find filters in sunscreens that keep out ultraviolet radiation can generate compounds that attack skin cells, UC-R Press Release of August 26, 2006, accessed at http://www.newsroom.ucr.edu/cgi-bin/display.cgi?id=1399

[32]Environmental Working Group. Which Sunscreens are Safest? First-ever online database rates sunscreen safety and effectiveness. June 19, 2007

[33]Antonia M. Calafat, Lee-Yang Wong, et al. Concentrations of the Sunscreen Agent, Benzophenone-3, in Residents of the United States: National Health and Nutrition Examination Survey 2003–2004. *Environmental Health Perspectives*, Volume 116, Number 3, March 2008, accessed at http://www.ehponline.org/docs/2008/11269/abstract.html

[34]Elizabeth Olson. The Rub On Sunscreens. *New York Times*, June 19, 2006 http://www.csgrr.com/csgrr-cgi-bin/mil?templ=cases/sunscreen/signup.html

[35]Robert Langreth. D is For Debate. *Forbes*, March 10, 2008

[36]Elizabeth T Jacobs, David S Alberts, et al. Vitamin D insufficiency in southern Arizona. *American Journal of Clinical Nutrition*, Vol. 87, No. 3, 608-613, March 2008

[37]Ginde AA, Liu MC, Camargo CA Jr. Demographic differences and trends of vitamin D insufficiency in the US population, 1988-2004. *Arch Intern Med*. 2009 Mar 23;169(6):626-32.

[38]Jane Brody. An Oldie Vies for Nutrient of the Decade. *New York Times*, February 19, 2008

[39]Gailon Totheroh. What's the Real Story on Vitamin D? *Canadian Broadcasting Network*, November 17, 2007, accessed March 2008 at http://www.cbn.com/CBNnews/269033.aspx

[40]HA Bischoff-Ferrari, B Dawson-Hughes, et al. Fall prevention with supplemental and active forms of vitamin D: a meta-analysis of randomised controlled trials. *British Medical Journal*, 2009 Oct 1;339:b3692. doi: 10.1136/bmj.b3692.

[41]Ceglia L. Vitamin D and its role in skeletal muscle. *Curr Opin Clin Nutr Metab Care*. 2009 Nov;12(6):628-33.

[42]Cria Perrine. Adherence to Vitamin D Recommendations Among US Infants. *Pediatrics*, March 22, 2010; vol 125: pp 627-632.

[43]Salynn Boyles. CDC: Babies Don't Get Enough Vitamin D. *WebMD Health News*, March 22, 2010

[44]American Academy of Pediatrics Committee on Environmental Health. Ultraviolet light: a hazard to children. *Pediatrics* 1999;104:328-33.

Epilogue

*W*hat would it look like if we made it priority to have a healthier population in America? What if we shifted our emphasis from disease management to prevention?

Let's get past the idea that "prevention" is lots of expensive tests for "early" diagnosis. By the time a test shows an illness, it's too late for prevention – the train has left the station, disease has already set in. An inconvenient truth of the disease management system is that sick people generate money for the industry. So-called "health" insurance only pays for treating damaged organs, not generally for the education and therapies which could prevent the damage in the first place.

Prevention, as we homeopathic physicians use the term, is a fundamentally different approach to medicine.

Our chemically-saturated environments and our way of eating are the big white elephants in the room when health care is discussed. According to the CDC, more than 75 percent of health care spending now goes to treat preventable chronic diseases. Most of these diseases have their roots in diet and environment.[1] We have not seen the political will to take a much firmer stand on what constitutes "food," and on what the government is willing to pay for with food stamps. Chemicals still are not tested for safety. Industry-sponsored tests delay government regulation on EMF pollution.

Research from Harvard University found that low omega-3 intake plays a role in about 84,000 deaths annually.[2] Contrast that with the estimate of 40,610 who were predicted to die from breast cancer in 2009. More Americans die of an omega-3 deficiency than breast cancer. Yet we are awash in pink ribbons asking us to take an annual mammogram test with its annual dose of cancer-causing radiation. What is wrong with this picture?

University of California-Berkeley scientists demonstrated that vitamins and natural supplements can repair DNA damage. They said, "There are many genetic differences that make people's enzymes less efficient than normal, and simple supplementation with vitamins can often restore some of these deficient enzymes to full working order." Who lobbies for Mother Nature's own good nutrients?

Prevention is a cost effective answer, but it was not part of the recent overhaul of America's health care system. Preventive medicine is a different way of thinking.

Patients want change. They want front-line practitioners to use something more than a prescription pad. In August, 2010, the American Medical Association reported there are 95 lawsuits for every 100 doctors.[3] An estimated 68 percent of Americans have opted for Complementary and Alternative Medicine for at least a part of their medical care.

There is a new paradigm emerging: we call it green medicine. It recognizes that healthy food and healthy environments beget healthy bodies – no matter what the genetics suggest. Good health is more than what happens in the medical office. Good health occurs best within the context of a healthy environment. When we measured mercury in the air originating from smoke stacks in the Far East, we began to realize how what we do can affect the entire world. A green lifestyle supports a healthier body. Consumers are driving change there too.

When parents got educated about the dangers of BPA in plastic baby bottles, they demanded BPA-free baby bottles and the marketplace responded. When people learned about the health effects of high fructose corn syrup and synthetic sugars, they demanded products without them. Despite industry pressure, the city of San Francisco put the country on notice that cell phones emit hazardous radiation. A June 27, 2008 letter from David Mackay, CEO of Kellogg's, to Ronnie Cummins, National

Director, Organic Consumers Association, reveals just how sensitive manufacturers can be to genetically modified foods:

> Consumer preference is the critical factor Kellogg uses in determining the products being provided in each market ... Public acceptance of biotechnology in Europe is lower than in the United States. As a result, all Kellogg products sold in Europe are free of any ingredients derived from biotech sources.[4]

Consumer demand gains traction when consumers are educated. They can change the marketplace faster than government regulation.

But let's be careful what we call "green." It sounded "green" to move to hybrid vehicles. But then we began to realize that the flow of electrical current to the motor produces unnatural magnetic fields, not unlike WiFi networks. How does this affect our biological electromagnetic energy, our body's information systems?

It sounds green to move toward wind energy, for example. But early reports suggest the acoustics of all that whooshing air have caused maladies ranging from sleep deprivation and nausea to strokes and epilepsy. The sound apparently causes bats to become confused and run into the turbines.

We need to consider the downside and the side effects of everything that we do – just as we need to consider them with pharmaceutical medications, radiation exposures, and surgery. Remember all the children who had their thymus gland shrunk by radiation in the 1930s to 1950s – a medical fad that was supposed to prevent crib death. Many of these children developed thyroid cancer and other immune system dysfunctions, all because we thought we knew enough to interfere with a natural phenomenon that we simply did not understand.

Green medicine also means the medical community advocates for change. When Dr. Ronald M. Davis was president of the American Medical Association in 2008, he pointed out that seven out of every 10 Americans today dies of a chronic disease and many of those diseases are linked to toxic pollutants. He called upon physicians to become more aware and involved in environmental issues. He called upon medical schools to offer an elective course on the connection between environmental issues and human health. He pointed to pollutants like dioxin, mercury, plastics, and he gave a thumbs up to organic food. And then, in an ironic twist, he died of pancreatic cancer.

A good place to start reducing our exposure to toxins is in our own back yard. For doctors, medical waste is something we all can reduce. We can make every effort to use recyclable glass bottles instead of non-recyclable plastic bags. We can recycle our office trash. When we build out our offices, if we ask for non-out gassing materials, our architects and builders will find them and use them.

We can set the example, starting within our own practices. We can bring healthy food for lunch. We can provide healthy snacks for our staff – fruit and vegetables rather than doughnuts and candy bars. We can provide filtered water. We can offer supplements and nutritional counseling as part of their benefits package.

And most of all, we can remember that a doctor's most important job is to teach – ourselves and our patients.

---

[1] CDC Publications. Chronic Diseases – The Power to Prevent, The Call to Control: At A Glance 2009
[2] G Danaei, EL Ding, et al. The Preventable Causes of Death in the United States: Comparative Risk Assessment of Dietary, Lifestyle, and Metabolic Risk Factors. *PLoS Medicine*, 2009 Apr 28;6(4):e1000058.
[3] Carol Kane. Policy Research Perspectives – Medical Liability Claim Frequency: A 2007-2008 Snapshot of Physicians. The American Medical Association. August, 2010
[4] Organic Consumers Association. June 27, 2008. Accessed at www.organicconsumers.org/ge/Kelloggsresponse.pdf

For more information:

THE ARIZONA CENTER FOR ADVANCED MEDICINE
9328 East Raintree Drive
Scottsdale, Arizona 85260
Phone: 480-240-2600
Facsimile: 480-240-2601

www.ArizonaAdvancedMedicine.com

info@ArizonaAdvancedMedicine.com

Index

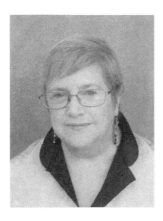

MARTHA GROUT, M.D., M.D.(H) is Vice-President of the Arizona Board of Homeopathic and Integrated Medicine Examiners and a member of the advisory board of the American Academy of Environmental Medicine. She has almost three decades in emergency medicine and a decade in homeopathic medicine. Her Scottsdale, Arizona clinic was built with environmentally friendly materials. She specializes in reversing chronic illness.

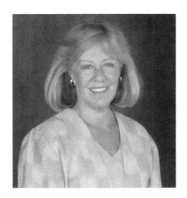

MARY BUDINGER is an Emmy award-winning journalist. After a decade in broadcast news, she moved to Phoenix and worked for the Arizona judicial system, AT&T Wireless, Sumco (formally Sumitomo Sitix), and consulted on the preparation of an application to the Arizona Corporation Commission for a merchant power plant. She focuses her efforts now on complementary and alternative medicine.

CPSIA information can be obtained at www.ICGtesting.com
Printed in the USA
BVOW020133170512

290280BV00001B/3/P